Cardiac Arrhythmias

Practical notes on interpretation and treatment

Seventh edition

David H. Bennett MD, FRCP, FACC, FESC
Consultant Cardiologist,
Regional Cardiac Centre,
Wythenshawe Hospital,
Manchester, UK

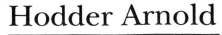

Hodder Arnold

A MEMBER OF THE HODDER HEADLINE GROUP

First published in Great Britain in 1981
Second edition 1985
Third edition 1989
Fourth edition 1993
Fifth edition 1997
Sixth edition 2002
This seventh edition published in 2006 by
Hodder Arnold, an imprint of Hodder Education, a member of the Hodder Headline Group,
338 Euston Road, London NW1 3BH

http://www.hoddereducation.com

Distributed in the United States of America by
Oxford University Press Inc.,
198 Madison Avenue, New York, NY10016
Oxford is a registered trademark of Oxford University Press

Hodder Headline's policy is to use papers that are natural, renewable and recyclable products
and made from wood grown in sustainable forests. The logging and manufacturing processes
are expected to conform to the environmental regulations of the country of origin.

Whilst the advice and information in this book are believed to be true and accurate at the date of
going to press, neither the author nor the publisher can accept any legal responsibility or liability
for any errors or omissions that may be made. In particular (but without limiting the generality
of the preceding disclaimer) every effort has been made to check drug dosages; however it is
still possible that errors have been missed. Furthermore, dosage schedules are constantly being
revised and new side-effects recognized. For these reasons the reader is strongly urged to
consult the drug companies' printed instructions before administering any of the drugs
recommended in this book.

British Library Cataloguing in Publication Data
A catalogue record for this book is available from the British Library

Library of Congress Cataloging-in-Publication Data
A catalog record for this book is available from the Library of Congress

ISBN-10   0 340 92562 0
ISBN-13   978 0 340 92562 1

1 2 3 4 5 6 7 8 9 10

Commissioning Editor: Philip Shaw
Project Editor: Heather Fyfe
Production Controller: Karen Tate
Cover Designer: Tim Pattinson

Typeset in 10/12 pts Minion by Charon Tec Ltd (A Macmillan Company), Chennai, India
www.charontec.com
Printed and bound in Spain

What do you think about this book? Or any other Hodder Arnold title?
Please send your comments to www.hoddereducation.com

Cardiac Arrhythmias

CONTENTS

There are several large textbooks which comprehensively cover the field of cardiac arrhythmias with thorough referencing of scientific papers. This book does not attempt to replicate these texts. The purpose of this seventh edition remains the same as its predecessors: to provide a concise, practical guide to the diagnosis, investigation and management of the main cardiac arrhythmias with particular emphasis on the problems commonly faced in practice.

Much new information in the areas of sudden cardiac death, heart failure, cardiac pacing and implantable defibrillators has been acquired since the last edition. Accordingly, the text has been updated.

In order to gain confidence in interpretation of arrhythmias it is necessary to examine a variety of examples of each rhythm disturbance. For this reason, it has always been a purpose of this book to present a large number of electrocardiograms. In this edition there are many new additional electrocardiograms and the quiz section has been revised and enlarged to provide a challenge to those who may be familiar with previous editions.

In recent years there has been a trend to sub-specialization in cardiology. Whatever the sub-specialty, cardiac arrhythmias will frequently be encountered. A thorough appreciation of the significance and management of cardiac arrhythmias is required of all who treat patients with cardiac disease.

I am most grateful to my technical and medical colleagues for their help, and to the staff at Hodder Arnold for their expertise.

D.H.B.

The purpose of this book is to describe the main cardiac arrhythmias, with particular emphasis on the problems commonly encountered in their interpretation, and to discuss the practical aspects of current methods of investigation and treatment. Information of purely academic value has not been included.

This book is intended to fill the gap between those textbooks that cover only the basics of arrhythmias and those that are written for the cardiac electrophysiologist. It has been written with junior hospital doctors in mind. They receive little formal training in the management of cardiac arrhythmias and yet, because prompt action is often required, the onus of diagnosis and treatment usually falls on them. It should also be of interest to medical students, who themselves will soon be responsible for dealing with arrhythmias, to nurses working in coronary and intensive care units and to physicians who want a brief review of the practical aspects of cardiac arrhythmias.

I would like to thank the cardiac technicians, coronary care nurses and medical staff at Wythenshawe Hospital for their help. I am particularly grateful to my colleagues, Dr Colin Bray and Dr Christopher Ward. Thanks are also due to Mrs Mary Rooney for typing the manuscript and to the Wythenshawe Hospital Medical Illustration Department.

Finally, I would like to acknowledge the distractions provided by my family, Irene, Samantha and Sally, to whom this book is dedicated.

D.H.B.

The subject of cardiac arrhythmias may appear complex; and indeed some enjoy making it look complicated! However, there are only a dozen important disturbances of cardiac rhythm. They all have characteristic electrocardiographic appearances that in most cases are easily identifiable. So do not lose heart!

Remember, when assessing a cardiac rhythm, that only atrial and ventricular activity register on the surface electrocardiogram (ECG). The site of impulse formation, sequence of cardiac chamber activation and functions of the sinus node and atrioventricular junction have to be deduced from analysis of the atrial and ventricular electrograms.

A single 'rhythm strip' may be inadequate for diagnosis. Scrutiny of several ECG leads, preferably recorded simultaneously, may be necessary. For example, atrial activity is often the key to diagnosis but may not be clearly shown in all ECG leads: it is often best seen in leads II and V1. Often, a '12-lead ECG' will provide much more information than a rhythm strip.

The electrocardiograms in this book have been recorded at the conventional paper speed of 25 mm/s, unless otherwise indicated. At this speed, each large square represents 0.2 s and each small square represents 0.04 s. Heart rate (beats/min) can therefore be calculated by dividing the number of large squares between two consecutive complexes into 300, or by dividing the number of small squares between two complexes into 1500.

An ECG recorded during an arrhythmia that is of diagnostic importance should always be safely stored in the patient's notes. This guideline, which may be very important to the long-term management of a patient, is often ignored, particularly on intensive care units!

Sinus rhythm

ECG CHARACTERISTICS

The sinus node initiates the electrical impulse that activates atrial and then ventricular myocardium during each normal heart beat. Sinus node activity itself does not register on the electrocardiogram (ECG).

P WAVE

Atrial activity, the P wave, is usually apparent in most ECG leads (Figure 1.1). However, sometimes the P wave is not visible or is of low amplitude and it may be necessary to inspect all leads of the ECG to establish that there is sinus rhythm (Figure 1.2).

The sinus node lies at the junction of the superior vena cava and right atrium. Atrial activation spreads from the sinus node inferiorly (that is towards the feet) to the atrioventricular (AV) junction. The P wave, therefore, is upright in those leads that are directed to the inferior surface of the heart (i.e. II, III and aVF), and is inverted in aVR, which faces the superior heart surface (Figure 1.1). If a P wave does not have these characteristics then, even though a P wave precedes each ventricular complex, the sinus node has not activated the atria and the rhythm is abnormal (Figure 1.3).

PR INTERVAL

The AV node delays conduction of the atrial impulse to the ventricles. Conduction through the AV node does not register on the ECG. The PR interval, which is measured from the onset of the P wave to the onset of the ventricular complex, indicates the time taken for an atrial impulse to reach the ventricles. The normal PR interval ranges from 0.12 to 0.21 s. It should shorten during sinus tachycardia.

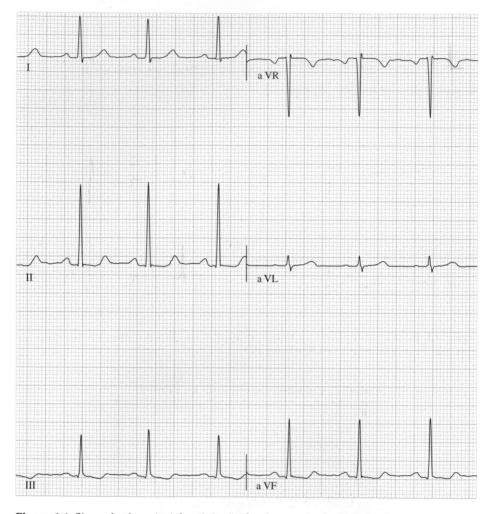

Figure 1.1 Sinus rhythm. Atrial activity is clearly seen in the limb leads.

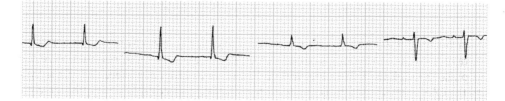

Figure 1.2 Sinus rhythm with low-amplitude P waves (leads I, II, III and V1). Atrial activity is only clearly seen in V1.

QRS COMPLEX

After traversing the AV node, the activating impulse reaches the bundle of His, which divides into the right and left bundle branches. The bundle of His, the bundle

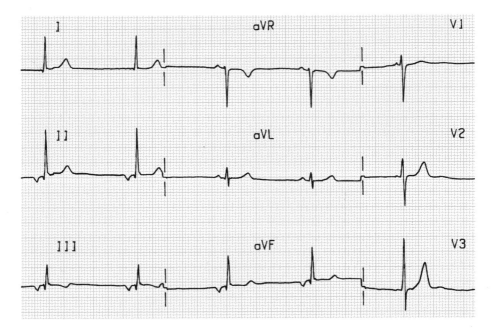

Figure 1.3 Junctional rhythm: a P wave precedes each QRS complex but is superiorly directed: it is negative in leads II, III and aVF.

Table 1.1 Characteristics of normal sinus rhythm

P wave:
    Precedes each QRS complex
    Upright in leads III, aVF
    Inverted in lead aVR

PR interval:
    Duration 0.12–0.21 s

QRS complex:
    Duration less than 0.10 s

branches and their ramifications, the Purkinje fibres, constitute the 'specialized intraventricular conducting system', which facilitates very rapid conduction of the impulse through the ventricular myocardium. Ventricular activation is represented by the QRS complex which is normally less than 0.10 s in duration. The characteristics of normal sinus rhythm are summarized in Table 1.1.

SINUS BRADYCARDIA

Sinus bradycardia is sinus rhythm at a rate less then 60 beats/min (Figure 1.4). It may be physiological, as in athletes or during sleep, or result from acute myocardial

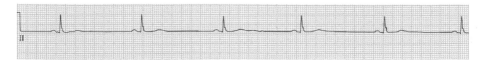

Figure 1.4 Sinus bradycardia (lead II): rate 34 beats/min.

infarction, sick sinus syndrome or from drugs such as beta-adrenoceptor blocking drugs (beta-blockers). Non-cardiac disorders such as hypothyroidism, jaundice and raised intracranial pressure can also cause sinus bradycardia.

Atropine or pacing can be used to increase the rate but are only necessary when sinus bradycardia causes symptoms, marked hypotension or leads to tachyarrhythmia.

SINUS TACHYCARDIA

Sinus tachycardia is defined as sinus rhythm at a rate greater than 100 beats/min (Figure 1.5). Exercise, anxiety or any disorder that increases sympathetic nervous system activity may cause sinus tachycardia.

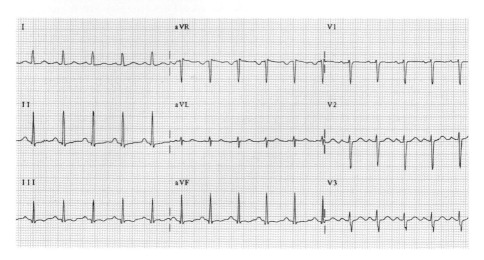

Figure 1.5 Sinus tachycardia during exercise. The rate is 136 beats/min.

Occasionally, sinus tachycardia can be inappropriate. Hyperthyroidism is a possible cause but often no cause is found. Young females are most commonly affected. Fast rates are usually persistent and there is an exaggerated response to exercise with rates increasing rapidly almost immediately exertion begins.

Rarely, inappropriate sinus tachycardia is due to a primary disorder of the sinus node (sinus node re-entry).

Since sinus tachycardia is usually a physiological response, there is rarely a need for specific treatment. However, if sinus tachycardia is inappropriate, the rate may be slowed by a beta-blocker.

At rest, the sinus node rate is seldom above 100 beats/min unless the patient is very ill. If there is apparent sinus tachycardia at rest alternative diagnoses such as atrial tachycardia or atrial flutter should be considered.

SINUS ARRHYTHMIA

Normally there are only minor changes in rate during sinus rhythm. In sinus arrhythmia, which is of no pathological significance, there are alternating periods of slowing and increasing sinus node rate. Usually the rate increases during inspiration (Figure 1.6). Sinus arrhythmia is most commonly seen in the young.

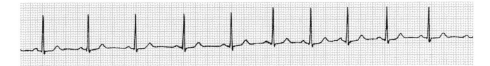

Figure 1.6 Sinus arrhythmia.

Main points

- During sinus rhythm, an inferiorly directed P wave (i.e. upright in leads III and aVF) precedes each QRS complex.

- If AV conduction is normal, the duration of the PR interval will be between 0.12 and 0.21 s.

- Normal intraventricular conduction results in a QRS complex with a duration less than 0.10 s.

- In cases of apparent sinus tachycardia at rest, it is important to exclude atrial flutter or tachycardia.

Ectopic beats

PREMATURITY

The terms ectopic beat, extrasystole and premature contraction are, for practical purposes, synonymous. They refer to an impulse originating from the atria, AV junction (i.e. AV node plus bundle of His) or ventricles that arises prematurely in the cardiac cycle (Figures 2.1–2.3).

By definition, an ectopic beat must arise earlier in the cardiac cycle than the next normally timed beat would be expected. Thus the interval between the ectopic beat and the preceding beat (i.e. the coupling interval) is shorter than the cycle length of the dominant rhythm. If this fact is ignored, other beats with abnormal configurations

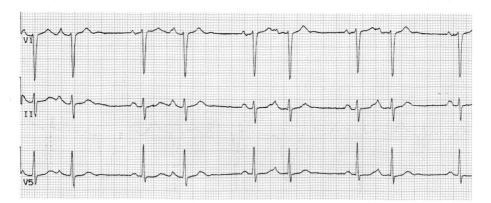

Figure 2.1 The second, fourth, sixth and eighth complexes are atrial ectopic beats. The ectopic P waves are premature and differ slightly in shape from those of sinus origin (the PR intervals of the atrial ectopic beats are prolonged).

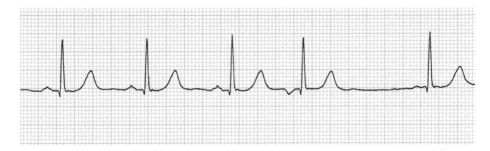

Figure 2.2 The fourth beat is a junctional ectopic beat (lead III). The junctional focus has activated the atria as well as the ventricles, resulting in an inverted P wave which precedes the QRS complex.

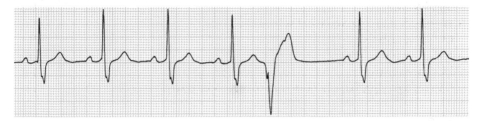

Figure 2.3 The fifth beat is a ventricular ectopic beat.

such as escape beats (see Chapter 3) and intermittent bundle branch block (see Chapter 4) may be misinterpreted as ectopic beats.

The site of origin of an ectopic beat can be determined by careful examination of the ECG. A single rhythm strip may be inadequate. Scrutiny of simultaneous recordings of several ECG leads is often necessary to detect the diagnostic clues (Figures 2.4 and 2.5).

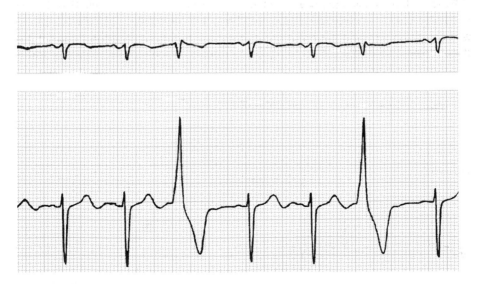

Figure 2.4 Simultaneous recording of leads V1 and V2. The third and sixth beats are unifocal ventricular ectopic beats. Their ventricular origin is not apparent in lead V1 because the complexes are narrow but is obvious in V2.

ATRIAL ECTOPIC BEATS

P WAVE

An atrial ectopic beat results in a P wave that is premature. The site of origin and therefore direction of atrial activation will differ from that during sinus rhythm, so a premature P wave will usually differ in shape to a P wave of sinus node origin (Figure 2.1).

Because atrial ectopic beats are premature, they may be superimposed on and thus deform the T wave of the preceding beat. Careful examination of the ECG is essential to detect ectopic P waves; often, lead V1 is the best lead (Figures 2.5 and 2.6).

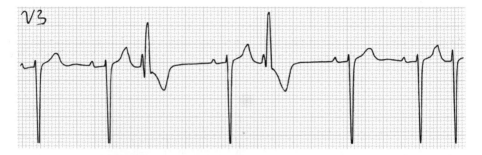

Figure 2.5 Atrial ectopic beats are superimposed on the T waves of the second, fourth and seventh ventricular complexes (lead V3). It can be seen how the T waves of these beats are modified by comparing them with the T wave of the first and sixth ventricular complexes, which are not followed by an atrial ectopic. The first two atrial ectopic beats are conducted with right bundle branch block.

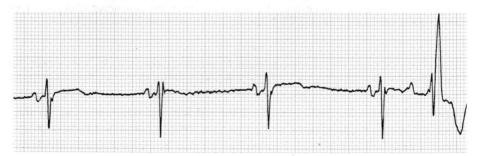

Figure 2.6 The last beat is an atrial ectopic beat conducted with a prolonged PR interval and right bundle branch block.

ATRIOVENTRICULAR AND INTRAVENTRICULAR CONDUCTION

Usually the AV junction and bundle branches will conduct an atrial ectopic beat to the ventricles in the same manner as if the sinus node had activated the atria. Thus the PR interval and QRS complex of the ectopic beat will be identical with those during sinus rhythm (Figure 2.1). If the QRS complex during sinus rhythm is abnormal due to bundle branch block, then so will be the QRS complex of the ectopic beat.

Sometimes, however, atrial ectopic beats, especially those that arise very early in the cardiac cycle, may encounter either an AV junction or a bundle branch which has not yet recovered from conduction of the last atrial impulse and is, therefore, partially or completely refractory to excitation. Partial and complete refractoriness of the AV junction will result in prolongation of the PR interval and blocked atrial ectopic beats, respectively (Figures 2.1, 2.6–2.8). Blocked atrial ectopics have been wrongly taken as an indication for cardiac pacing!

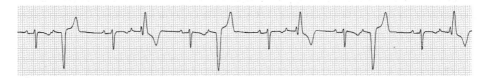

Figure 2.7 Lead V1. Atrial ectopic beats follow each sinus beat. The second, sixth and tenth complexes are atrial ectopic beats conducted with left bundle branch block. The fourth, eighth and twelfth complexes are conducted with right bundle branch block.

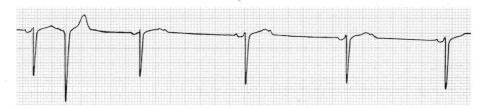

Figure 2.8 Lead V1. Atrial ectopic beats are superimposed on the terminal portion of the T wave of each ventricular complex. The first atrial ectopic is conducted with partial left branch block. The other atrial ectopic beats are not conducted to the ventricles.

Partial or complete refractoriness of one or other bundle branch (it is usually the right bundle) will correspondingly lead to partial or complete bundle branch block (Figures 2.6 and 2.7). This phenomenon of functional bundle branch block is referred to by some as 'phasic aberrant intraventricular conduction'. The resultant QRS complexes are broad and can therefore be confused with ventricular ectopic beats if the premature P wave preceding the ventricular complex is not detected.

The ECG characteristics of atrial ectopic beats are summarized in Table 2.1.

Table 2.1 Characteristics of atrial ectopic beats

The P wave of atrial ectopic beats:
is premature
may be superimposed on and distort the preceding T wave
is usually followed by a normal QRS complex
is sometimes not conducted to the ventricles, or is conducted with a bundle branch block pattern

SIGNIFICANCE

Atrial ectopic beats occur in many cardiac disorders but are also commonly found in individuals with normal hearts, particularly the elderly. They are usually benign. However, if they are frequent they may herald atrial fibrillation or atrial tachycardia.

ATRIOVENTRICULAR JUNCTIONAL ECTOPIC BEATS

AV junctional beats used to be called 'nodal' beats. It is now recognized that at least part of the AV node is not capable of pacemaker activity and that it is not possible to distinguish between beats originating from the AV node and those from the bundle of His. Hence the more general term 'AV junction' is used. AV junctional ectopic beats are not as common as atrial or ventricular ectopics. Treatment is rarely necessary.

ECG APPEARANCE

AV junctional ectopic beats are recognized by a premature QRS complex that is similar in appearance to that occurring in sinus rhythm. The junctional focus may activate the atria as well as the ventricles, leading to a retrograde P wave (i.e. negative in leads II, III and aVF). The retrograde P wave may precede, follow or be buried within the QRS complex, depending on the relative speeds of conduction of the premature junctional impulse to the ventricles and to the atria (Figure 2.2).

VENTRICULAR ECTOPIC BEATS

The impulse of a ventricular ectopic beat is not conducted through the ventricles via the specialized, rapidly conducting tissues. The abnormal course and consequent slowing of ventricular activation result in ventricular complexes that are bizarre in shape and of prolonged duration.

ECG APPEARANCE

The complexes are premature, broad (>0.12s), bizarre in shape and, in contrast to atrial ectopic beats, are obviously not preceded by an ectopic P wave (Figures 2.3 and 2.4).
    The characteristics of ventricular ectopic beats are summarized in Table 2.2.

Table 2.2 Characteristics of ventricular ectopic beats

The QRS complex of a ventricular ectopic beat:
is premature
is broad (>0.12s)
is abnormal in shape
is not preceded by a premature P wave

Several terms are used to describe the origin, timing and quantity of ventricular ectopic beats. These are explained below.

Focus

Ectopic beats with the same shape and coupling intervals are assumed to arise from the same focus and are termed 'unifocal' (Figure 2.4), whereas differing shapes and coupling intervals suggest more than one focus. These are called 'multifocal' or 'multiform' (Figure 2.9).

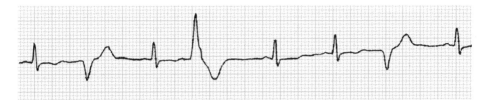

Figure 2.9 Multifocal ventricular ectopic beats. The second ventricular ectopic beat has a different shape and coupling interval from the first and third ectopic beats.

Timing

Beats that occur very early in the cardiac cycle will be superimposed on the T wave of the preceding beat and are described as 'R on T' (Figure 2.10). Most episodes of ventricular fibrillation and many episodes of ventricular tachycardia are initiated by 'R on T' ectopics; though by no means do all 'R on T' ectopic beats precipitate these arrhythmias.

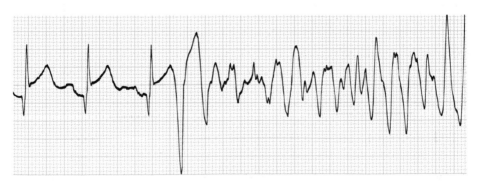

Figure 2.10 An 'R on T' ventricular ectopic beat, which in this case initiates ventricular fibrillation.

A ventricular ectopic beat that occurs only slightly prematurely in the cardiac cycle may fall, by chance, immediately after a P wave initiated by normal sinus node activity: the P wave will not, therefore, in contrast to an atrial ectopic beat, be premature. Such a ventricular ectopic beat is described as 'end-diastolic' (Figures 2.11 and 2.12).

Usually there is a pause after a ventricular ectopic beat. When there is no such pause and the ectopic beat is thus sandwiched between two normal beats, the ectopic beat is said to be 'interpolated' (Figure 2.13).

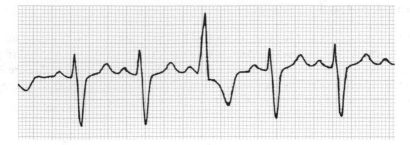

Figure 2.11 The third beat is an end-diastolic ventricular ectopic beat. It is preceded by a normally timed P wave.

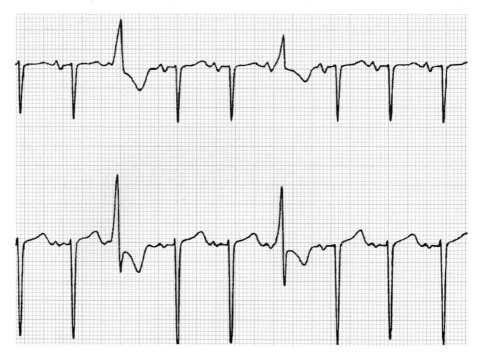

Figure 2.12 Simultaneous recording of leads V1 and V2. Two end-diastolic ventricular ectopic beats. The second mimicking the Wolff–Parkinson–White syndrome.

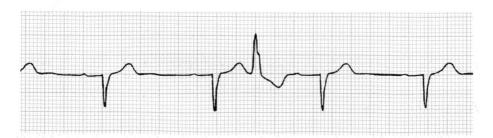

Figure 2.13 Interpolated ventricular beat. (The subsequent PR interval is prolonged owing to retrograde concealed conduction.)

Quantification

Ventricular ectopic beats are often quantified by the number occurring each minute. When an ectopic beat follows each sinus beat the term 'bigeminy' is applied (Figure 2.14). If an ectopic follows a pair of normal beats it is called 'trigeminy' (Figure 2.15). When two ectopics occur in succession (Figure 2.16) they are referred to as a 'couplet'. A 'salvo' refers to more than two ectopic beats in succession.

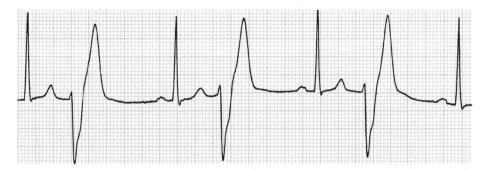

Figure 2.14 Ventricular bigeminy.

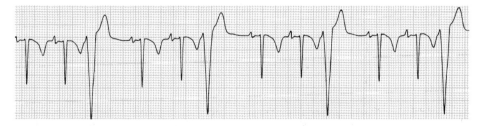

Figure 2.15 Ventricular trigeminy.

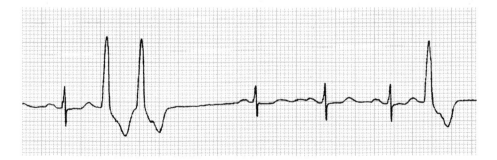

Figure 2.16 The first sinus beat is followed by a couplet of ventricular ectopic beats.

Atrial activity

The pattern of atrial activity following a ventricular ectopic beat depends on whether the AV junction transmits the ventricular impulse to the atria. If this occurs, the result is an inverted P wave which is often superimposed on and may therefore be concealed by the ventricular ectopic beat (Figure 2.17). When the AV junction does not transmit the ventricular impulse to the atria, atrial activity continues independently of ventricular activity; it is only in these cases that a ventricular impulse is followed by a full compensatory pause (i.e. the lengths of the cycles before and after the ectopic beat will equal twice the sinus cycle length) (see Figures 2.3 and 2.4).

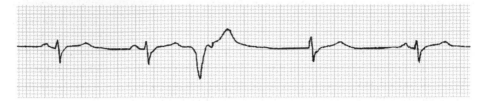

Figure 2.17 The third beat is a ventricular ectopic beat that has been conducted back to the atria, resulting in an inverted P wave (lead aVF). (The ectopic beat is followed by a junctional escape beat.)

Sometimes a ventricular impulse only partially penetrates the AV junction. The next impulse arising from the sinus node may therefore encounter an AV junction that is partially refractory and be conducted with a prolonged PR interval (Figure 2.13). This phenomenon of 'retrograde concealed conduction' often occurs following interpolated ventricular extrasystoles.

Parasystole

Parasystole, which is uncommon, is an exception to the rule that unifocal ectopic beats have a constant coupling interval. The ventricular ectopic focus discharges regularly and is undisturbed by the dominant rhythm. It will capture the ventricles provided the ectopic discharge does not occur when the ventricles have just been activated by the dominant rhythm and are therefore refractory. Thus ventricular parasystole is characterized by a variable coupling interval, inter-ectopic intervals that are multiples of a common factor and, because the ventricles may by chance be simultaneously activated by both ectopic and normal pacemakers, fusion beats (i.e. a complex which is a composite of normal and ectopic beat).

CAUSES AND SIGNIFICANCE OF VENTRICULAR ECTOPIC BEATS

The causes of ventricular ectopic beats include acute myocardial infarction, myocardial ischaemia, myocardial damage caused by previous infarction, myocarditis, cardiomyopathy, mitral valve prolapse, valvular heart disease and digoxin toxicity.

Occasional ventricular ectopic beats at rest and even frequent unifocal ectopic beats on exercise can occur in otherwise normal individuals and are not necessarily pathological or of prognostic significance. However, a survey of middle-aged men did show that frequent ventricular ectopic beats (more than 10 per cent of all ventricular complexes) occurring during exercise was associated with a 2.5 increase in mortality over the 23-year period of the survey. In a population of adult patients referred for exercise testing, frequent ventricular ectopic beats (7 or more per minute) immediately after exercise have also been shown to be a risk factor.

The frequency of ectopic beats in the adult population increases with age.

'Complex' ventricular ectopic beats (i.e. frequent, multifocal, 'R on T' or those that occur in salvos) are rarely found in the absence of cardiac disease and are associated with an increased cardiovascular mortality. In patients who have sustained myocardial damage from coronary heart disease, there is a correlation between severity of damage and frequency of ventricular ectopic beats. Recent evidence, however, points to the presence of ectopic beats as an added and independent risk factor but there is no evidence to show that suppression of ectopic beats by antiarrhythmic therapy improves prognosis. Indeed, several antiarrhythmic drugs have been shown to increase mortality in patients with ventricular ectopic beats after myocardial infarction.

Ectopic beats do not usually cause symptoms. Some patients, however, experience distressing symptoms. They may be upset by the irregularity resulting from the premature beats or by the compensatory pause or 'thump' caused by increased myocardial contractility associated with the post-ectopic beat. They may be anxious that their irregular heart rhythm is a sign of impending heart attack or other major cardiac problem.

There is a group of patients with structurally normal hearts who have distressing symptoms caused by ventricular ectopic beats in whom reassurance is inadequate. In these patients, antiarrhythmic therapy may be necessary for symptomatic purposes. Beta-blockers may help, particularly in patients whose symptoms are related to exertion. Flecainide is useful, provided the patient has a structurally normal heart and there is no evidence of coronary disease.

The significance of ventricular ectopic beats in acute myocardial infarction is discussed in Chapter 18.

Main points

- Ectopic beats are premature and therefore have a coupling interval shorter than the cycle length of the dominant rhythm.

- The P waves of atrial ectopic beats are often superimposed on and distort the preceding T wave and can easily be missed. They are usually best seen in lead V1.

- Sometimes atrial ectopic beats are not conducted to the ventricles or are conducted with a bundle branch block pattern.

- Ventricular ectopic beats cause premature, broad and bizarrely shaped QRS complexes.

- Chronic ventricular ectopic beats that are frequent, multifocal, 'R on T' or occur in salvos are associated with an increased cardiovascular mortality, but there is no evidence to show that their suppression improves prognosis.

Escape beats

TIMING

When the sinus node fails to discharge, escape beats may arise from subsidiary sites in the specialized conducting system. In contrast to ectopic beats, escape beats are always late (i.e. the coupling interval is greater than the cycle length of the dominant rhythm) (see Figures 3.1 and 3.3). Distinction between escape and ectopic beats is important because the former indicate impaired pacemaker function. Escape beats themselves require no treatment. If treatment is necessary, it is to accelerate the basic rhythm.

ORIGINS

Escape beats usually arise from the AV junction (Figures 3.1–3.3); less commonly, they originate from the ventricles (Figures 3.4 and 3.5). The ventricular complexes of

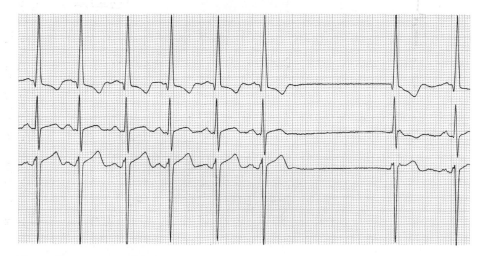

Figure 3.1 Leads I, II and III. After the sixth complex there is a pause in sinus node activity followed by a junctional escape beat.

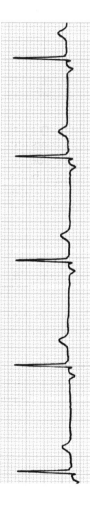

Figure 3.2 Junctional escape rhythm (lead II). The junctional focus has also activated the atria as indicated by the inverted P wave preceding each QRS complex. (The rhythm has also been termed 'coronary sinus' rhythm.)

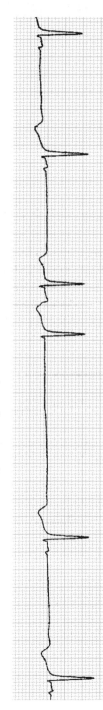

Figure 3.3 The third ventricular complex is a junctional escape beat which arises during sinus arrest. The escape beat is followed by an atrial ectopic beat.

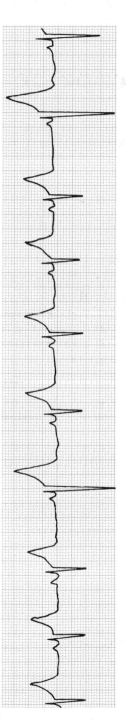

Figure 3.4 The fourth and ninth ventricular complexes are escape beats arising from the ventricles that result from slowing of the sinus node. Though P waves precede the escape beats, they are unlikely to have captured the ventricles since the PR intervals are shorter than those during sinus rhythm.

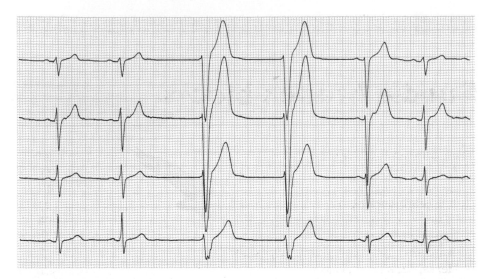

Figure 3.5 Ventricular escape rhythm during sinus bradycardia. After two normally timed sinus beats there are two ventricular escape beats. These are followed by a complex intermediate in appearance between normal sinus and ventricular escape beats which is the result of simultaneous ventricular activation by the sinus node and the ventricular escape focus: a 'fusion beat'.

junctional escape beats are similar to those during normal rhythm. As with junctional ectopic beats, the junctional focus may activate the atria as well as the ventricles, leading to a retrograde P wave (i.e. negative in leads II, III and aVF). The retrograde P wave may precede, follow or be buried within the QRS complex, depending on the relative speeds of conduction of the premature junctional impulse to the ventricles and to the atria.

Ventricular escape beats have a configuration similar to that of ventricular ectopic beats (Figures 3.4 and 3.5).

Main points

- In contrast to ectopic beats, the coupling interval of escape beats is greater than the cycle length of the dominant rhythm.

- As with ectopic beats, the configuration of escape beats indicates whether they are of supraventricular or ventricular origin.

- Escape beats should not be suppressed by drugs.

Bundle branch blocks

The bundle of His divides into left and right bundle branches. These facilitate very rapid activation of the left and right ventricles. The left bundle branch has two main subdivisions: the anterior and posterior fascicles.

Block in conduction through one or other bundle branch results in a ventricular complex that is prolonged in duration with an abnormal configuration.

RIGHT BUNDLE BRANCH BLOCK

ECG APPEARANCE

In right bundle branch block there is delay in activation of the right ventricle, while activation of the interventricular septum and free wall of the left ventricle is normal (Figure 4.1). Delayed right ventricular activation results in:

1. an increase in duration of the QRS complex ($\geqslant$0.12 s);
2. a secondary R wave in leads facing the right ventricle (V1 and V2) and hence an 'M' shaped complex in these leads; and
3. a broad S wave in left ventricular leads and lead I.

Partial right bundle branch block results in a similar ECG appearance but the QRS duration is 0.11 s or less.

CAUSES AND SIGNIFICANCE

Right bundle branch block may be an isolated congenital lesion. It often occurs in congenital heart disease, in other causes of right ventricular hypertrophy or strain

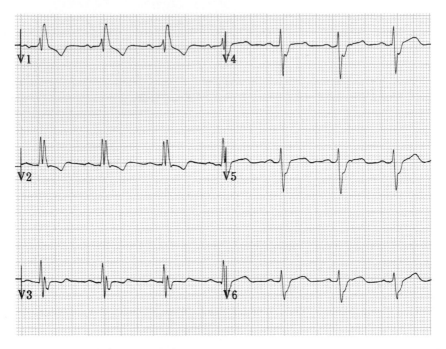

Figure 4.1 Right bundle branch block. There is an M-shaped complex in V1 and a deep slurred S wave in lead V6.

and where there is myocardial damage. Right bundle branch block is common when there is disease of the specialized conducting tissues.

Based on limited data, neither pre-existing nor acquired right bundle branch block are of prognostic significance. However, a recent long-term survey has demonstrated a four-fold risk of developing AV block.

Supraventricular extrasystoles and tachycardias may encounter a right bundle branch that is refractory to excitation and be conducted to the ventricles with a right bundle branch block pattern.

LEFT BUNDLE BRANCH BLOCK

ECG APPEARANCE

In left bundle branch block, activation of the interventricular septum is in the opposite direction to normal (i.e. from right to left), being initiated by an impulse arising from the right bundle branch. Thus:

1. The initial small, negative q wave normally seen in left ventricular leads (V5, V6, I and aVL) is replaced by a larger, positive R wave.
2. Activation of the left ventricle will be delayed, resulting in a broad and usually notched R wave in left ventricular leads, and prolongation of the duration of the QRS complex ($\geq$0.12 s) (Figure 4.2).

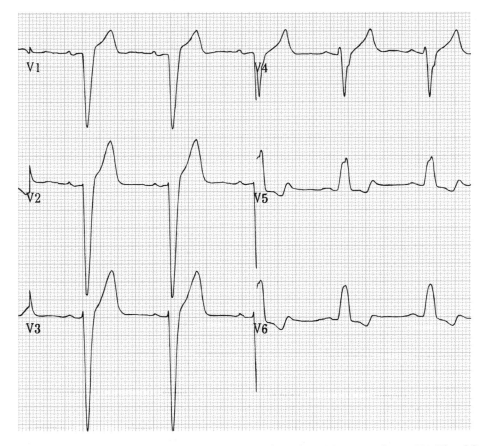

Figure 4.2 Left bundle branch block. There is a broad positive complex in V6. The QS complex in V1 is also characteristic of left bundle branch block.

Partial left bundle branch block has a similar ECG appearance to complete left bundle branch block, but the QRS duration is 0.10 or 0.11 s.

CAUSES AND SIGNIFICANCE

Causes of left bundle branch block include myocardial damage due to coronary artery disease or cardiomyopathy, and left ventricular hypertrophy. Left bundle branch block can also be caused by disease of the specialized conduction tissues. Rarely, left bundle branch block may occur in an otherwise normal heart.

Recently acquired left bundle branch block is associated with an increased risk of death: mainly sudden death from coronary disease. In addition, an 18-fold risk of developing AV block in the long term has recently been reported.

Supraventricular extrasystoles and tachycardias may encounter a left bundle branch that is refractory to excitation and be conducted to the ventricles with a left bundle branch block pattern.

Left bundle branch block can be intermittent.

LEFT ANTERIOR AND POSTERIOR FASCICULAR BLOCKS

The anterior and posterior fascicles of the left bundle branch conduct impulses to the anterosuperior and posteroinferior regions of the left ventricle, respectively. Block can occur in either anterior or posterior fascicles and is known as fascicular block or hemiblock. Left anterior and posterior fascicular blocks are common in conduction tissue disease (see Chapter 15).

Diagnosis of the fascicular blocks is based on the hexaxial reference system.

HEXAXIAL REFERENCE SYSTEM

The hexaxial reference system is a method of displaying the orientation of the six ECG limb leads to the heart in the frontal plane (Figure 4.3). For example, a superiorly directed impulse will move away from leads II, III and aVF, producing a negative wave in these leads, and towards aVL, producing a positive wave in this lead. The direction of an impulse can be expressed by the number of degrees clockwise (positive) or anticlockwise (negative) of lead I, which is the zero reference point. For example, an impulse towards lead aVL has an axis of −30 degrees and an impulse towards lead III has an axis of +120 degrees (Figure 4.3).

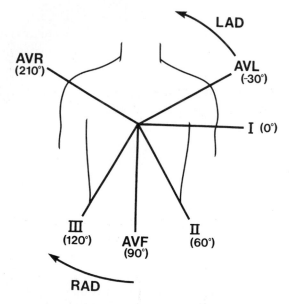

Figure 4.3 Hexaxial reference system. LAD, left axis deviation; RAD, right axis deviation.

Mean frontal QRS axis

The mean frontal QRS axis describes the dominant or average direction of the various electrical forces that develop during ventricular activation. Normally, the mean frontal QRS axis lies between aVL (i.e. −30 degrees) and aVF (i.e. +90 degrees).

If the axis is to the left of aVL (i.e. less than −30 degrees), it is termed abnormal left axis deviation. If the axis is to the right of aVF (i.e. more than +90 degrees), there is right axis deviation.

Using the hexaxial reference system, the mean frontal QRS axis may be calculated to within a few degrees. However, this degree of precision is unnecessary and most people get it wrong when trying to calculate the axis! It is easier to diagnose left and right axis deviation from a simple rule of thumb, as follows.

- In left axis deviation, lead I is mainly positive and both leads II and III are mainly negative (Figure 4.4). Contrary to some older texts, *both* II and III must be mainly negative (i.e. if in lead II the S wave is smaller than the R wave, abnormal left axis deviation is not present) (Figure 4.5). If lead II is equiphasic, there is borderline left axis deviation (Figure 4.5).

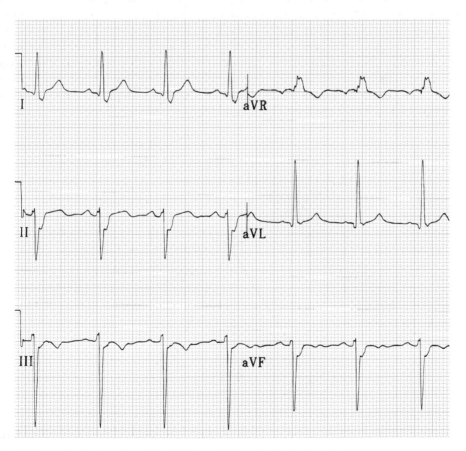

Figure 4.4 Left axis deviation due to left anterior fascicular block.

- In right axis deviation, lead I is mainly negative and *both* leads II and III are predominantly positive (Figure 4.6).

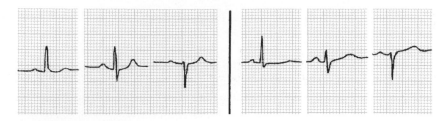

Figure 4.5 Leads I, II and III from two patients. In the first, the mean frontal QRS axis is normal. In the second, lead II is equiphasic and thus there is borderline left axis deviation.

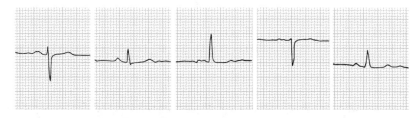

Figure 4.6 Right axis deviation due to left posterior fascicular block (leads I, II, III, aVL and aVF).

LEFT ANTERIOR FASCICULAR BLOCK

Block in the anterior fascicle of the left bundle branch causes delay in activation of the anterosuperior portion of the left ventricle. Initial left ventricular activation will be via the posterior fascicle to the posteroinferior region and will therefore be directed inferiorly and to the right. This results in an initial small positive deflection (i.e. r wave) in inferiorly orientated leads (II, III and aVF) (Figure 4.4).

The anterosuperior region will be activated by conduction from the posteroinferior region. The resultant wave will, therefore, be superiorly directed (R wave in I and aVL; S in II, III and aVF). Because conduction is through ordinary myocardium rather than the specialized conducting tissues, it will be relatively slow. As a result, activation of the anterosuperior region will be delayed and thus unopposed by activity from the rest of the ventricles. Thus the resultant superiorly directed wave is larger than the initial inferiorly directed wave and the mean frontal QRS axis will also be superiorly directed (i.e. there will be left axis deviation).

Left anterior fascicular block is a common cause of left axis deviation. The other cause is inferior myocardial infarction (Figure 4.7).

To diagnose left anterior fascicular block two criteria must be satisfied:

1. There must be left axis deviation, i.e. lead I must be predominantly positive and both leads II and III predominantly negative.
2. The initial direction of ventricular activation must be inferior and to the right, i.e. there must be an initial r wave in leads II, III and aVF.

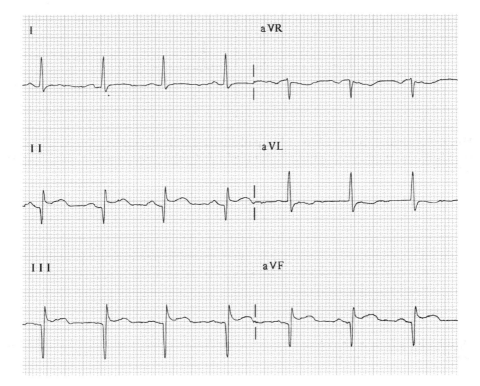

Figure 4.7 Inferior myocardial infarction. There is left axis deviation but not left anterior fascicular block.

LEFT POSTERIOR FASCICULAR BLOCK

In left posterior fascicular block, activation of the posteroinferior portion of the left ventricle is delayed. As a result, there will be an initial positive r wave in leads I and aVL and an initial negative q wave in leads II, III and aVF; and there will be right axis deviation (i.e. lead I will be predominantly negative and leads II and III predominantly positive) (Figure 4.6).

A diagnosis of left posterior fascicular block can only be made in the absence of other causes of right axis deviation such as right ventricular hypertrophy or strain, lateral myocardial infarction or a young person with a tall, thin build.

Main points

- Complete bundle branch block prolongs QRS duration to 0.12 s or greater. In incomplete block QRS duration is 0.10–0.11 s.

- With right bundle branch block, there will be a secondary R wave in lead V1, resulting in an M-shaped complex in this lead.

- With left bundle branch block, there will be an M-shaped or notched complex in left ventricular leads and no M-shaped complex in lead V1.

- In abnormal left axis deviation, lead I is predominantly positive and *both* leads II and III are predominantly negative.

- In right axis deviation, lead I is predominantly negative and *both* leads II and III positive.

- The criteria for left anterior hemiblock are left axis deviation together with a small initial r wave in leads II and aVF.

- Left posterior hemiblock should be considered when there is right axis deviation in the absence of other causes (e.g. right ventricular hypertrophy or strain).

CHAPTER 5

The supraventricular tachycardias

MAIN TYPES

Several tachycardias originate from the atria or AV junction and are therefore, by definition, supraventricular in origin (Table 5.1). They have one thing in common: because they arise from above the level of the bundle branches, ventricular activation is via the rapidly conducting specialized intraventricular system and thus normal, and therefore narrow, ventricular complexes will usually result. However, it is very important to appreciate that there are significant differences in mechanism, ECG characteristic and treatment. It is necessary to identify the type of tachycardia and not merely treat all tachycardias with narrow QRS complexes as 'supraventricular tachycardia'.

Table 5.1 Types of supraventricular tachycardias

1. Atrioventricular re-entrant tachycardia
2. Atrioventricular nodal re-entrant tachycardia
3. Atrial fibrillation
4. Atrial flutter
5. Atrial tachycardia
6. Sinus tachycardia (see Chapter 1)

ATRIAL ORIGIN VERSUS ATRIOVENTRICULAR RE-ENTRY

Supraventricular tachycardia are of two main types: AV junctional re-entrant tachycardias and atrial tachyarrhythmias.

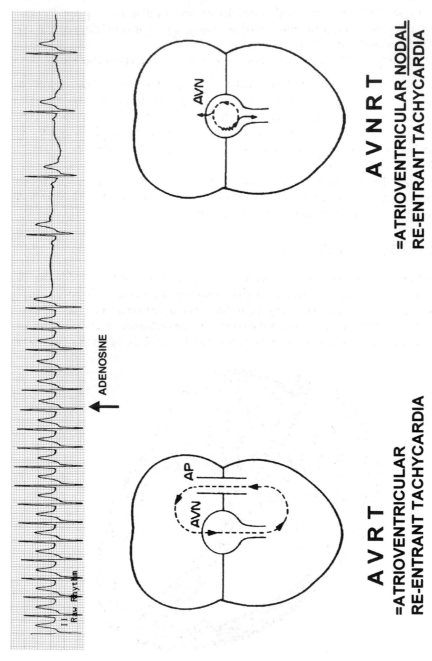

Figure 5.1 The two mechanisms of junctional re-entrant tachycardia: atrioventricular re-entrant tachycardia (AVRT) due to an accessory atrioventricular pathway and atrioventricular nodal re-entrant tachycardia (AVNRT) due to dual atrioventricular nodal pathways. Both typically result in a rapid, narrow QRS tachycardia that can be terminated by adenosine. (AVN, AV node; AP, accessory pathway.)

Atrioventricular junctional re-entrant tachycardias

In AV junctional re-entrant tachycardias (see Chapter 9) there is an additional electrical connection between atria and ventricles so an impulse can repeatedly and rapidly circulate between atria and ventricles along a circuit consisting of the AV junction and the additional AV connection.

There are two types of additional connection between atria and ventricles:

- In atrioventricular re-entrant tachycardia (AVRT), the additional connection is an accessory AV pathway which is a strand of myocardium that straddles the groove between atria and ventricles and therefore bypasses the AV node (Figure 5.1). (If the accessory AV pathway can conduct anterogradely, i.e. from atria to ventricles, then the patient will have the features of the Wolff–Parkinson–White syndrome (see Chapter 10).)
- In atrioventricular nodal re-entrant tachycardia (AVNRT), the AV node and its adjacent atrial tissues are functionally dissociated into fast and slow AV nodal pathways (i.e. dual AV nodal pathways) (Figure 5.1).

Atrial tachyarrhythmias

The second group of supraventricular tachycardias comprises those caused by rapid, abnormal atrial activity, i.e. atrial tachycardia, flutter and fibrillation. The mechanism responsible for the tachycardia is *confined* to the atria. In contrast to the first group, the AV node is not an integral part of the tachycardia mechanism but simply transmits some or all the atrial impulses to the ventricles (Figure 5.2). Arrhythmias in this

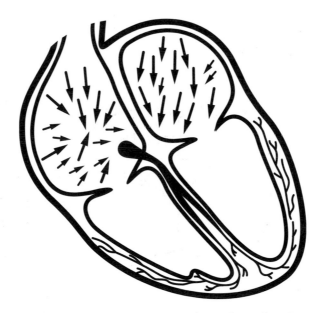

Figure 5.2 Diagram illustrating the supraventricular tachycardias that are caused by rapid abnormal activity originating from within the atria. The atrioventricular node is not an integral part of the arrhythmia mechanism but merely conducts some or all of the atrial impulses to the ventricles.

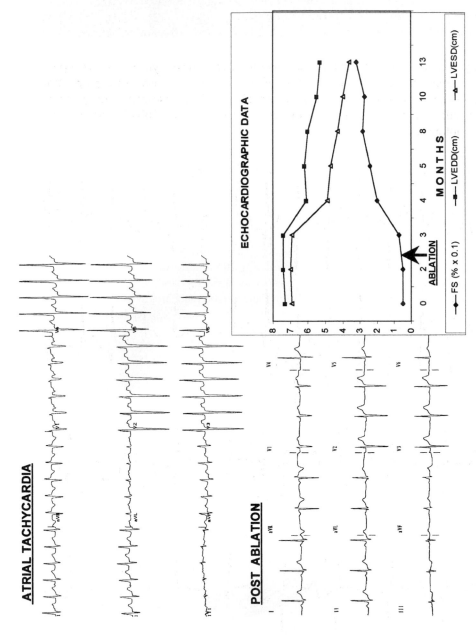

Figure 5.3 ECGs before and after ablation of incessant atrial tachycardia in a patient who presented with severe heart failure. Over the months, left ventricular end-diastolic (LVEDD) and end-systolic (LVESD) dimensions and fractional shortening (FS) returned to normal.

group are atrial fibrillation (see Chapter 6), atrial flutter (see Chapter 7) and atrial tachycardia (see Chapter 8).

EFFECTS OF SUPRAVENTRICULAR TACHYCARDIAS

Paroxysmal supraventricular tachycardias may cause major symptoms: syncope or near-syncope, particularly at the onset of the arrhythmia; distressing palpitation; angina, even in the absence of coronary artery disease; dyspnoea; fatigue and polyuria. Other patients will merely be aware of but not distressed by palpitation or may even be asymptomatic.

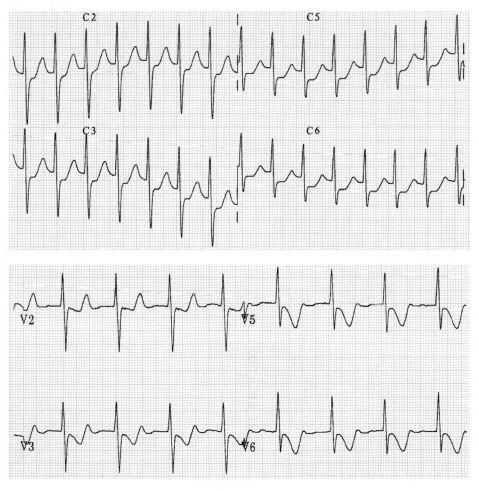

Figure 5.4 Leads V2–V6 during and soon after atrioventricular re-entrant tachycardia showing marked ST depression and T wave inversion in a young woman with normal coronary arteries.

Patients may be distressed not only by the symptoms caused by their tachycardia but by the unpredictable nature of the arrhythmia. Some live in dread of their next attack and may be frightened to travel or even to go out, for fear that a tachycardia might occur.

Most patients do not have structural heart disease but they may fear that the arrhythmia is a sign of impending heart attack or other major cardiac catastrophe. They need to be reassured that they have an 'electrical' rather than 'plumbing' or structural cardiac problem.

If sustained, supraventricular arrhythmias, especially atrial tachycardia, AVRT and atrial fibrillation with a very rapid ventricular response, can lead to heart failure. The term 'tachycardiomyopathy' is applied. Restoration of normal rhythm will reverse the failure (Figure 5.3).

Sometimes tachycardia can lead to marked ECG changes typical of those caused by myocardial ischaemia in patients without coronary heart disease (Figure 5.4). An elevated troponin level is widely regarded as evidence of acute myocardial infarction. However, small increases are sometimes seen in patients with prolonged tachycardias who have angiographically normal coronary arteries or whose age and coronary risk profile make the possibility of coronary disease most unlikely.

Atrial fibrillation

This is the most common of all cardiac arrhythmias. Indeed, as a result of increased life expectancy in the population and in particular in patients with heart disease its incidence is increasing. It is important to be familiar with the many causes, clinical manifestations and treatments of this heart rhythm disturbance.

ECG CHARACTERISTICS

During atrial fibrillation, the atria discharge at a rate between 350 and 600 beats/min. The arrhythmia is due to multiple wavelets of electrical activity randomly circulating within the atrial myocardium. The very rapid electrical activity results in loss of effective atrial contraction.

ATRIAL ACTIVITY

The rapid and chaotic atrial activity during atrial fibrillation results in small, irregular waves at a rate of 350–600 beats/min. The amplitude of these 'f' waves varies from patient to patient, and also from ECG lead to lead: in some leads, 'f' waves may not be apparent, whereas in other leads, especially lead V1, the waves may appear so coarse that atrial flutter is suspected (Figures 6.1 and 6.2).

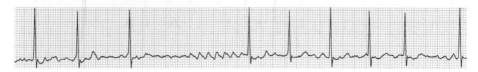

Figure 6.1 Typical 'f' waves of atrial fibrillation.

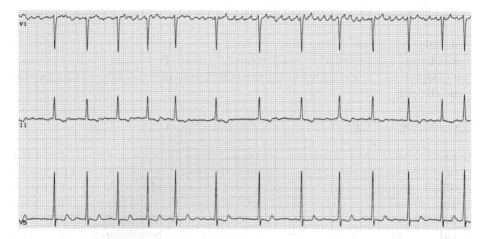

Figure 6.2 Atrial fibrillation. 'f' waves appear coarse in V1, fine in II and are not seen in V5. There is a totally irregular ventricular rhythm.

ATRIOVENTRICULAR CONDUCTION

Fortunately, the AV node cannot conduct every atrial impulse to the ventricles: if it could, ventricular fibrillation would result! Some impulses are totally blocked. Others only partially penetrate the AV node. They will not therefore activate the ventricles but may block or delay succeeding impulses. This process of 'concealed conduction' is responsible for the totally irregular ventricular rhythm that is the hallmark of this arrhythmia.

In the absence of P waves, even if 'f' waves are not seen, a totally irregular ventricular rhythm is indicative of atrial fibrillation. Atrial fibrillation with a rapid ventricular rhythm is often misdiagnosed. If the characteristic irregular rhythm is remembered, errors will not be made (Figure 6.3). If, however, there is complete AV block, ventricular activity will, of course, be slow and regular (Figure 6.4).

The ventricular rate during atrial fibrillation is dependent on the conducting ability of the AV node, which is itself influenced by the autonomic nervous system. Atrioventricular conduction will be enhanced by sympathetic activity and depressed by high vagal tone. Typically, ventricular rates are rapid, up to 200 beats/min, when the patient is active and are slow when the patient is at rest or asleep.

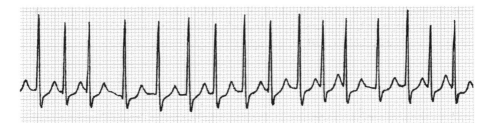

Figure 6.3 Atrial fibrillation with rapid ventricular response.

INTRAVENTRICULAR CONDUCTION

Ventricular complexes during atrial fibrillation are normal in duration unless there is established bundle branch block (Figure 6.5), Wolff–Parkinson–White syndrome (see Chapter 10), or aberrant intraventricular conduction (i.e. rate-related bundle branch block).

Aberrant intraventricular conduction

Aberrant conduction is the result of unequal recovery periods of the two bundle branches. An early atrial impulse may reach the ventricles when one bundle branch is still refractory to excitation following the previous cardiac cycle but the other is capable of conduction. The resultant ventricular complex will have a bundle branch block configuration. Because the right bundle usually has the longer refractory period, aberrant conduction commonly leads to right bundle branch block. The duration of the refractory periods of the bundle branches is related to the preceding cycle length. Thus, aberration is likely to occur when a short cycle succeeds a long cycle (Figure 6.6). Sometimes a series of aberrantly conducted beats will be misdiagnosed as paroxysmal ventricular tachycardia (see Figure 6.10). However, even though the rate is rapid there will be marked irregularity in the cycle length, and why should there be 'bursts' of a second arrhythmia during atrial fibrillation?

INITIATION

Atrial fibrillation is usually initiated by an atrial extrasystole (Figure 6.7). Sometimes atrial flutter or AV re-entrant tachycardia degenerate into atrial fibrillation.

The ECG characteristics of atrial fibrillation are summarized in Table 6.1.

Table 6.1 ECG characteristics of atrial fibrillation

Ventricular activity: Totally irregular

Atrial activity:
    P waves absent
    'f' waves to be seen in at least some leads

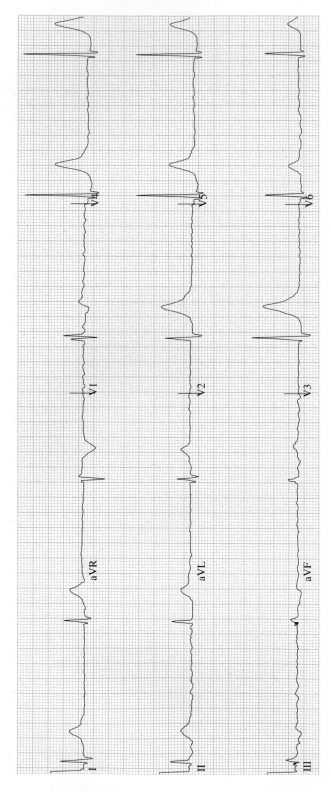

Figure 6.4 Atrial fibrillation with complete atrioventricular block. The ventricular rhythm is regular: rate 39 beats/min.

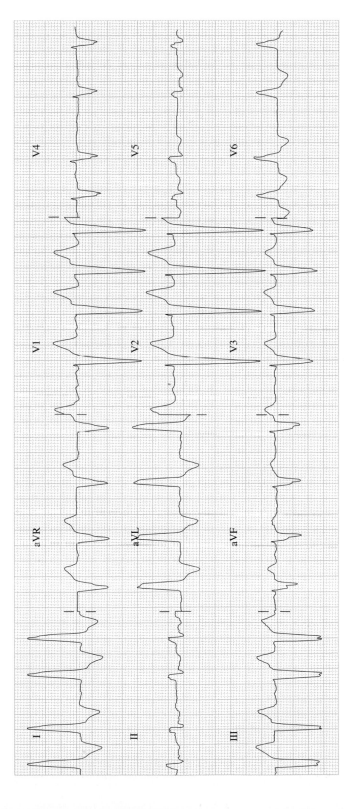

Figure 6.5 Atrial fibrillation with established left bundle branch block. The ventricular rhythm is totally irregular.

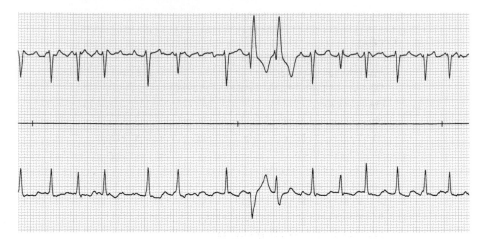

Figure 6.6 Atrial fibrillation. After seven normally conducted ventricular complexes, there are two complexes with right bundle branch block configuration.

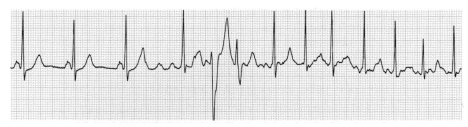

Figure 6.7   Atrial ectopic beat superimposed on T wave of third sinus beat initiates atrial fibrillation. Second and third complexes during atrial fibrillation are aberrantly conducted.

CAUSES

The most common causes are heart muscle damage due to coronary artery disease, hypertension or cardiomyopathy; heart valve disease; hyperthyroidism; and sick sinus syndrome (Table 6.2). In a substantial proportion of cases, atrial fibrillation is idiopathic (i.e. there is no demonstrable cause).

Coronary artery disease per se does not cause atrial fibrillation. However, the arrhythmia often results from myocardial infarction, both acutely and in the long term, and is an indicator of extensive myocardial damage.

A cause for atrial fibrillation should be sought. Many of the causes can be identified or excluded by clinical examination, electrocardiography and echocardiography. measurement of serum thyroxine is often necessary to exclude hyperthyroidism. Ambulatory electrocardiography may be required where sick sinus syndrome is a possibility.

PROGNOSIS

A major determinant of prognosis is the presence or absence of organic heart disease. For example, in patients with coronary artery disease, because atrial fibrillation is

Table 6.2   Causes of atrial fibrillation

Cardiac:
  Acute myocardial infarction
  Past myocardial infarction
  Dilated and hypertrophic cardiomyopathies
  Hypertension
  Myocarditis and pericarditis
  Heart valve disease especially rheumatic mitral valve disease
  Atrial septal defect
  Coronary bypass surgery
  Constrictive pericarditis
  Sick sinus syndrome
  Atrioventricular junctional re-entrant arrhythmias
  Wolff–Parkinson–White syndrome

Non-cardiac:
  Hyperthyroidism
  Chronic obstructive airways disease
  Chest infection
  Carcinoma lung
  Pulmonary embolism
  Acute and chronic alcohol abuse
  Idiopathic, i.e. no recognized cause (common)
  Familial, i.e. genetically determined (rare)

usually a result of extensive myocardial damage, it indicates a poor prognosis. Most studies have shown that idiopathic atrial fibrillation has a very good prognosis.

PREVALENCE

Prevalence increases with age. In a survey of male civil servants in the United Kingdom, atrial fibrillation was found in 0.16 per cent, 0.37 per cent and 1.13 per cent of those aged 40–49 years, 50–59 years and 60–64 years, respectively. In a British general practice 3.7 per cent of patients over 65 years were found to have the arrhythmia.

The Framingham study found that 7.8 per cent of men aged between 65 and 74 years had atrial fibrillation. The prevalence increased to 11.7 per cent in men aged 75–84 years. There is a 26 per cent 'life-time' likelihood of atrial fibrillation. Even in people without a history of heart failure or myocardial infarction the risk is in the order of 15 per cent. The arrhythmia was 1.5 times more common in men than in women.

CLASSIFICATION

The arrhythmia can be classified in terms of its duration:

- **Paroxysmal** – atrial fibrillation terminates spontaneously in less than seven days.

- **Persistent** – atrial fibrillation would continue indefinitely but normal rhythm can be restored by cardioversion.
- **Permanent** – restoration of normal rhythm is impossible.

LONE ATRIAL FIBRILLATION

Lone (i.e. idiopathic) atrial fibrillation is a common problem. While the prognosis is good and the risk of systemic embolism is low, lone atrial fibrillation can cause very troublesome symptoms and great anxiety. Like secondary atrial fibrillation, it may be paroxysmal or, less commonly, persistent.

PAROXYSMAL LONE ATRIAL FIBRILLATION

Some patients will experience only a single or a very occasional episode. Others will experience frequent recurrences; perhaps several times in a day. Paroxysms may last for many hours or stop after only a few seconds (Figure 6.8). With time, in some but not all patients, atrial fibrillation will become persistent. Some studies have shown that an episode of atrial fibrillation can lead to alterations in the electrical properties of the atria that encourage perpetuation of atrial fibrillation. This process is termed 'electrical remodelling'.

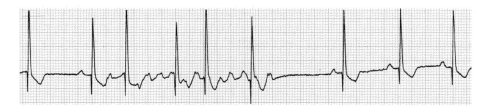

Figure 6.8 A brief episode of atrial fibrillation.

Patients often suffer major symptoms. Others, including some with frequent episodes and rapid ventricular rates, will be asymptomatic or merely aware of but not distressed by palpitation.

In a minority of patients there will be an identifiable precipitating event such as exercise, vomiting, alcohol or fatigue. One form of paroxysmal lone atrial fibrillation has been attributed to high vagal activity: the arrhythmia always starts at rest during bradycardia (Figure 6.9).

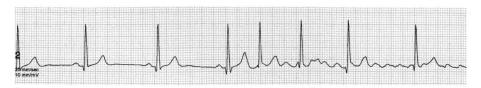

Figure 6.9 Onset of atrial fibrillation at rest during sinus: rate 50 beats/min.

MANAGEMENT OF ATRIAL FIBRILLATION

Management involves ascertaining the cause of the arrhythmia, protecting the patient from systemic embolism and either restoring normal rhythm or controlling the heart rate during atrial fibrillation.

SYSTEMIC EMBOLISM

During atrial fibrillation, stasis of blood in the left atrium and its appendage can lead to thrombus formation and hence systemic embolism. Of particular concern is the risk of stroke.

Increased levels of plasma fibrinogen and fibrin D-dimer have been found in atrial fibrillation. Levels return to normal after cardioversion, suggesting that it may be atrial fibrillation itself that causes a 'hypercoagulable' state.

RISK

Atrial fibrillation caused by rheumatic mitral valve disease leads to a very high (15-fold) risk of stroke. 'Non-rheumatic' causes of atrial fibrillation, mainly cardiac failure and hypertension, are associated with a moderately high (five-fold) risk of embolism with an incidence of approximately 5 per cent per annum. Furthermore, computerized tomography has demonstrated a 14 per cent incidence of asymptomatic cerebral infarction in these patients.

PREVENTION

Warfarin

Warfarin markedly reduces the risk of embolism but at a small increased risk of intracranial haemorrhage and other forms of bleeding. Studies have shown that very low dose warfarin is ineffective and have indicated that the ideal international normalized ratio of the prothrombin time (INR) is 2.0–3.0.

Aspirin

Aspirin is a more convenient alternative to warfarin for many patients and is less likely to cause haemorrhage but is less effective. The appropriate dose is 150–300 mg daily. The 'coronary prevention' dose of 75 mg daily has not been shown to reduce embolism due to atrial fibrillation.

Some patients with non-rheumatic atrial fibrillation are at risk from stroke from causes other than left atrial thrombus: for example, patients with myocardial damage caused by coronary disease may also have carotid artery stenosis. Atrial fibrillation in these patients may be a 'marker' of vascular disease; aspirin will be beneficial. The widely held belief that the combination of aspirin and warfarin increases the risk of bleeding has not been confirmed in recent studies though clearly aspirin must be avoided if there is a specific contraindication to this drug.

Warfarin or aspirin?

High embolic risk

All patients who are at high risk of embolism (Table 6.3) should receive warfarin provided they have no major contraindication. Risk in these patients appears to continue if sinus rhythm returns, perhaps because there is asymptomatic paroxysmal atrial fibrillation. Warfarin should be continued.

Table 6.3 Causes of atrial fibrillation leading to high risk of systemic embolism

Rheumatic mitral valve disease
Previous embolism
Thyrotoxicosis
Heart failure
Patients older than 75 years who are female, hypertensive or diabetic

Low embolic risk

Patients with idiopathic atrial fibrillation below 65 years of age are at low risk: approximately 1 per cent per annum. It is recommended that they receive aspirin. However, some of those patients may find even this low risk to be unacceptable and they may elect to receive warfarin for maximum protection.

Intermediate embolic risk

A somewhat greyer area is the patient who is at intermediate risk (Table 6.4): both warfarin and aspirin are reasonable options, and the merits of each therapy should be discussed with the patient.

Table 6.4 Patients at intermediate risk of systemic embolism

Age ⩾65 years
Diabetes
Coronary disease
Peripheral vascular disease

Newer treatments

Ximelagatran, an oral thrombin inhibitor, has been shown to be as effective as warfarin in preventing embolism, with no significant difference in risk of major haemorrhage. It has the major advantages that it can be prescribed in a fixed dose (typically 36 mg twice daily) and therefore blood tests are not required. Unlike warfarin it does not have the major risks of interaction with other drugs or alcohol. However, it has had to be withdrawn because of significant risk of liver damage.

Recently, the combination of aspirin and clopidogrel has been shown to be less effective than warfarin.

A percutaneous technique for closure of the left atrial appendage is currently being evaluated in patients in whom anticoagulants are contraindicated.

RHYTHM MANAGEMENT

Choice of treatment depends on whether the purpose is to control the ventricular response to atrial fibrillation or to maintain sinus rhythm. These strategies are termed 'rate control' and 'rhythm control', respectively.

Atrial fibrillation results in loss of atrial contraction prior to ventricular systole and often an inappropriate heart rate. Consequently, cardiac output usually falls. One would expect that patients would fare better if normal rhythm could be maintained rather than allowing persistent or paroxysmal atrial fibrillation to continue. However, several large studies have shown that a strategy of rhythm control is no better than one of rate control in terms of mortality, hospital admission and quality of life. The patients studied were mainly older and had cardiovascular disease. The results cannot be applied to all patients; for example younger patients with paroxysmal idiopathic atrial fibrillation are often highly symptomatic and benefit greatly from maintenance of normal rhythm.

Though these studies showed that the *strategy* of trying to maintain normal rhythm was no better than that of rate control, long-term normal rhythm was not achieved in many patients in the rhythm control groups. It is very likely that patients in whom normal rhythm is achieved do benefit. This is supported by both recent and old studies that have shown that maintenance of sinus rhythm improves quality of life and exercise capacity.

Not all patients with atrial fibrillation are the same. Some experience troublesome symptoms in spite of effective rate control and feel very much better when in normal rhythm. Others, including those who are asymptomatic prior to treatment, do well with a rate control approach. Treatment has to be tailored to the individual patient.

Not infrequently a rhythm control strategy will fail and a rate control approach will have to be accepted, but in highly symptomatic patients an 'aggressive' approach to maintaining normal rhythm is justified.

RATE CONTROL

Digoxin

Oral digoxin is widely used to control the ventricular response to atrial fibrillation. It has the advantages that it has long duration of action and may be positively inotropic. However, digoxin sometimes fails to control the heart rate at rest and is very often ineffective at controlling the rate during exertion in spite of appropriate plasma concentrations. Unwanted effects are common (see Chapter 19). Increasing age, renal or electrolyte disturbance, or the introduction of other drugs can lead to digoxin toxicity in patients who had been established on an appropriate therapeutic dose.

Intravenous digoxin is often ineffective at promptly reducing the ventricular response to atrial fibrillation. As stated below, digoxin has been shown to be ineffective at terminating or preventing atrial fibrillation.

In view of the many limitations of the drug and the fact that calcium channel blockers or beta-blockers can be used to slow the ventricular response to atrial fibrillation, there is a case for no longer using this drug.

Calcium channel blockers

Intravenous verapamil quickly and effectively depresses AV conduction and will thereby control a rapid ventricular response to atrial fibrillation within a few minutes. However, it is unlikely to restore sinus rhythm and indeed there is some evidence to suggest that verapamil will encourage the arrhythmia to persist.

Oral verapamil (120–240 mg daily) is usually effective in controlling the ventricular rate during atrial fibrillation, both at rest and on exertion.

Diltiazem (but not the dihydropyridine calcium channel blockers, i.e. nifedipine or amlodipine) has similar actions to verapamil.

When digoxin alone is inadequate, the addition of verapamil is extremely effective in controlling the ventricular response to atrial fibrillation. Verapamil increases digoxin concentrations but this mechanism is not thought to be responsible for its beneficial effect.

Beta-blockers

Beta-blocking drugs have similar benefits to the calcium antagonists.

Fast and slow ventricular rates

Some patients demonstrate both very fast and slow ventricular responses to atrial fibrillation. Ventricular pacing may occasionally be required to allow introduction of AV nodal blocking drugs (Figures 6.10 and 6.11).

Some patients with atrial fibrillation, presumably due to impaired AV nodal conduction, are unable to increase their heart rate adequately in response to exercise: 'chronotropic incompetence' (see Chapter 16). A pacemaker with the facility to increase heart rate when its sensor detects activity will enable an improvement in the ability to exercise.

Heart failure

Particular attention should be applied to patients with heart failure and atrial fibrillation. Sustained rapid ventricular rates may worsen or indeed may be the cause of heart failure. It is important to ensure that the ventricular rate is controlled not only at rest but also on exertion.

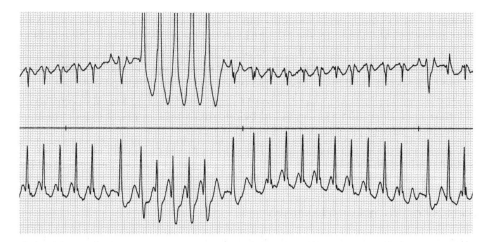

Figure 6.10 Very fast ventricular response to atrial fibrillation. There is aberrant conduction of the seventh to eleventh ventricular complexes.

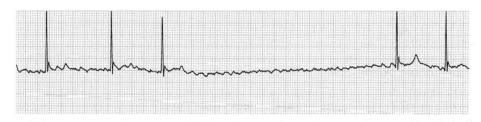

Figure 6.11 Very slow ventricular response during the night in the same patient as in Figure 6.10.

As stated above, some patients may have chronotropic incompetence due to impaired AV nodal conduction, whether spontaneous or due to medication such as beta-blockers. It is therefore important to ensure that the heart rate does increase appropriately on exertion.

RHYTHM CONTROL

Antiarrhythmic drugs

Intravenous therapy

Intravenous flecainide, propafenone, sotalol and amiodarone may restore normal rhythm (i.e. achieve chemical cardioversion) provided atrial fibrillation is of recent onset (i.e. within seven days). Only the latter drug should be used in patients with heart failure or who have marked impairment of ventricular function: the others may worsen myocardial function and, in patients with damaged myocardium, may cause ventricular arrhythmias.

Flecainide and propafenone can sometimes fail to restore normal rhythm but slow the atrial rate and thus convert atrial fibrillation to atrial flutter or tachycardia.

Paradoxically, the *lower* atrial rate can lead to a marked acceleration of the ventricular rate because the AV node can conduct a greater proportion of atrial impulses – occasionally necessitating electrical cardioversion.

Dofetilide and ibutilide are new drugs with a class III antiarrhythmic action (see Chapter 19) that have been shown to be effective at terminating atrial fibrillation of recent onset. However there is a significant risk of precipitating torsade de pointes ventricular tachycardia (see Chapter 13). These drugs are not currently available in the United Kingdom.

Digoxin is ineffective and there is evidence to show that it may actually help perpetuate the arrhythmia by shortening the refractory period of atrial myocardium. It should not be used.

It should be borne in mind that approximately half of episodes of recent onset atrial fibrillation will terminate spontaneously within 8 hours. Thus, an antiarrhythmic drug may not necessarily get the credit for restoring normal rhythm in every case!

Oral therapy

Flecainide and propafenone are moderately effective in preventing a recurrence of atrial fibrillation but the same contraindications as for intravenous therapy apply. They should not be used in patients with myocardial dysfunction or with coronary artery disease and ideally should be combined with a beta-blocker or calcium antagonist in case atrial flutter occurs, which might lead to a very fast ventricular rate. The author favours flecainide and would recommend it as a first-line drug in patients whose fibrillation usually starts at rest, provided there is normal ventricular function.

Beta-blockers may sometimes prevent atrial fibrillation and are the drug of choice if the history suggests that fibrillation is induced by exertion. Some, but not all, studies show that sotalol with its class III antiarrhythmic action (see Chapter 19) is more effective than other beta-blockers but must be avoided in patients with a prolonged QT interval.

Amiodarone is the most effective drug in preventing atrial fibrillation, but because of the high incidence of unwanted effects it should be reserved for patients with troublesome symptoms who fail to respond to the drugs above. It is a drug of choice in patients with heart failure.

Quinidine had been used for many years to prevent paroxysmal atrial fibrillation. However, a meta-analysis of studies of the efficacy of quinidine in preventing recurrence of atrial fibrillation found that the drug was associated with a significant increase in mortality, presumably due to a proarrhythmic effect.

In order to avoid daily medication, a 'pill in the pocket' approach to paroxysmal atrial fibrillation has been assessed. A single oral dose of flecainide (200 mg) or propafenone (600 mg) is taken by the patient at the onset of rapid palpitation. A return to normal rhythm can be expected in many patients within 2–3 hours. This approach may be useful in patients prone to prolonged episodes of atrial fibrillation and may avoid the need for hospital admission. However, many patients with paroxysmal atrial fibrillation experience incapacitating symptoms: abbreviation of an episode using a 'pill in the pocket' will be inadequate. Furthermore, these drugs must be avoided in patients with coronary artery disease or poor ventricular function, and, because of the significant risk of them leading to atrial flutter with a very fast ventricular response, should ideally be combined with an AV nodal blocking drug (i.e. a beta-blocker or calcium antagonist).

Digoxin shortens the atrial refractory period and may thereby increase the tendency to atrial fibrillation. There is no evidence that it prevents the arrhythmia.

Angiotensin-converting enzyme (ACE) inhibitors, angiotensin receptor blocking (ARB) drugs, statins, omega-3 fatty acids and eating oily fish have all been shown to be associated with a lower incidence of atrial fibrillation.

Electrical cardioversion

Sinus rhythm can be restored by electrical cardioversion in most patients with atrial fibrillation. However, the arrhythmia frequently returns. Risk factors for recurrence include a long duration of atrial fibrillation, heart failure, marked left atrial enlargement and age. No more than a third of patients will remain in normal rhythm in the long term.

High-energy shocks are often required for successful cardioversion of atrial fibrillation (see Chapter 21). Drugs such as flecainide, sotalol, propafenone and particularly amiodarone reduce the relapse rate after cardioversion. These drugs may have unwanted effects and in many patients should be reserved for repeat cardioversion when restoration of normal rhythm had resulted in major benefit and dictated the need for a further attempt at restoring and maintaining normal rhythm. Digoxin may actually increase the recurrence rate.

While cardioversion only leads to long-term sinus rhythm in a minority of patients, an attempt at restoring sinus rhythm should be considered in those patients with recent atrial fibrillation (less than 12 months) where no cause has been identified or in whom the disorder that has caused the arrhythmia has resolved or is self-limiting. If there is a recurrence, a further attempt at cardioversion, after initiation of antiarrhythmic therapy, should be undertaken in those with troublesome symptoms attributable to the arrhythmia.

There are reports of restoring and maintaining normal rhythm by cardioversion in up to one-third of patients with atrial fibrillation that has persisted for over 12–24 months. In patients with atrial fibrillation that is difficult to treat, even if long-standing, cardioversion should also be considered because there is a small chance that normal rhythm will be achieved and maintained.

Transvenous cardioversion is now an established means of restoring normal rhythm (see Chapter 21). A low-energy shock is delivered between transvenous electrodes positioned in the right atrium and either the coronary sinus or pulmonary artery. Higher success rates than for transthoracic cardioversion, especially in very large patients, have been reported.

Most patients undergo cardioversion as an elective procedure but occasionally urgent cardioversion is required in haemodynamically unstable patients.

Anticoagulation before and after cardioversion

Cardioversion can result in immediate systemic embolism because of dislodgement of pre-existing thrombus. Also new atrial thrombus can develop after cardioversion because atrial mechanical activity often does not return for up to three weeks after the procedure and because cardioversion itself can increase blood hypercoagulability. Hence embolism can also occur in the few weeks following cardioversion. It is therefore important that non-urgent cardioversion in patients who have been in atrial fibrillation for more than 24–48 hours is preceded by warfarin to achieve an INR of 2.5 for at least three weeks, and that anticoagulation is continued for at least four weeks after restoration of normal rhythm.

If urgent cardioversion is required, transoesophageal echocardiography can be used to exclude left atrial thrombus or stasis. The echocardiographic signs of left atrial stasis are spontaneous echo contrast and reduced left atrial appendage flow velocity. If cardioversion has to be carried out urgently it should be preceded by heparin and succeeded by warfarin.

'Refractory' atrial fibrillation

Amiodarone

Amiodarone is a very potent antiarrhythmic drug that will often maintain sinus rhythm or at least control the ventricular response to atrial fibrillation when other drugs have failed. However, in view of the high incidence of major unwanted effects, the drug should be reserved for patients in whom other drugs have failed and for patients in whom the risk of side-effects in the long term may not be a major consideration because their prognosis is poor (e.g. the elderly and those with severe myocardial damage).

Catheter ablation

Transvenous radiofrequency ablation of the AV junction should be considered in patients with severe symptoms in whom antiarrhythmic drugs are ineffective or cannot be tolerated (see Chapter 26). It necessitates pacemaker implantation and in many cases oral anticoagulation, but it is very effective at controlling symptoms and has been demonstrated in several studies to improve patients' quality of life. It also avoids the need for antiarrhythmic therapy.

Recently, radiofrequency ablation has been shown to be effective in preventing paroxysmal atrial fibrillation. This is discussed in Chapter 26.

There is interest in atrial pacing to prevent paroxysmal atrial fibrillation. Stimulation of the atrial septum or simultaneous stimulation of the right atrial appendage and coronary os has been shown to abbreviate the duration of atrial activation – an important determinant of predisposition to paroxysmal atrial fibrillation. Studies have shown that in some patients the arrhythmia can be prevented by these pacing modes, though in the author's experience it is usually necessary to continue an antiarrhythmic drug such as flecainide that without pacing was ineffective.

An implantable atrial defibrillator is available for control of paroxysmal atrial fibrillation. The device is usually activated by the patient rather than discharging a shock automatically. Shock delivery is painful and clearly the device is only suitable for patients with infrequent episodes. Apart from the pain, concerns include the unpredictable nature of paroxysmal atrial fibrillation and the high rate of early or even immediate recurrence of the arrhythmia. For these reasons implantation rates are low and the explantation rate is substantial!

The most aggressive approach to dealing with very troublesome atrial fibrillation is the 'maze procedure'. Lines of conduction block in the atria are created by incision, radiofrequency energy, ultrasound or cryothermy, resulting in barriers in atrial conduction such that the multiple wavelets of electrical activity circulating within the atria that cause the atrial fibrillation cannot be sustained. Cardiac surgery or a very prolonged catheter procedure is required, with their associated significant risks.

Main points

- Atrial fibrillation is characterized by a totally irregular ventricular rhythm and absence of P waves. The chaotic atrial activity results in rapid, small, irregular 'f' waves which may not be seen in all ECG leads.

- The main causes are heart muscle damage from coronary artery disease or cardiomyopathy, rheumatic heart valve disease, hyperthyroidism, sick sinus syndrome, thoracotomy, obstructive airways disease and alcohol abuse. Often, atrial fibrillation is idiopathic.

- Prevalence increases with age.

- The arrhythmia may be paroxysmal, persistent or permanent.

- Treatment has to be tailored to the individual patient according to the causes, clinical effects and risks of the arrhythmia.

- Sotalol, flecainide and amiodarone but not digoxin may terminate and/or prevent paroxysmal atrial fibrillation.

- Though cardioversion usually restores sinus rhythm, there is a high relapse rate. High-energy shocks are required.

- The ventricular response to atrial fibrillation can be controlled by calcium antagonists and beta-blocking drugs that slow conduction in the AV node. Digoxin may fail to control the rate, particularly during exercise.

- Atrial fibrillation may cause systemic embolism that can be prevented by warfarin. Rheumatic mitral valve disease leads to a very high risk of stroke. 'Non-rheumatic' causes of atrial fibrillation are associated with a moderately high risk. The risk in non-rheumatic atrial fibrillation increases with age: it is small in those less than 60 years. Embolism is rare in idiopathic atrial fibrillation.

Atrial flutter

In the typical form of atrial flutter the atria discharge at a rate between 240 and 350 beats/min. Usually, the atrial rate is close to 300 beats/min. The arrhythmia is caused by a re-entrant circuit within the right atrium. Usually, the impulse circulates in an inferior direction along the lateral border of the right atrium and returns in a superior direction along the interatrial septum (Figure 7.1). The left atrium is activated by the impulses arising from the right atrium.

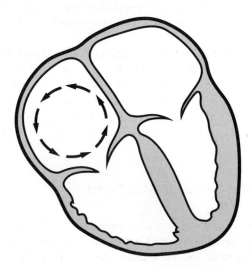

Figure 7.1 Common atrial flutter: counterclockwise circuit within the right atrium.

ECG CHARACTERISTICS

Atrial flutter may be paroxysmal or sustained. It is usually initiated by an atrial extrasystole. It may degenerate into atrial fibrillation.

ATRIAL ACTIVITY

During the typical form of atrial flutter, the atria discharge regularly at a rate of approximately 300 beats/min. In many leads there will be no isoelectric line between atrial deflections or 'F' waves, leading to the characteristic sawtooth appearance that is usually best seen in leads II, III and aVF. However, in some leads, especially lead V1, atrial activity will be seen in the form of discrete waves (Figure 7.2).

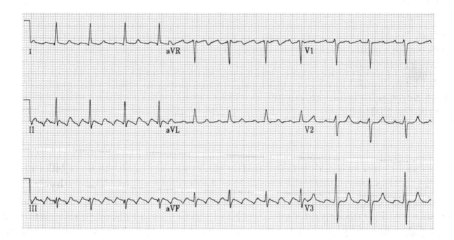

Figure 7.2 Typical atrial flutter: negative sawtooth pattern in the inferior leads and positive, discrete F waves in lead V1 as is seen in the common form of typical atrial flutter.

Commonly in typical atrial flutter, the atrial impulse circulates counterclockwise within the right atrium in which case the F waves are negative in leads II, III and aVF, of very low amplitude in lead I and positive in V1 (Figure 7.2). Uncommonly, the impulse circulates in a clockwise direction (Figure 7.3).

In atypical atrial flutter, the atrial rate is faster, ranging from 350 to 450 beats/min. It is not amenable to isthmus ablation (see below) and cannot be terminated by rapid atrial pacing.

ATRIOVENTRICULAR CONDUCTION

As with atrial fibrillation, the ventricular response to atrial flutter is determined by the conducting ability of the AV junction. Commonly, alternate 'F' waves are conducted to the ventricles with a resultant ventricular rate close to 150 beats/min (Figure 7.4). Drugs or impaired AV nodal function may lead to a higher degree of AV block

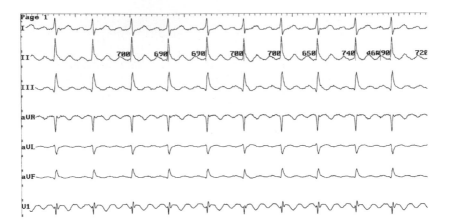

Figure 7.3 Uncommon form of typical atrial flutter due to clockwise rotation within the right atrial re-entrant circuit.

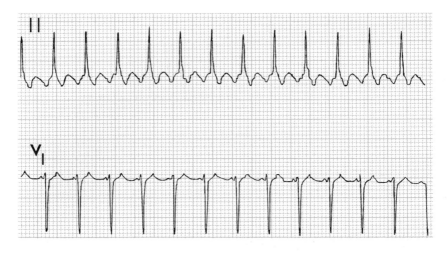

Figure 7.4 Atrial flutter with 2:1 atrioventricular block. Lead II shows a classic sawtooth appearance while V1 shows discrete atrial waves. In V1 each QRS complex is immediately preceded by an F wave and is followed by an F wave which is superimposed on the T wave.

(Figure 7.5). High levels of sympathetic nervous system activity, as may occur during exercise, may enhance AV nodal conduction and result in 1:1 conduction and a ventricular rate of approximately 300 beats/min (Figure 7.6).

With high degrees of AV block, atrial activity is clearly discernible and the arrhythmia is easy to diagnose (Figure 7.7). However, during a rapid ventricular response, ventricular T waves may be superimposed on alternate 'F' waves and may obscure the characteristic atrial activity: sinus tachycardia may be mistakenly diagnosed (Figure 7.8). Atrial flutter should be suspected if the heart rate is 150 beats/min at rest. Carotid sinus massage or adenosine can transiently impair AV conduction and aid diagnosis (Figure 7.9).

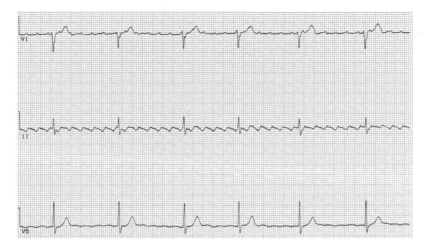

Figure 7.5 Atrial flutter with slow ventricular response.

INTRAVENTRICULAR CONDUCTION

Ventricular complexes will be normal in duration unless there is bundle branch block, ventricular preexcitation or aberrant intraventricular conduction.

The ECG characteristics of atrial flutter are summarized in Table 7.1.

Table 7.1 ECG characteristics of atrial flutter

Atrial activity:
   'F' waves at rate of 300 beats/min
   'Sawtooth' appearance in limb leads
   Discrete atrial waves in V1
Ventricular activity:
   Rarely, 1:1 atrioventricular conduction resulting in ventricular rate of 300 beats/min
   Usually, 2:1 or higher degrees of atrioventricular block

CAUSES

Atrial flutter has similar aetiologies to atrial fibrillation, including idiopathic.

PREVALENCE

Atrial flutter is less common than atrial fibrillation. A recent survey reports an annual incidence of 88 per 100 000.

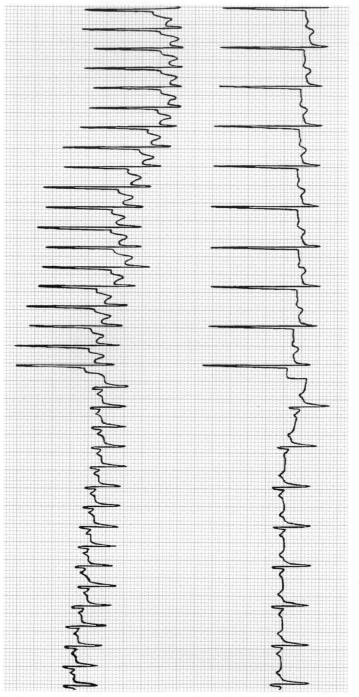

Figure 7.6 Continuous recordings of leads V1 and V4. In the upper trace the ventricular rate is 300 beats/min, suggesting atrial flutter with 1:1 atrioventricular conduction. The lower trace shows the effect of carotid massage. The ventricular rate is halved and F waves can be seen in V1 immediately before the QRS complex and superimposed on the T wave.

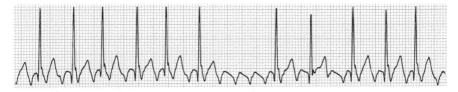

Figure 7.7 Atrial flutter only clearly seen during transient increase in atrioventricular block.

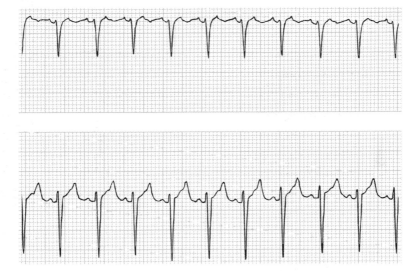

Figure 7.8 Simultaneous recording of leads V1 and V2. Atrial flutter can be diagnosed from V1 (alternate F waves are superimposed on the beginning of the ventricular T wave)

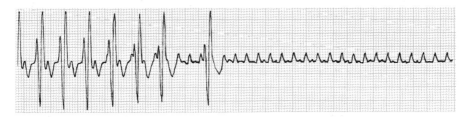

Figure 7.9 Atrial flutter revealed during several seconds of complete atrioventricular block induced by adenosine.

TREATMENT

Attempts to control a rapid ventricular response to atrial flutter by drugs are often unsuccessful. Where possible, the aim should be to restore and maintain sinus rhythm.

CARDIOVERSION

Sustained atrial flutter can almost always be terminated with a low-energy DC shock (e.g. 50 J). The consensus is that, where possible, cardioversion should be preceded by anticoagulation as for atrial fibrillation (see Chapter 6). In patients with idiopathic atrial flutter the case for warfarin may be less compelling.

ANTIARRHYTHMIC DRUGS

Drugs such as sotalol, flecainide, disopyramide and propafenone may be effective in terminating atrial flutter. However, it should be borne in mind that these drugs, if unsuccessful in restoring sinus rhythm, may possibly lead to higher ventricular rates. First, some drugs, particularly disopyramide, have a vagolytic effect that might enhance conduction through the AV node. Second, drugs often slow the atrial rate, facilitating a reduction in the AV conduction ratio and thereby paradoxically leading to an increase in ventricular rate (Figure 7.10).

Ibutilide may be effective but may cause torsade de pointes tachycardia.

Drugs that may prevent a recurrence of atrial fibrillation, as discussed above, may be effective in preventing recurrence of atrial flutter. Amiodarone can be very

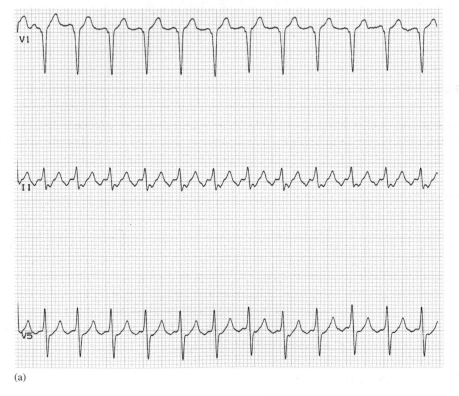

(a)

Figure 7.10 (a) Atrial flutter prior to intravenous flecainide; (b) Same patient as in (a) after intravenous flecainide which slowed the atrial rate and thereby facilitated a faster ventricular response.

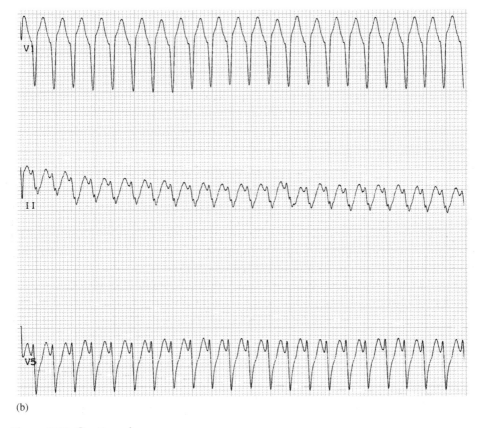

(b)

Figure 7.10 Continued.

successful in maintaining sinus rhythm when other drugs have failed. Even if atrial flutter persists, the drug's actions in both slowing the atrial rate and depressing AV conduction can lead to a substantial slowing of the ventricular rate.

RAPID ATRIAL PACING

Rapid atrial pacing at a rate approximately 25 per cent in excess of the atrial rate (not the ventricular rate!) for 30s will often restore sinus rhythm: pacing may have to be repeated several times before atrial flutter is terminated. Atrial fibrillation may sometimes be precipitated, but usually sinus rhythm returns within a few hours.

Pacing is generally carried out transvenously. Stimulation of the low right atrium is more likely to lead to successful termination of the arrhythmia. It is important to ensure that pacing stimuli do capture the atria: capture is usually reflected by an increase or decrease in the ventricular rate.

CATHETER ABLATION

Catheter ablation can be used to interrupt the re-entrant circuit in the right atrium and thereby terminate and prevent typical atrial flutter (see Chapter 26). Radiofrequency energy is usually delivered to the isthmus between the posterior portion of the tricuspid valve and the inferior vena cava. Success rates are not quite as high as in ablation of other arrhythmias but do compare very favourably with antiarrhythmic therapy. Atrial fibrillation can sometimes result in the longer term.

In the long term, atrial flutter will return in 50 per cent of cases after cardioversion and further cardioversion or alternative treatment will be required. Radiofrequency ablation should be considered if atrial flutter does recur. Some would recommend ablation for a first episode of atrial flutter. However, there is a fair chance that either atrial flutter will not recur after cardioversion or there is a very long interval between episodes, in which case the patient may opt for further cardioversion. Not infrequently, coronary bypass surgery causes atrial flutter: it is the author's impression that recurrence in this situation is less likely.

CONTROL OF VENTRICULAR RESPONSE

If normal rhythm cannot be restored or maintained, AV nodal blocking drugs may be required to control the rapid ventricular response to atrial flutter. Intravenous verapamil or diltiazem will promptly slow the ventricular rate during atrial flutter.

An oral calcium antagonist or beta-blocking drug can be employed as with atrial fibrillation. Amiodarone may also be effective. Sometimes, it is not possible to control the ventricular response to atrial flutter with oral drugs.

SYSTEMIC EMBOLISM

As with atrial fibrillation, atrial flutter can cause systemic embolism. Current evidence suggests that the risk is low but patients with atrial flutter who have clinical or echocardiographic findings that would indicate high risk if they had atrial fibrillation should receive warfarin. It is possible that embolism in cases of atrial flutter is due to these patients also experiencing paroxysmal atrial fibrillation.

Main points

- The diagnosis of atrial flutter is based on the finding of atrial activity at a rate of approximately 300 beats/min.

- In typical atrial flutter, atrial activity will be in the form of a sawtooth pattern in leads II, III and aVF, but discrete F waves will be seen in lead V1.

- Lead V1 is often the best lead for demonstrating atrial flutter: when there is 2:1 AV conduction, alternate F waves will be superimposed on ventricular T waves.

- Where possible, a return to sinus rhythm should be sought.

- Cardioversion with low energy will usually terminate atrial flutter but there is a substantial recurrence rate that may necessitate catheter ablation.

Atrial tachycardia

The practical difference between atrial tachycardia and flutter is that in the former the atrial rate is slower, being between 120 and 240 beats/min. Again, sometimes the AV node can conduct all atrial impulses but often there is a degree of AV block. Atrial tachycardia can originate from either the right or left atrium.

ECG CHARACTERISTICS

Because the atrial rate is slower, there is no sawtooth appearance to the baseline. Abnormally shaped P waves are inscribed at a regular rate (Figures 8.1 and 8.2). The ventricular complexes will be narrow unless there is pre-existent bundle branch block, or aberrant intraventricular conduction. Again as for atrial flutter, atrial activity is often best seen in lead V1.

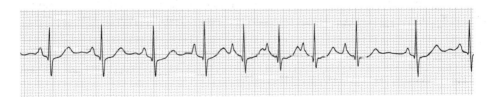

Figure 8.1 After three sinus beats there is a short episode of atrial tachycardia: the rate abruptly increases and there is a change in P wave morphology.

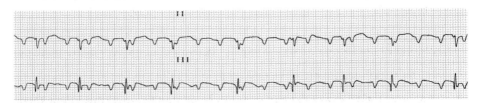

Figure 8.2 Atrial tachycardia with atrioventricular block. The atrial rate is 150 beats/min.

Atrial tachycardia with 1:1 AV conduction may occur (Figure 8.3). As in atrial flutter, carotid sinus massage is often helpful in the diagnosis (Figure 8.4). However, it should be noted that in some patients adenosine will terminate atrial tachycardia without causing transient AV block.

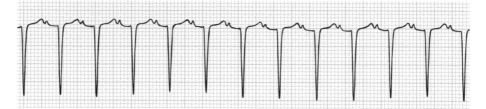

Figure 8.3 Lead V1. Atrial tachycardia with 1:1 atrioventricular conduction.

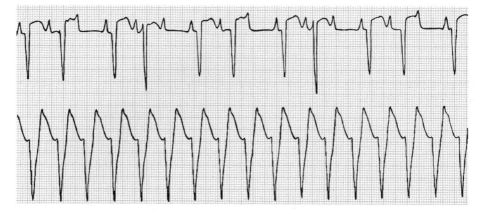

Figure 8.4 Lead V1. Atrial tachycardia before (lower trace) and during carotid sinus massage (upper trace). The atrial rate in the upper trace is the same as the ventricular rate in the lower trace: showing that without carotid massage there is 1:1 atrioventricular conduction.

Sometimes, when there is 1:1 AV conduction there can be doubt as to whether the rhythm is atrial or sinus tachycardia. Usually, the PR interval is short during sinus tachycardia so a long PR interval points to atrial rather than sinus tachycardia (Figure 8.3).

A positive P wave in lead V1 points to a left atrial origin while a positive P wave in lead aVL points to a right atrial origin (Figure 8.5).

With fairly high grades of AV block, because the ventricular rate is relatively slow, the rhythm may be misdiagnosed as complete heart block and an inappropriate request made for cardiac pacing!

Atrial tachycardia is often paroxysmal (Figure 8.6). If incessant, however, it may lead to heart failure (see Figure 5.3).

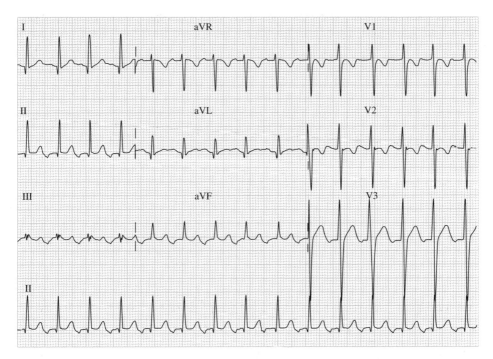

Figure 8.5 Right atrial tachycardia with 1:1 atrioventricular conduction. P waves are inverted in inferior leads and positive in aVL.

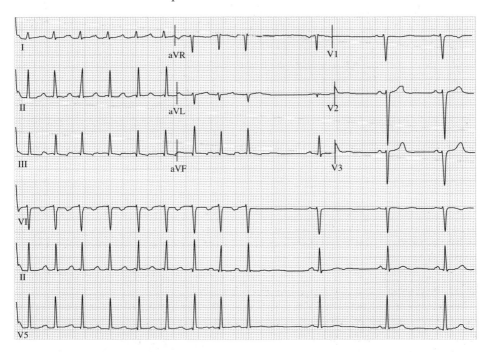

Figure 8.6 Paroxysmal atrial tachycardia terminates after nine beats. During tachycardia there is a P wave superimposed on each T wave.

CAUSES

Causes of atrial tachycardia include cardiomyopathy, chronic ischaemic heart disease, rheumatic heart disease, chronic obstructive airways disease and sick sinus syndrome. Not infrequently, no cause is found.

Atrial tachycardia with AV block may be due to digoxin toxicity (Figure 8.7). The arrhythmia is often referred to as 'paroxysmal atrial tachycardia with block', abbreviated to PATB. The term paroxysmal is inappropriate, particularly in the context of digoxin toxicity, because the arrhythmia is usually sustained.

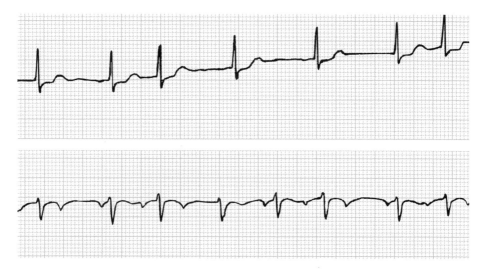

Figure 8.7 Atrial tachycardia (leads II and V1) in a patient with digoxin toxicity. Lead II suggests atrial fibrillation but V1 clearly shows atrial tachycardia with Mobitz I atrioventricular block.

TREATMENT

If the patient is receiving digoxin, toxicity should be suspected and the drug discontinued.

If a return to sinus rhythm is required, cardioversion or rapid atrial pacing should be performed.

Antiarrhythmic drugs such as sotalol, flecainide and amiodarone may be effective in maintaining normal rhythm.

Radiofrequency catheter ablation to the site of origin, which is often in the lateral or low septal wall of the right atrium or near the pulmonary veins in the left atrium, should be considered in refractory cases.

Main points

- The atrial rate is between 120 and 240 beats/min.

- The AV node may conduct all atrial impulses or there may be a degree of AV block.

- Carotid massage or adenosine may aid diagnosis when there is doubt as to whether there is an atrial tachycardia.

- Treatments include antiarrhythmic drugs, cardioversion and catheter ablation.

CHAPTER 9

Atrioventricular junctional re-entrant tachycardias

In these supraventricular arrhythmias, as stated earlier, there is an additional connection between atria and ventricles so an impulse can repeatedly travel along a circuit consisting of the AV junction and the additional AV connection. This is in contrast to the atrial arrhythmias discussed in the previous three chapters, where the mechanism responsible for the tachycardia is confined to the atria and the AV node merely transmits some or all of the atrial impulses to the ventricles.

MECHANISM

In most cases the heart is structurally normal (i.e. there is no valve, myocardial or coronary disease). The impulse is usually conducted from atria to ventricles by the AV junction and then re-enters the atria via the additional connection (Figure 9.1).

The additional connection can be of one of two types: an accessory AV pathway or a dual AV nodal pathway.

ACCESSORY ATRIOVENTRICULAR PATHWAY

An accessory AV pathway is a strand of myocardium that straddles the groove between atria and ventricles and therefore bypasses the AV node. A re-entrant

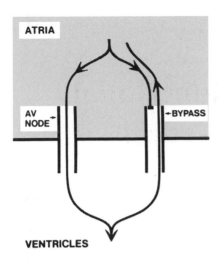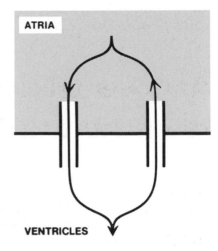

Figure 9.1 Initiation of atrioventricular junctional re-entrant tachycardia. An atrial extrasystole arrives at the atrioventricular junction while the bypass tract is still refractory to excitation following the last cardiac cycle. The extrasystole is therefore only conducted to the ventricles via the atrioventricular node. By the time the extrasystole has traversed the atrioventricular node and reached the ventricles, the bypass tract has recovered and can conduct the impulse back to the atria (left-hand panel), thereby initiating the re-entrant mechanism (right-hand panel).

tachycardia involving an accessory AV pathway is termed an AV junctional re-entrant tachycardia (AVRT).

DUAL ATRIOVENTRICULAR NODAL PATHWAYS

The other type of additional connection occurs when the AV node and its adjacent atrial tissues are functionally dissociated into fast and slow AV nodal pathways (i.e. dual AV nodal pathways). Conduction from atria to ventricles is usually via a relatively slowly conducting AV nodal pathway while ventriculo-atrial conduction is via a fast AV pathway. A tachycardia due to dual AV nodal pathways is termed an AV nodal re-entrant tachycardia (AVNRT).

ECG CHARACTERISTICS

The tachycardia is regular and usually the QRS complexes are normal and therefore narrow (Figure 9.2). Occasionally pre-existing bundle branch block or bundle branch block caused by the tachycardia will lead to broad ventricular complexes (Figure 9.3).

The rate during tachycardia can range from 120 to 250 beats/min and is influenced by the sympathetic nervous system. For example, sympathetic activity and consequently the speed of AV nodal conduction increase on standing or during exertion so the tachycardia becomes faster.

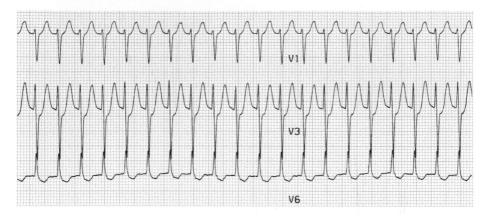

Figure 9.2 Atrioventricular junctional re-entrant tachycardia. A regular tachycardia with narrow ventricular complexes.

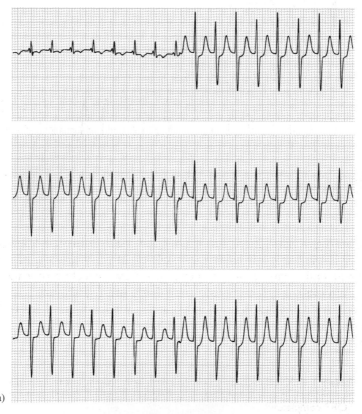

(a)

Figure 9.3 Atrioventricular re-entrant tachycardia, leads V1–V6. (a) With narrow complexes.

Clearly, normal P waves will not occur during this arrhythmia. Since the circulating impulse re-enters the atria after ventricular activation, each QRS complex will be followed by a P wave, though this wave is not always detectable (Figures 9.4–9.6, pages 68–69). If the atrial rate exceeds the ventricular rate, whether spontaneously

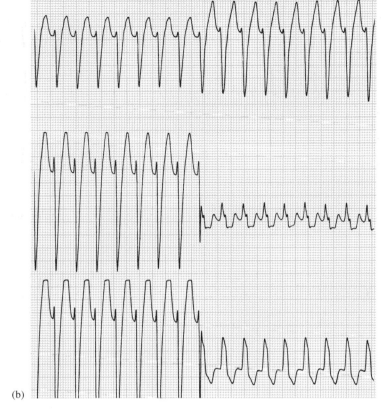

(b)

Figure 9.3 (b) A few minutes later, broad complexes have developed due to functional left bundle branch block.

or due to a drug or manoeuvre which slows AV node conduction, then the rhythm is not AV re-entrant tachycardia, it is probably atrial tachycardia or flutter.

ST segment and T wave changes can be caused by the tachycardia and persist for some time after its cessation: they are of no diagnostic significance.

The ECG during sinus rhythm is usually normal unless there is the Wolff–Parkinson–White syndrome (see Chapter 10).

The ECG characteristics of AVRTs are summarized in Table 9.1.

Table 9.1 ECG characteristics of atrioventricular re-entrant tachycardias

QRS complexes:
   Regular
   Rate 130–250 beats/min
   Usually narrow
P waves:
   Inverted, during or after each QRS complex

TIMING OF ATRIAL ACTIVITY DURING TACHYCARDIA

The timing of atrial activity, if identifiable, will indicate whether the tachycardia is due to an accessory AV pathway (i.e. AVRT), or due to dual AV nodal pathways (i.e. AVNRT). The distinction is relevant if the patient is a candidate for radiofrequency ablation.

With typical AVNRT, a P wave *immediately* follows or is actually superimposed on the QRS complex because the length of the re-entrant circuit is small (Figures 9.4–9.6).

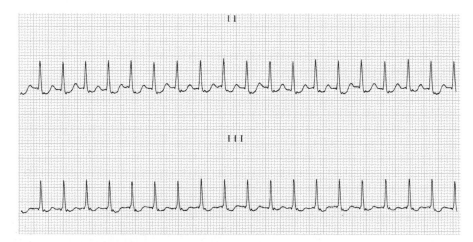

Figure 9.4 Atrioventricular nodal re-entrant tachycardia. A small P wave immediately follows each QRS complex.

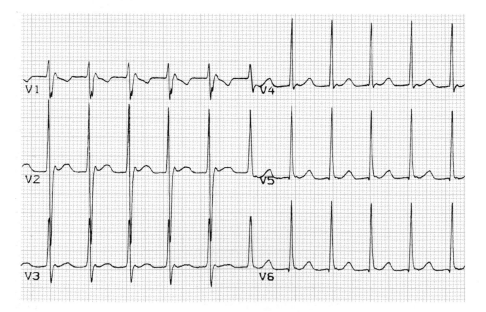

Figure 9.5 Atrioventricular nodal re-entrant tachycardia. A small P wave can be seen after each QRS. In leads V1 and V2 it could be mistaken for a secondary R wave.

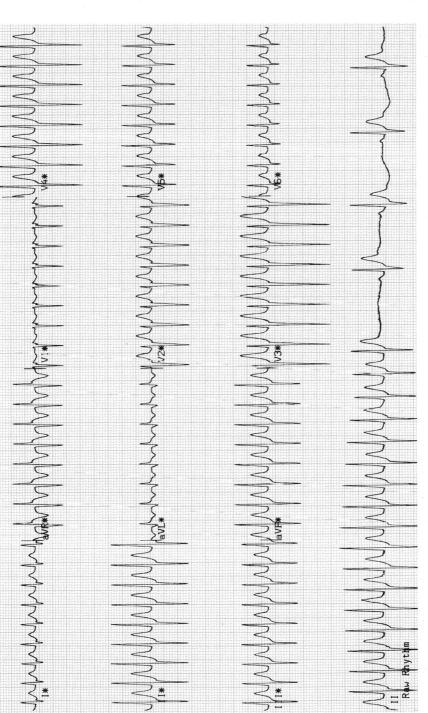

Figure 9.6 Atrioventricular nodal re-entrant tachycardia. The retrograde P wave can be seen superimposed on the terminal part of lead V1. Sinus rhythm returns during recording of rhythm strip (lead II).

The P wave is often best seen in lead V1. It might be mistaken for the secondary R wave of right bundle branch block but if this were the case the same wave should be present in lead V1 during sinus rhythm (Figures 9.5 and 9.6).

The length of the re-entrant circuit is greater in AVRT because the accessory AV pathway is some distance from the AV junction. It therefore takes longer for an impulse to circulate and re-enter the atria. Hence the inverted P wave occurs roughly halfway between QRS complexes and will therefore usually be superimposed on the T wave (Figure 9.7). It can be identified because superimposition of the P wave on the T wave usually leads to a pointed appearance of the T wave (Figures 9.7–9.9).

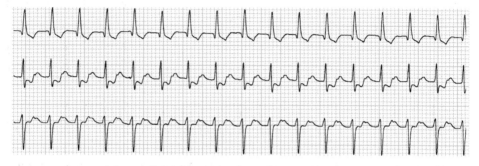

Figure 9.7 Atrioventricular re-entrant tachycardia. There is a P wave after each QRS complex that is superimposed on the T wave, resulting in its pointed appearance. An inverted P wave in lead I suggests a left-sided accessory pathway.

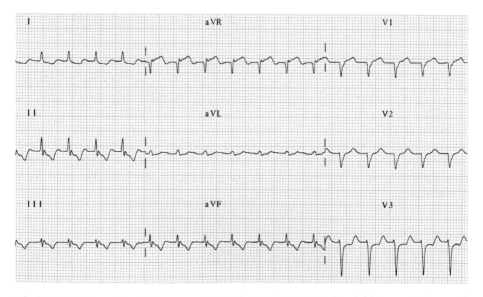

Figure 9.8 Atrioventricular re-entrant tachycardia (due to left posterior accessory atrioventricular pathway).

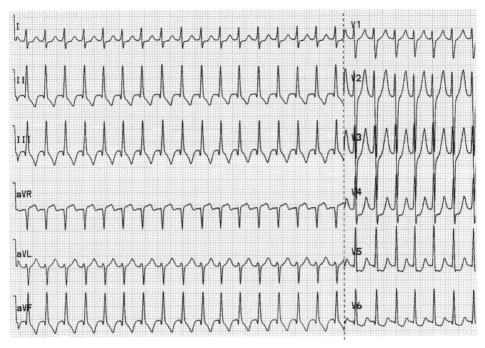

Figure 9.9 Atrioventricular re-entrant tachycardia. There is a P wave after each QRS complex that is superimposed on the T wave, resulting in its pointed appearance. The inverted P wave in leads II, III and aVF indicates a posteroseptal pathway.

CLINICAL FEATURES

The arrhythmia is common. Attacks may start in infancy, childhood or adult life and often recur. Though AVRT is due to a congenitally acquired abnormality the first attack can occur in adult life. AVNRT can occur at any age but typically starts after the second decade and is more common in females.

The duration and frequency of attacks varies from patient to patient. They may last for a few minutes or for many hours, and may occur several times per day or be separated by many months. In some patients, attacks are precipitated by exertion. In most, episodes can occur at rest or on exertion and can be brought on by trivial activities such as bending down.

TREATMENT

The patient should be reassured the tachycardia is not dangerous and that it is due to an electrical rather than structural cardiac abnormality: patients often fear the arrhythmia is due to coronary disease and that they are at risk from a heart attack.

Treatment is unnecessary for short episodes of tachycardia that do not cause distress.

Several treatments can be used to terminate or to prevent recurrence of the arrhythmia (Table 9.2).

Table 9.2 Summary of treatments for atrioventricular re-entrant tachycardias

Termination:
Vagal stimulation
Intravenous drugs, e.g. adenosine, verapamil
Cardioversion
Pacing (overdrive or programmed stimulation)
Prevention:
Ablation of additional connection
Drugs, e.g. sotalol, flecainide

VAGAL STIMULATION

The first approach to termination is vagal stimulation. An increase in vagal tone may temporarily slow conduction through the AV node and thereby interrupt the tachycardia circuit.

The Valsalva manoeuvre and carotid sinus massage are the best methods: they should be carried out with the patient lying down. The former is performed by the patient attempting to forcefully exhale for 10–15 s while sealing the nose and mouth, and then breathing normally. Carotid massage is performed by firm digital pressure over one carotid artery at the level of the upper border of the thyroid cartilage for 5 s (Figure 9.10a).

Eyeball pressure is widely quoted as a method for vagal stimulation but is very painful and should not be used.

INTRAVENOUS DRUGS

If vagal stimulation fails, the tachycardia can almost certainly be terminated by an intravenous injection of one of several drugs. Adenosine is the treatment of choice.

Adenosine

Adenosine is a potent blocker of AV nodal conduction that has an extremely short duration of action: 20 s. It is very effective in terminating AVNRT and AVRT (Figure 9.10b).

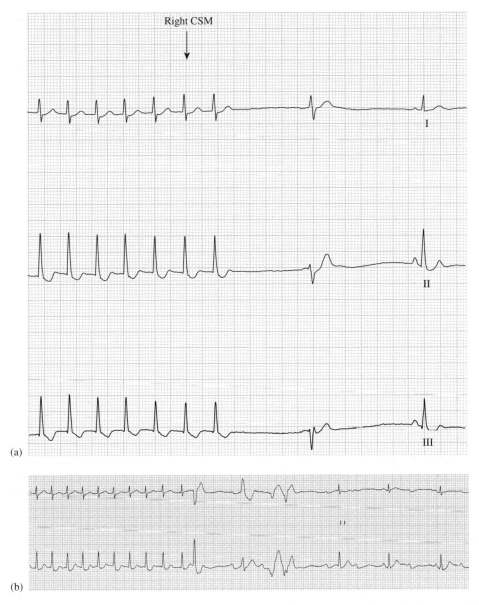

Figure 9.10 Termination of atrioventricular junctional re-entrant tachycardia. By carotid sinus massage (a) and by adenosine (b). There are some ventricular ectopic beats and a short period of atrioventricular block after adenosine as commonly occurs.

It should be given as a rapid (2 s) intravenous bolus, followed by a saline flush. The recommended initial dose in adults and in children is 3 mg and 0.05 mg/kg, respectively. If ineffective, further dosages of 6 mg (0.10 mg/kg) and, if necessary, 12 mg can be given after 1 min intervals up to a recommended maximum of 12 mg

(0.25 mg/kg). A dose of 3 mg is rarely effective and there is a good case for starting with 6 mg. Doses as high as 18 mg have been given without significant unwanted effect. If a patient has received adenosine in the past, it would be sensible to start with the dose that was previously shown to be effective.

Many patients will experience chest tightness, dyspnoea and flushing but the symptoms last less than 30 s. There may be complete AV block for a few seconds following termination of the tachycardia. A few ventricular ectopic beats may also occur. The drug does not have a negative inotropic action.

Adenosine can cause bronchospasm and avoidance is recommended in asthmatics.

Verapamil

Intravenous verapamil (5–10 mg over 30 s) will usually restore sinus rhythm within a couple of minutes.

Verapamil must not be used if the patient has recently received an oral or intravenous beta-blocking drug (see Chapter 19).

Other drugs

Drugs such as sotalol, disopyramide and flecainide may also be effective (see Chapter 19).

ELECTRICAL METHODS

Pacing

Various pacing methods may terminate AV re-entrant tachycardias. The simplest is pacing the right atrium at a rate 20–30 per cent faster than the tachycardia (overdrive pacing). On abrupt termination of pacing, sinus rhythm will often return: if unsuccessful, pacing should be repeated (Figure 9.11). There is a small risk of precipitating atrial fibrillation that usually will not last for many minutes before sinus rhythm is restored. However, in patients with the Wolff–Parkinson–White syndrome atrial fibrillation might lead to a very fast ventricular response.

More sophisticated methods require a programmable pacemaker which allows the introduction of precisely timed extra stimuli (Figure 9.12). These methods can also be used on a long-term basis by implanting a pacemaker (Figure 9.13) but pacing has now been superseded by radiofrequency catheter ablation.

Cardioversion

If drugs are ineffective or if clinical circumstances necessitate an immediate return to sinus rhythm, cardioversion should be carried out (see Chapter 21).

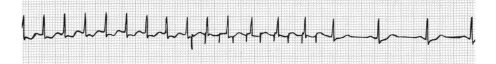

Figure 9.11 Termination of atrioventricular re-entrant tachycardia by rapid atrial pacing.

PREVENTION

There are two main approaches: drug therapy or ablation of part of the re-entry circuit.

DRUGS

Selection of a drug which is both effective and well tolerated is often a process of trial and error. Sotalol (160 mg daily) and flecainide (100 mg twice daily) are good first-line drugs. The patient should keep a record of the date and duration of any attacks so that the effect of therapy can be assessed.

Amiodarone is likely to be effective where other drugs have failed, but should be reserved for refractory cases where the need for tachycardia control outweighs the drug's possible unwanted effects.

CATHETER ABLATION

Radiofrequency energy, delivered by a catheter introduced via a vein or artery, can be used to ablate an accessory pathway responsible for AVRT, or to modify the slow or fast AV nodal tract involved in AVNRT (see Chapter 26). For most patients, this is the treatment of choice, offering a cure and obviating the need for antiarrhythmic drugs. Success rates over 90 per cent are being widely achieved and the risks are very low.

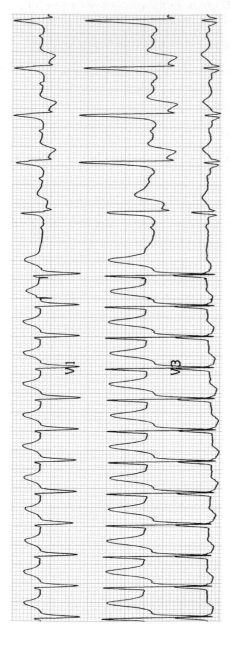

Figure 9.12 Termination of atrioventricular re-entrant tachycardia by a couplet of precisely timed atrial premature stimuli, best seen in lead V1, revealing Wolff–Parkinson–White syndrome on return to sinus rhythm.

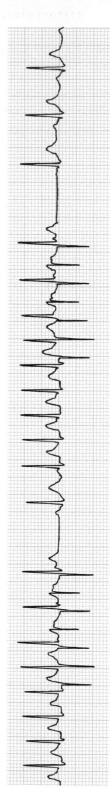

Figure 9.13 Implanted antitachycardia pacemaker. Automatic detection and termination of two episodes of atrioventricular re-entrant tachycardia.

Main points

- AV junctional re-entrant tachycardias require the presence of a second connection between atria and ventricles in addition to the AV node.

- AV re-entrant tachycardia (AVRT) is due to an accessory AV pathway.

- AV nodal re-entrant tachycardia (AVNRT) is caused by dual AV nodal pathways.

- Usually structural heart disease is absent.

- The ventricular rhythm is regular and QRS complexes usually normal.

- Atrial activity, if seen, will be in the form of an inverted P wave after each QRS complex.

- Tachycardia can be terminated by vagal stimulation or adenosine.

- Radiofrequency ablation is a first-line choice for the prevention of troublesome tachycardias.

Wolff–Parkinson–White syndrome

This syndrome is due to an accessory AV pathway: the same pathway which, as discussed earlier, is the cause of an AV re-entrant tachycardia (AVRT). The connection is a strand of normal myocardium. It is also referred to as a bundle of Kent.

Normally the atria become electrically isolated from the ventricles during fetal development, apart from the AV junction (i.e. AV node plus bundle of His). Incomplete separation leads to an accessory AV pathway. The pathway may be situated anywhere across the groove between atria and ventricles. The most common site is the left free wall of the heart. Other locations are postero-septal, right free wall and rarely antero-septal. In a minority of patients there is more than one accessory pathway.

Approximately 1.5–3 per 1000 of the population have the electrocardiographic signs of Wolff–Parkinson–White syndrome, two-thirds of whom will experience cardiac arrhythmias. One survey reported 4 per 100 000 newly diagnosed cases per annum. The syndrome is more common in young people. With age, fibrosis may occasionally develop in the AV groove and block an accessory pathway.

To facilitate the common form of AV re-entrant tachycardia it is only necessary for the accessory pathway to conduct in a retrograde direction (i.e. from ventricles to atria). Many patients with AV re-entrant tachycardia have an accessory AV pathway which is only capable of ventriculo-atrial conduction. In patients with the Wolff–Parkinson–White syndrome the pathway is *also* capable of anterograde conduction (i.e. from atria to ventricles). Unlike the AV node, the accessory connection does not delay conduction between atria and ventricles.

ECG CHARACTERISTICS

The characteristics of the Wolff–Parkinson–White syndrome are a short PR interval, a widened QRS complex due to the presence of a delta wave, and paroxysmal tachycardia (Figure 10.1).

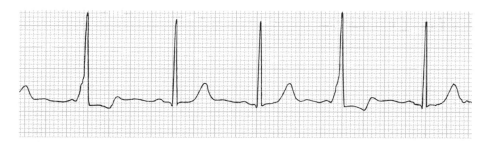

Figure 10.1 Wolff–Parkinson–White syndrome. In this patient, the accessory pathway conducts intermittently. The second, third and fifth complexes are normal whereas the first and fourth complexes show the characteristic short PR interval and delta wave. By comparing pre-excited and normal beats, it can be seen how the delta wave both shortens the PR interval and broadens the ventricular complex.

During sinus rhythm, an atrial impulse will reach the ventricles via both the accessory pathway and the normal AV node. The AV node conducts relatively slowly. Therefore initial ventricular activation is solely due to accessory pathway conduction that results in a shortened PR interval: ventricular pre-excitation. Because the accessory pathway is not connected to specialized conducting tissue (i.e. the His-Purkinje system), early ventricular activation will be slow, leading to slurring of the ventricular complex (i.e. a delta wave) rather than the brisk upstroke that would result from rapid ventricular activation via the specialized conducting tissues. Once the atrial impulse has traversed the AV node, further ventricular activation will proceed normally. During sinus rhythm, therefore, the ventricular complex is a fusion between delta wave and normal QRS complex (Figure 10.1).

LOCATION OF ACCESSORY PATHWAY

The syndrome is classified into types A and B, depending on the ventricular complex in lead V1. If predominantly positive, it is type A and if negative, type B (Figures 10.2 and 10.3, see pages 80 and 81).

Type A is caused by a left-sided accessory pathway. However, type B is not necessarily due to a right-sided pathway, especially if the delta wave is small.

Complex electrocardiographic algorithms have been devised for precise location of accessory pathways but none are very reliable. There are a few simple guides. A positive delta wave in lead V1 indicates a left-sided pathway. A negative delta wave in leads III and aVF together with positive waves in leads V2 and V3 points to a posteroseptal pathway (see Figure 10.6b) while a right free wall pathway is usually associated with positive waves in leads II and III and a negative wave in lead V1.

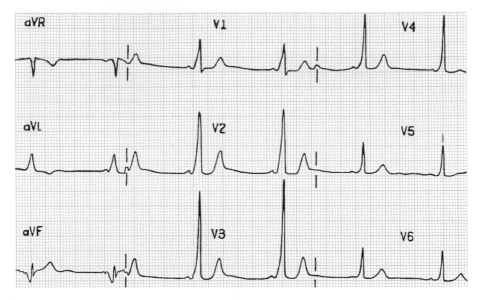

Figure 10.2 Type A Wolff–Parkinson–White syndrome (the negative delta wave in lead aVF could be misinterpreted as a Q wave due to inferior myocardial infarction).

ARRHYTHMIAS

Two main arrhythmias can occur in patients with the Wolff–Parkinson–White syndrome: atrial fibrillation and, more commonly, AV re-entrant tachycardia.

ATRIAL FIBRILLATION

In patients without pre-excitation the AV node protects the ventricles from the rapid atrial activity during atrial fibrillation (350–600 impulses/min). In the Wolff–Parkinson–White syndrome, the accessory pathway provides an additional route of access to the ventricles and can in some patients conduct very frequently. As a result, ventricular rates during atrial fibrillation are often very fast. Usually, most conducted impulses reach the ventricles via the accessory pathway and therefore lead to delta waves. The minority of impulses that reach the ventricles via the AV node produce normal QRS complexes. The resultant ECG will show the totally irregular ventricular response that is characteristic of atrial fibrillation. Some ventricular complexes will be normal, but most will be delta waves (Figures 10.4–10.6).

A very rapid ventricular response to atrial fibrillation may occasionally cause heart failure or shock. If the ventricles are stimulated at a very fast rate there is a risk of ventricular fibrillation. The risk of ventricular fibrillation is small and mainly affects those patients where the minimum interval between delta waves during atrial fibrillation is less than 250 ms (Figure 10.6). The risk is very low in asymptomatic patients and in those with intermittent accessory pathway conduction (see Figure 10.1).

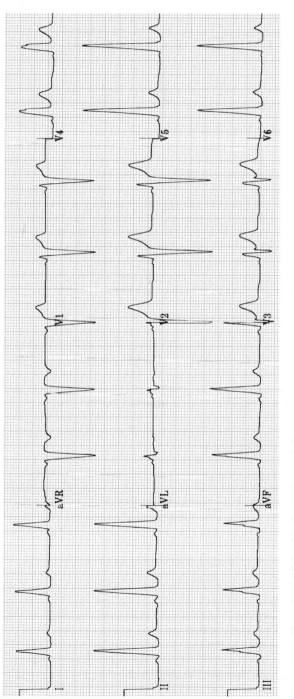

Figure 10.3 Type B Wolff–Parkinson–White syndrome.

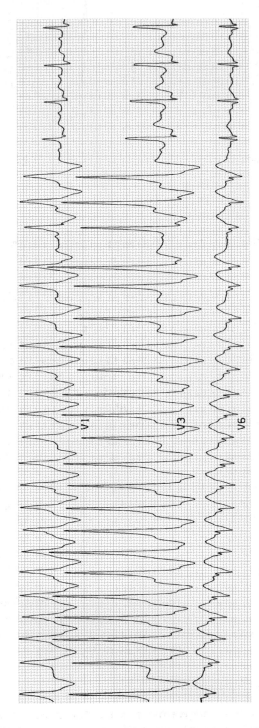

Figure 10.4 Atrial fibrillation. Irregular, rapid succession of complexes with large delta waves; then return of sinus rhythm.

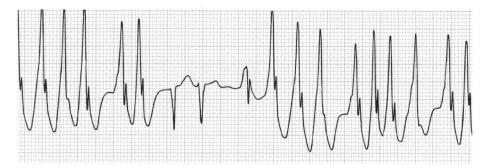

Figure 10.5 Atrial fibrillation. Most complexes are delta waves; the seventh and eighth complexes are narrow due to conduction via the atrioventricular node.

ATRIOVENTRICULAR JUNCTIONAL RE-ENTRANT TACHYCARDIA

The AV node and accessory pathway differ in the time they take to recover after excitation. Usually, the AV node recovers first. If an atrial ectopic beat arises during sinus rhythm when the AV node has recovered but the accessory pathway is not yet capable of conduction, the resultant ventricular complex will clearly not have a delta wave and will be narrow. By the time the premature atrial impulse has traversed the AV junction and stimulated the ventricles, the accessory pathway will have recovered and will be able to conduct the impulse back to the atria. When the impulse reaches the atria the AV junction will again be able to conduct and hence the impulse can repeatedly circulate between atria and ventricles, leading to an AV re-entrant tachycardia (see Figure 9.1). Similarly, a ventricular ectopic beat during sinus rhythm can be conducted to the atria via the accessory pathway and thereby initiate AV re-entrant tachycardia.

The ECG during tachycardia will show narrow ventricular complexes (unless there is rate-related bundle branch block) in rapid, regular succession (Figure 10.7).

Unlike atrial fibrillation, there will be no delta waves and thus there will be no clue from the ventricular complexes during tachycardia that the patient has Wolff–Parkinson–White syndrome. However, as discussed above, the timing of atrial activity during tachycardia, if identifiable, may point to the tachycardia mechanism. An accessory AV pathway is some distance from the AV junction. It therefore takes longer for an impulse to circulate and re-enter the atria. Hence the inverted P wave occurs roughly halfway between QRS complexes (Figure 10.8). If inverted in lead I, the accessory pathway is likely to be left-sided. If inverted in leads II, III and aVF it is likely the pathway is postero-septal (see Figure 9.9).

Antidromic tachycardia

Antidromic AV re-entrant tachycardia is much less common than the above-mentioned form of AV re-entrant tachycardia (which is termed orthodromic). The

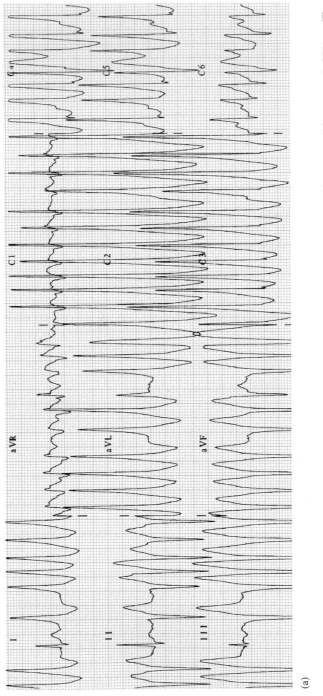

Figure 10.6 (a) Atrial fibrillation with a very rapid ventricular response. The minimum interval between delta waves is 200 ms. The totally irregular response excludes a diagnosis of ventricular tachycardia.

(a)

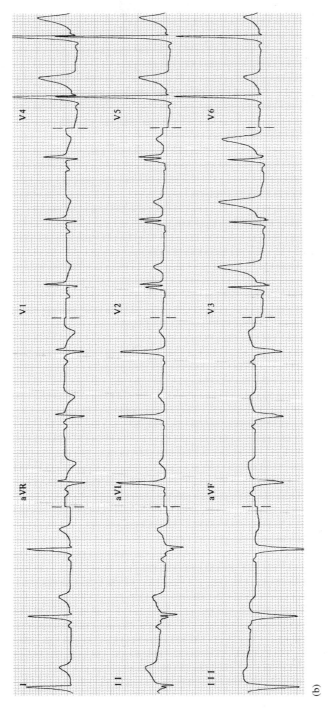

Figure 10.6 (b) Same patient in sinus rhythm. ECG suggests postero-septal accessory pathway.

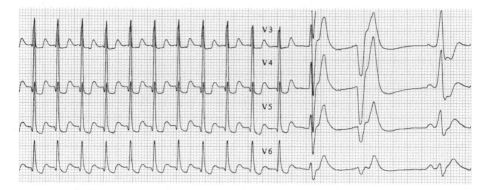

Figure 10.7 Atrioventricular re-entrant tachycardia terminated by adenosine. After two ventricular ectopic beats there is a sinus beat with short PR interval and delta wave.

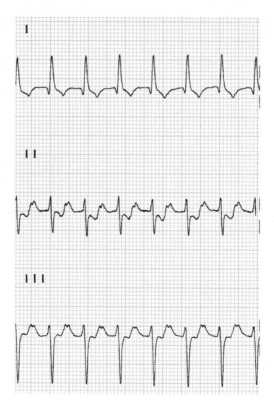

Figure 10.8 Atrioventricular re-entrant tachycardia due to Wolff–Parkinson–White syndrome. Inverted P waves can be seen halfway between QRS complexes. (The P wave is negative in lead I, suggesting a left-sided pathway.)

circulating impulse travels in the opposite direction: conduction from atria to ventricles is over the accessory AV pathway and return to the atria is via the AV node. Consequently, ventricular complexes will be in the form of large delta waves (Figure 10.9).

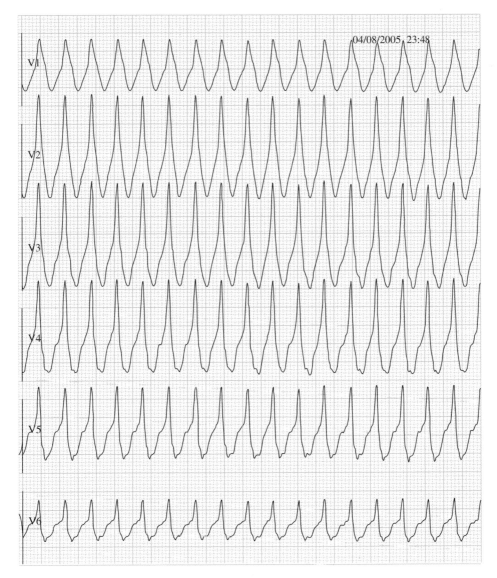

04/08/2005 23:48

Figure 10.9 Antidromic tachycardia resulting in large type A delta waves.

TREATMENT

Radiofrequency ablation of the accessory pathway (see Chapter 26) should be considered in all symptomatic patients, particularly if drugs are ineffective or cannot be tolerated, or if there is a fast ventricular response to atrial fibrillation. Occasionally, ablation may be indicated in some asymptomatic patients by reason of their profession, such as a pilot.

ATRIOVENTRICULAR RE-ENTRANT TACHYCARDIA

Methods for the termination and prevention of AV re-entrant tachycardia are appropriate whether or not the patient has pre-excitation during sinus rhythm (see Chapter 9).

ATRIAL FIBRILLATION

During atrial fibrillation, most atrial impulses reach the ventricles via the accessory AV pathway. Thus AV nodal-blocking drugs such as digoxin and verapamil are of little use during atrial fibrillation in the Wolff–Parkinson–White syndrome. Indeed, both digoxin and verapamil can increase the frequency of conduction in the accessory pathway and therefore lead to a faster ventricular rate. These drugs must not be used in those patients who are capable of a rapid ventricular response in case a dangerously fast ventricular rate develops. In patients in whom atrial fibrillation has never occurred, and thus a fast response has not been excluded, the drugs should be avoided.

Intravenous sotalol, flecainide, disopyramide or amiodarone, drugs that slow conduction in the accessory pathway, should be used. These drugs will slow the ventricular response to atrial fibrillation and will often restore sinus rhythm. A simple alternative method of terminating atrial fibrillation is cardioversion, but this is not appropriate if the arrhythmia is frequently recurrent.

For prevention of atrial fibrillation, oral sotalol, flecainide, disopyramide or amiodarone are often effective but catheter ablation is the treatment of choice.

Main points

- The Wolff–Parkinson–White syndrome is characterized by a short PR interval and a widened QRS complex due to presence of a delta wave. It is caused by an accessory AV pathway (bundle of Kent), which connects atrial and ventricular myocardium, bypassing the AV junction.

- Two main arrhythmias can occur: AV junctional re-entrant tachycardia and atrial fibrillation.

- During AV re-entrant tachycardia, there will be no delta waves and thus no evidence from the ventricular complex of pre-excitation. Treatment is the same whether or not there is pre-excitation.

- During atrial fibrillation, most ventricular complexes are broad due to the presence of large delta waves. The ventricular rate is often very fast and there is a risk of ventricular fibrillation when the minimum interval between delta waves during atrial fibrillation is less than 250 ms. If the hallmark of atrial fibrillation (i.e. a totally irregular rhythm) is ignored, the arrhythmia may be mistaken for ventricular tachycardia.

- Since most atrial impulses are conducted to the ventricles via the accessory AV pathway during atrial fibrillation, AV nodal-blocking drugs (digoxin, verapamil) are not helpful and may be dangerous. If a drug is used, it should slow conduction in the accessory pathway (e.g. sotalol, flecainide and amiodarone). Cardioversion is an alternative.

- Radiofrequency catheter ablation should be considered in all symptomatic patients. Success rates are high and the risks low.

CHAPTER 11

Ventricular tachyarrhythmias

Ventricular tachycardia is defined as four or more ventricular ectopic beats in rapid succession (Figure 11.1). Ventricular tachycardias vary in rate, duration and frequency of recurrence. The consequences also vary. Some patients will develop shock or ventricular fibrillation whereas others may tolerate ventricular tachycardia with few or no symptoms.

There are two main types of ventricular tachycardia: monomorphic and polymorphic. Monomorphic ventricular tachycardia (see Chapter 12) is usually due to heart muscle damage but there are two specific tachycardias which occur in patients with a structurally normal heart: namely, right ventricular outflow tract and fascicular tachycardia. Polymorphic ventricular tachycardia (see Chapter 13) is also but not always caused by heart muscle damage.

Sometimes, polymorphic ventricular tachycardia is associated with a prolonged QT interval when it is termed 'torsade de pointes tachycardia'. There may be no structural heart disease. The arrhythmia results from abnormalities in ventricular repolarization, which can be acquired or inherited.

Ventricular fibrillation (see Chapter 13) is usually a consequence of myocardial damage from either coronary disease or cardiomyopathy but occasionally is due to primary electrical disorders, including the recently described Brugada syndrome.

Difficulty is often encountered in distinguishing supraventricular from ventricular tachycardia. There are a number of pointers that can usually easily ascertain the origin of a tachycardia (see Chapter 14).

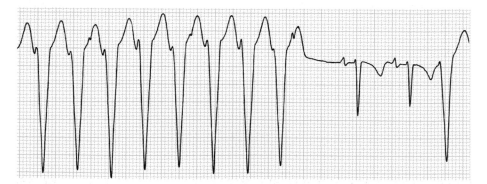

Figure 11.1　Ventricular tachycardia: a succession of ventricular ectopic beats, followed by two sinus beats and then a single ventricular ectopic beat.

CHAPTER 12

Monomorphic ventricular tachycardia

ECG CHARACTERISTICS

The arrhythmia consists of a rapid succession of ventricular ectopic beats each with the same configuration, hence the term monomorphic (Figure 12.1). As with single ventricular ectopic beats, the complexes will be abnormal in shape, and the duration

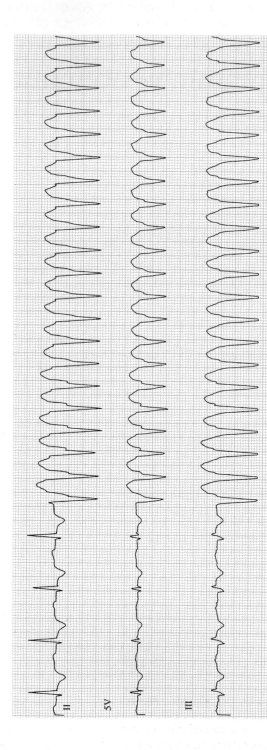

Figure 12.1 Monomorphic ventricular tachycardia. There is a rapid, regular succession of broad complexes after four sinus beats.

of each complex will be more than 0.12 s and usually greater than 0.14 s. The rhythm is regular unless there are capture beats (see below) which cause minor irregularities in the rhythm. The rate ranges from 120 to 250 beats/min.

ATRIAL ACTIVITY DURING VENTRICULAR TACHYCARDIA

With many ventricular tachycardias, the sinus node continues to initiate atrial activity which is therefore independent of, and slower than ventricular activity (Figure 12.2). In others, the AV node conducts each ventricular impulse to the atria so a P wave follows the ventricular complex. The P wave is often concealed by the superimposed terminal portion of the ventricular complex (Figure 12.3). Rarely, second-degree block may occur at the AV junction so only some ventricular impulses are conducted to the atria.

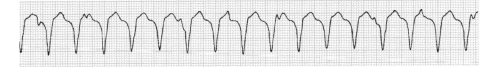

Figure 12.2 Ventricular tachycardia with direct evidence of independent atrial activity. P waves separated by intervals of 0.75 s, can be seen after the first, third, sixth, eighth, tenth, thirteenth, fifteenth and seventeenth ventricular complexes.

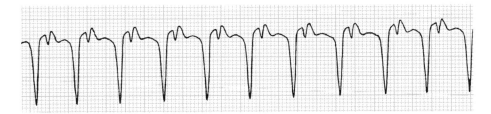

Figure 12.3 Ventricular tachycardia (lead aVF) with retrograde atrial activation. In this case, each P wave can be clearly seen to be superimposed on the T wave of each ventricular complex.

Identification of independent atrial activity during tachycardia excludes an origin at AV node level or above and will thus distinguish ventricular tachycardia from supraventricular tachycardia with broad ventricular complexes. There may be direct or indirect evidence of independent atrial activity.

Direct evidence of independent atrial activity

P waves at a slower rate than and dissociated from ventricular activity are direct evidence of independent atrial activity (Figure 12.2). Inevitably, some P waves will be concealed by superimposed ventricular complexes. Furthermore, not all leads will clearly show atrial activity. A rhythm strip is often inadequate and scrutiny of a simultaneous recording of several different leads may be necessary. Sometimes there will be doubt whether small waves on the ECG during tachycardia are caused by atrial activity. If they are, they will be separated by similar intervals, or multiples of that interval.

Indirect evidence of independent atrial activity

Capture or fusion beats are indirect evidence of atrial activity. Just one is sufficient to confirm ventricular tachycardia.

Capture beats occur when the timing of an atrial impulse during ventricular tachycardia is such that it can be transmitted via the AV junction and activate the ventricles before the next discharge from the ventricular focus. The resultant ventricular complex will be normal in shape and duration and will occur slightly earlier than the next ventricular ectopic beat would have been expected (see Figure 12.11). Fusion beats are caused by a similar process. However, the atrial impulse activates the ventricles slightly later in the cardiac cycle leading to simultaneous activation of the ventricles by the transmitted atrial impulse and the ventricular focus. The result is a ventricular complex with an appearance intermediate between a normal QRS complex and a ventricular ectopic beat (Figure 12.4).

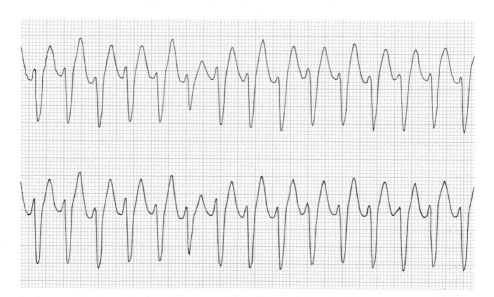

Figure 12.4 Ventricular tachycardia. The sixth complex is a fusion beat.

The ECG characteristics of monomorphic ventricular tachycardia are summarized in Table 12.1.

Table 12.1 ECG characteristics of monomorphic ventricular tachycardia

Regular rhythm
Broad complexes ($\geqslant$0.12 s and usually >0.14 s)
Ventricular complexes of uniform appearance
Independent P waves may be present
Capture or fusion beats may be present

CAUSES

Ventricular tachycardia is most often the result of myocardial damage from coronary heart disease or from cardiomyopathy. Ventricular tachycardia that is not due to an acute event such as within 24–48 hours of acute myocardial infarction is very likely to recur.

The main causes are listed in Table 12.2.

Table 12.2 Causes of ventricular tachycardia

Acute myocardial infarction or ischaemia
Past myocardial infarction
Dilated cardiomyopathy
Hypertrophic cardiomyopathy
Arrhythmogenic right ventricular dysplasia
Myocarditis
Mitral valve prolapse
Valvular heart disease
Repair of tetralogy of Fallot
Sarcoidosis
Idiopathic

CORONARY HEART DISEASE

The commonest cause of ventricular tachycardia, by far, is myocardial damage resulting from infarction. Ventricular tachycardia can occur days, weeks or even years after myocardial infarction. The worse the ventricular function the more susceptible the patient is to this arrhythmia. Usually, ventricular tachycardia occurs in patients whose left ventricular ejection fraction is less than 40 per cent (the normal value is >60 per cent). The lower the ejection fraction below this level the worse is the prognosis.

In patients with poor ventricular function, most antiarrhythmic drugs are negatively inotropic i.e. they may worsen ventricular function and are 'proarrhythmic', i.e. they are likely to cause or aggravate arrhythmias. Amiodarone is fairly safe and is widely used in this situation. However, though it may suppress some arrhythmias it is unlikely to improve a patient's prognosis. Hence the role of the implantable defibrillator whose functions and indications are discussed in Chapter 25.

In some patients, the arrhythmia is provoked not by the myocardial scar but by ischaemia. This is particularly likely if the arrhythmia has occurred during physical effort. Myocardial revascularization may be effective. Beta-blocking drugs may prevent the arrhythmia in this situation. Coronary angiography with a view to revascularization should always be considered in patients with coronary disease and ventricular tachycardia.

Acute myocardial infarction can cause ventricular tachycardia. This is discussed in Chapter 18.

DILATED CARDIOMYOPATHY

Dilated cardiomyopathy is an important cause of ventricular tachycardia. As with patients whose impaired ventricular function is due to coronary disease, negatively inotropic antiarrhythmic drugs should be avoided, beta-blockers and/or amiodarone may be required and defibrillator implantation considered.

HYPERTROPHIC CARDIOMYOPATHY

This is a common condition, which in many patients is asymptomatic and benign. However, it can cause sustained and non-sustained ventricular tachycardia and sudden death may be the first manifestation of the condition.

Sustained ventricular tachycardia is an indication for antiarrhythmic therapy, especially beta-blockers and amiodarone, and implantation of a defibrillator. Non-sustained ventricular tachycardia has been shown to be an important risk factor for sudden death. Other risk factors include syncope, family history of sudden cardiac death, severe left ventricular hypertrophy and failure to increase blood pressure during an exercise test. If more than one risk factor is present then amiodarone or an implantable defibrillator should be considered to improve the patient's prognosis.

ARRHYTHMOGENIC RIGHT VENTRICULAR DYSPLASIA

Arrhythmogenic right ventricular dysplasia (ARVD), also referred to as arrhythmogenic right ventricular cardiomyopathy (ARVC), is caused by fatty and/or fibrous infiltration of the right ventricle. Sometimes only localized areas of the ventricle are affected. Impaired function can be demonstrated by angiography, magnetic resonance imaging and sometimes by echocardiography. There is often some left ventricular impairment but it is less marked than right ventricular dysfunction.

ARVD is usually familial: the result of inheritance of an autosomal dominant gene. Thus females and males are equally likely to inherit the abnormal gene but males are more commonly affected by its clinical manifestations: arrhythmias and heart failure. ARVD is an important cause of sudden cardiac death in younger people.

Because the tachycardia arises from the right ventricle, it has left bundle branch block morphology (Figure 12.5a). Typically, during sinus rhythm there is T wave inversion in leads V1–V3 (Figure 12.5b). The QRS duration in these leads is often

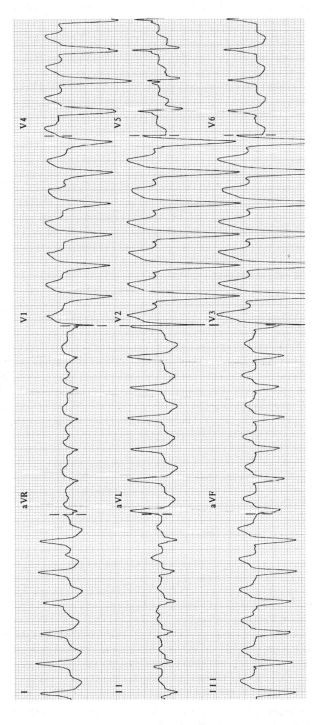

Figure 12.5 (a) Ventricular tachycardia caused by arrhythmogenic right ventricular dysplasia. The QRS complexes have a left bundle branch configuration.

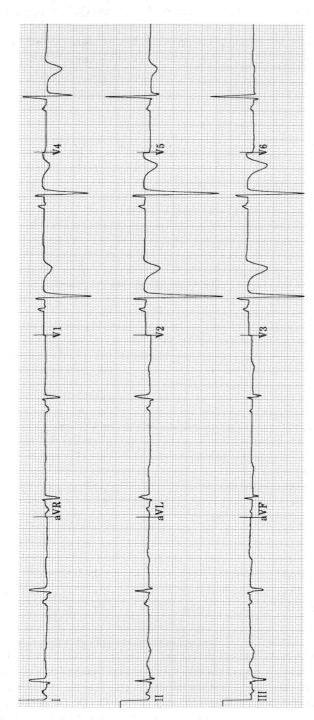

Figure 12.5 (b) The same patient with arrhythmogenic right ventricular dysplasia during sinus rhythm.

slightly increased. An epsilon wave is not infrequently seen (Figure 12.6). This is a low-amplitude wave seen in the terminal portion of the QRS complex in leads V1 and sometimes V2. It represents an area of delayed right ventricular activation. It is the surface manifestation of late potentials detected by signal-averaged electrocardiography (see below), which are often present in arrhythmogenic right ventricular dysplasia.

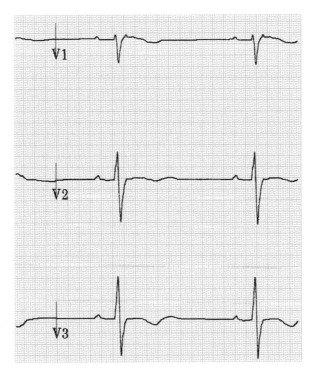

Figure 12.6 Patient with arrhythmogenic right ventricular dysplasia during sinus rhythm. An epsilon wave can be seen in lead V1 in the terminal portion of the QRS complex.

Patients usually present between the ages of 20 and 50 years with palpitation, syncope or near-syncope. Often the arrhythmia is provoked by effort. The disease is progressive and as time goes by lesser degrees of exertion may precipitate ventricular tachycardia. Sudden death can occur and may be the first manifestation of this disorder.

Patients should avoid severe exertion. Beta-blockers and/or amiodarone are often effective. Because of the significant risk and the progressive nature of the disease the implantation of an automatic cardiovertor defibrillator should be considered in patients presenting with ventricular tachycardia. A family history of sudden cardiac death is not a strong predictor of risk. On the other hand, if a family has already lost one member, it might be considered appropriate to have a lower threshold for defibrillator implantation.

MECHANISMS OF VENTRICULAR TACHYCARDIAS

Two main mechanisms cause tachycardias: re-entry, which is the commonest mechanism for ventricular tachycardia, and enhanced automaticity, which may be spontaneous or triggered.

RE-ENTRY

Two conditions are necessary for a re-entrant tachycardia to occur. The first is the presence of a potential circuit made up of two pathways of tissue with differing electrical characteristics. The second is transient or permanent block in one direction in one of the pathways so an impulse can be conducted along one pathway and return in the opposite direction via the other pathway, thereby re-entering the circuit. The activating impulse is repeatedly conducted around the circuit, exciting the surrounding myocardium at a rapid rate.

In ventricular tachycardia, fibrosis or ischaemia may cause delay in activation and hence recovery of an area of myocardium. Tachycardia results when a premature beat arrives at the abnormal area to find it is refractory to excitation following the last heart beat. The impulse is conducted around the damaged area by the adjacent, normally responsive myocardium. By the time the impulse has circumvented the damaged area, the abnormal myocardium has become excitable again and conducts the impulse in the opposite direction, giving rise to a re-entrant circuit. Perpetuation of this process results in ventricular tachycardia.

Ventricular re-entrant tachycardias can be initiated and terminated by precisely timed premature ventricular pacing stimuli.

ENHANCED AUTOMATICITY

Damage or disease can result in a group of myocardial cells acquiring enhanced automaticity (i.e. the cells discharge at a higher rate than the sinus node, taking over control of the heart rhythm). Enhanced automaticity can either be spontaneous or be triggered by after-depolarizations that lead to early reactivation of the myocardium.

INITIATION OF TACHYCARDIA

A re-entrant circuit or focus of enhanced automaticity provides the substrate for ventricular tachycardia. Initiation of the arrhythmia is usually triggered by an ectopic beat. Ischaemia, increased sympathetic nervous system activity or electrolyte imbalance may influence the arrhythmia substrate and may account for a tachycardia occurring at a particular time.

ACCELERATED IDIOVENTRICULAR RHYTHM

Monomorphic ventricular tachycardia with a rate less than 120 beats/min is termed accelerated idioventricular rhythm or slow ventricular tachycardia (Figure 12.7). Acute myocardial infarction is the most common cause; treatment is unnecessary.

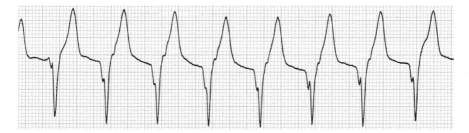

Figure 12.7 Accelerated idioventricular rhythm.

NON-SUSTAINED VENTRICULAR TACHYCARDIA

Non-sustained ventricular tachycardia is defined as three or more ventricular ectopic beats in succession at a rate in excess of 120 beats/min with return to normal rhythm within 30 s (Figure 12.8).

It rarely causes symptoms but it may be of prognostic significance. Many but not all studies have shown that patients with non-sustained ventricular tachycardia who have suffered a myocardial infarction and who have a left ventricular ejection fraction of less than 40 per cent have a marked increased risk of death either from ventricular arrhythmia or from heart failure. In dilated cardiomyopathy, there is a slight increase in risk of sudden death in those with non-sustained ventricular tachycardia. The arrhythmia is associated with a significant increased risk in symptomatic patients with hypertrophic cardiomyopathy.

Rarely, non-sustained ventricular tachycardia occurs in subjects without structural heart disease and is not associated with risk.

VENTRICULAR TACHYCARDIAS NOT DUE TO STRUCTURAL HEART DISEASE

There are two important ventricular tachycardias that can arise in structurally normal hearts. The more common one arises from the right ventricle and the other from the left ventricle. Recognition is important because they are associated with a good prognosis, their typical configurations point strongly to the heart being structurally normal, and because they are easily amenable to radiofrequency ablation if required for symptomatic purposes (see Chapter 26).

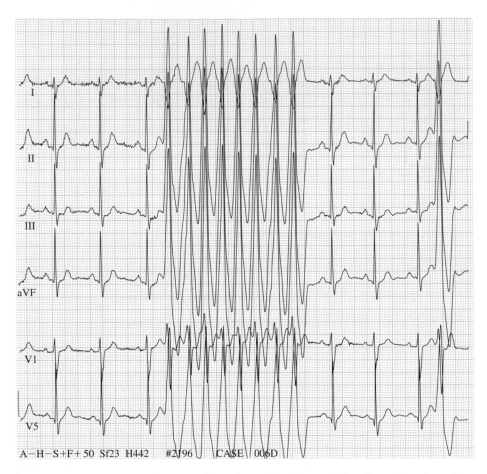

Figure 12.8 Non-sustained ventricular tachycardia followed after three sinus beats by a ventricular extrasystole with the same configuration.

RIGHT VENTRICULAR OUTFLOW TRACT TACHYCARDIA

This tachycardia has a characteristic ECG appearance that reflects its origin in the right ventricular outflow tract, just below the pulmonary valve. Because it arises in the right ventricle the complexes are similar to those seen during left bundle branch block, and because the impulse spreads inferiorly from beneath the pulmonary valve there is an inferior frontal QRS axis (i.e. right axis deviation) (Figure 12.9).

There are two types of clinical presentation. Either the tachycardia is paroxysmal and is provoked by effort, or it occurs at rest and is repetitive and non-sustained. In contrast to most ventricular tachycardias, it may be terminated by adenosine and verapamil.

In some patients, frequent ectopic beats rather than tachycardia arise from the right ventricular outflow tract, termed right ventricular outflow tract ectopia (Figure 12.10).

Rarely, a similar tachycardia arises from the left ventricular outflow tract. In contrast to right ventricular outflow tract tachycardia, leads V1–V3 are usually positive.

Some patients have been found to be prone to both right ventricular outflow tract and AV junctional re-entrant tachycardias.

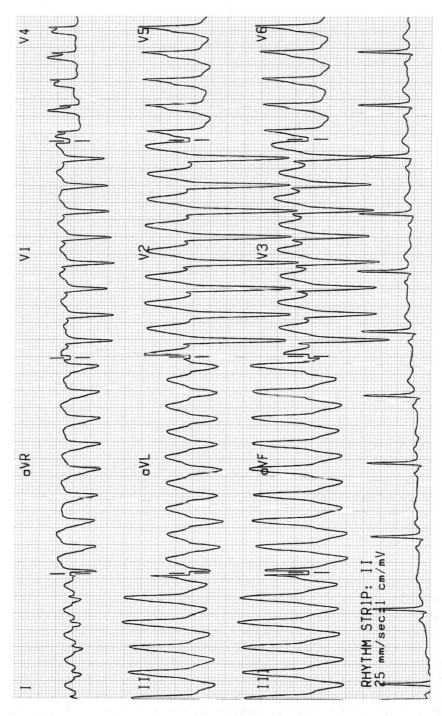

Figure 12.9 Right ventricular outflow tract tachycardia. There is an inferior axis and left bundle branch block configuration. Sinus rhythm returns as the rhythm strip (lead II) is recorded.

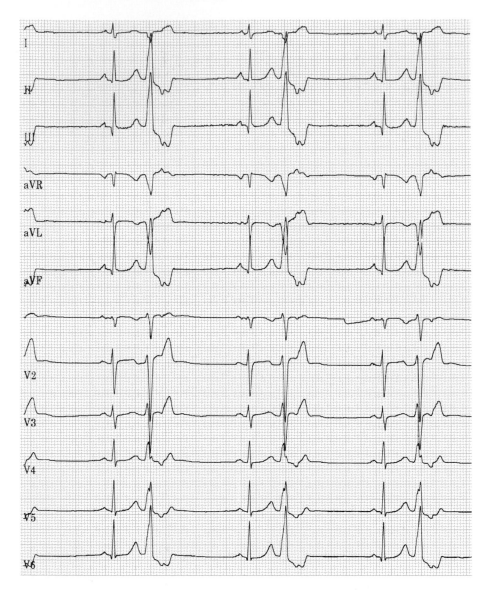

Figure 12.10 Ventricular bigeminy arising from right ventricular outflow tract.

FASCICULAR TACHYCARDIA

Fascicular tachycardia is an uncommon arrhythmia which arises from the posterior fascicle or, more rarely, from the anterior fascicle of the left bundle branch.

A posterior fascicular origin results in ventricular complexes during tachycardia with a right bundle branch block and left axis configuration (Figure 12.11), while an anterior fascicular origin leads to right bundle branch block with right axis deviation. Because the origin is within the specialized conducting system the

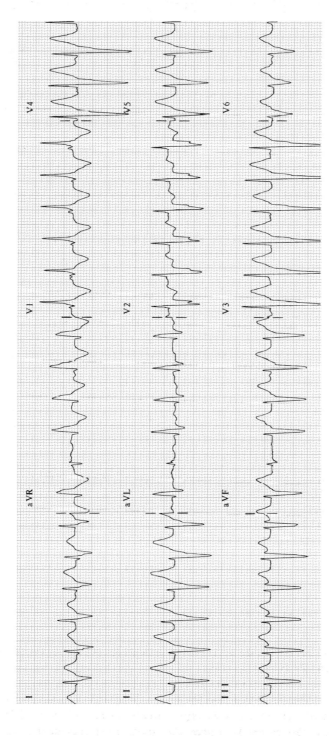

Figure 12.11 Fascicular tachycardia arising from the posterior fascicle. The complexes have a left axis and right bundle branch block configuration. The eighth complex is a capture beat.

ventricular complexes are of relatively short duration (0.12 s), sometimes leading to confusion with supraventricular tachycardia. The right bundle branch configuration may be atypical, for example there is a small q wave rather than a primary r wave.

Like right ventricular outflow tract tachycardia, it can be terminated by verapamil (but not adenosine).

INVESTIGATIONS

The nature and extent of investigations has to be tailored to the individual clinical situation. The aims should be to identify the cause, which may well be of therapeutic or prognostic importance, and to assess the role and efficacy of any therapy that may be indicated.

TWELVE-LEAD ECG

Whenever possible, a 12-lead ECG during tachycardia should be recorded and saved. It may point to the origin of the tachycardia. Furthermore, if electrophysiological studies are to be carried out, it is important to know that a tachycardia induced during the study has the same morphology and is therefore the same arrhythmia as has occurred spontaneously.

An ECG during sinus rhythm may reveal the cause of tachycardia (e.g. demonstrating myocardial infarction or a prolonged QT interval).

The configuration of the ventricular complex during tachycardia gives a clue as to its site of origin. A tachycardia with left bundle branch block morphology (i.e. a complex which is positive in V5 and V6 and which is akin to left bundle branch block in its appearance) will usually have a right ventricular origin (Figure 12.5a). A positive complex in lead V1 (i.e. with right bundle branch block morphology) points to a left ventricular free wall or septal source. If complexes are negative in V4–V6, a left ventricular apical origin is likely, while Q waves in the inferior leads suggest that the tachycardia is arising from the base of the left ventricle. The configurations of right ventricular outflow tract tachycardia and fascicular tachycardia are, of course, specific for those arrhythmias.

IMAGING

Echocardiography may help establish the cause of the arrhythmia. For example, by demonstrating dilated or hypertrophic cardiomyopathy, or right ventricular dysplasia.

Coronary angiography is often indicated, particularly if myocardial ischaemia might be the cause of the arrhythmia or if surgery is contemplated.

Magnetic resonance imaging is becoming used more widely. Some regard it as the 'gold standard' for the diagnosis of arrhythmogenic right ventricular dysplasia.

AMBULATORY ELECTROCARDIOGRAPHY

Ambulatory electrocardiography will help to assess the frequency and duration of episodes of ventricular tachycardia and the effect of therapy in those patients who have had frequent episodes.

Occasionally, ventricular tachycardia is triggered by bradycardia. This may be revealed by ambulatory electrocardiography. Prevention of bradycardia will often prevent ventricular tachycardia.

EXERCISE TESTING

Exercise-induced tachycardia is common. An exercise test can be useful in its diagnosis and response to therapy.

Most antiarrhythmic drugs can in some patients be proarrhythmic (see Chapter 19). A proarrhythmic effect may only be apparent during exercise. As a rule, patients who receive long-term therapy to prevent ventricular tachycardia should undergo exercise testing.

VENTRICULAR STIMULATION STUDY

Stimulation of the ventricles with up to three precisely timed premature stimuli delivered by a pacing lead, usually introduced via the femoral vein, will usually initiate ventricular tachycardia in patients who are prone to this arrhythmia (see Figure 13.11). Stimulation protocols involve progressively aggressive attempts to initiate ventricular tachycardia.

A typical protocol consists of a drive-train of eight paced beats (termed S1) at a cycle length of 600 ms followed by a single premature stimulus (S2) introduced after 350 ms. This is repeated with progressively shorter S1–S2 intervals until tachycardia is initiated, or S2 fails to activate the ventricles (i.e. the myocardial refractory period has been reached), or an interval of 200 ms has been arrived at. If ventricular tachycardia is not initiated, the process is then repeated with S1–S2 held at 10 ms greater than the refractory period, and a second premature stimulus (S3) is introduced: the S2–S3 interval is progressively reduced until the myocardium is refractory or the cycle length of 200 ms has been reached. If tachycardia has still not been initiated the process is repeated with the addition of a third stimulus (S4) and again S3–S4 is progressively reduced until tachycardia is initiated or the refractory period is reached. If tachycardia has not been induced the whole process is then repeated with the drive-train (S1) shortened to a cycle length of 400 ms.

If monomorphic ventricular tachycardia is induced it can normally be terminated by a burst of rapid pacing but sometimes cardioversion is required. Non-sustained tachycardia, or ventricular fibrillation initiated by a very aggressive stimulation protocol, is not of diagnostic significance.

The predictive value of a ventricular stimulation study in dilated cardiomyopathy is lower than for myocardial damage caused by coronary artery disease.

SIGNAL-AVERAGED ELECTROCARDIOGRAPHY

Late potentials are low-voltage, high-frequency signals in the terminal portion of the QRS complex. They indicate an area of delayed myocardial activation and are commonly found in patients subject to ventricular tachycardia caused by a re-entrant mechanism. They are demonstrated by signal-averaged electrocardiography. The ECG is recorded with an orthogonal system: leads are placed in the fourth intercostal space in both mid-axillary lines, on the front (lead V2 position) and back of chest, and top and bottom of the sternum. Computerized signal averaging and appropriate filtering of a series of QRS complexes eliminate electrical noise, which is random, and the main part of the QRS complex and thereby demonstrates late potentials (Figure 12.12).

Widely used criteria for late potentials are the presence of two of the following three observations:

1. Filtered QRS duration >110 ms
2. Root mean square of last 40 ms of QRS complex <25 µV
3. Duration of terminal portion of QRS complex <40 µV exceeds 32 ms.

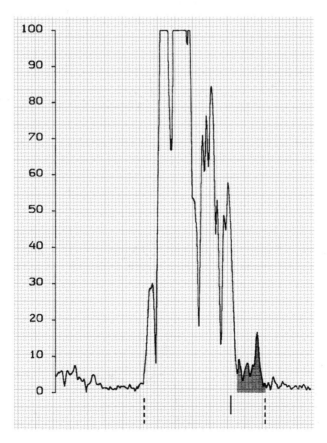

Figure 12.12 Signal-averaged ECG. Shaded area indicates late potential. Filtered QRS = 167 ms, root mean square of terminal 40 ms = 7 µV and duration of high-frequency, low-amplitude signals <40 µV = 48 µV.

Late potentials indicate the presence of the substrate for ventricular tachycardia (i.e. an area of slowed conduction), not that spontaneous ventricular tachycardia will necessarily occur. In patients who present with ventricular tachycardia, late potentials show the arrhythmia should be inducible at electrophysiological study. Late potentials after myocardial infarction point to a poor prognosis, particularly where there is evidence of extensive myocardial damage.

Rarely, a late potential may be apparent on routine electrocardiography; this is termed an epsilon wave (Figure 12.13).

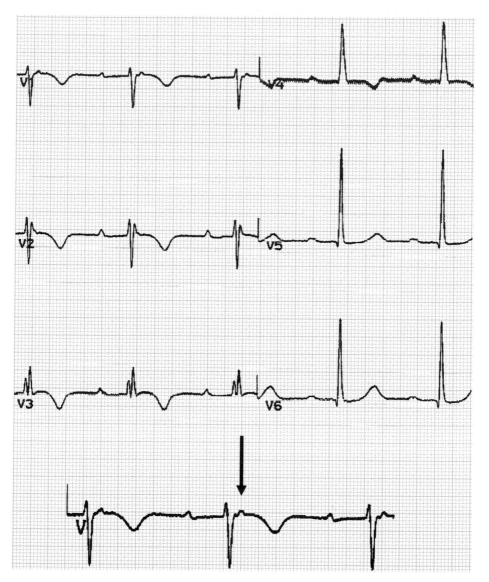

Figure 12.13 Patient with arrhythmogenic right ventricular dysplasia. An epsilon wave can be seen in the terminal portion of the QRS complex in lead V1. As commonly occurs, there is also first degree atrioventricular block and partial right bundle branch block.

TREATMENT

Choice of treatment depends on what symptoms the arrhythmia causes, whether the arrhythmia is likely to recur, and the prognosis.

TERMINATION OF TACHYCARDIA

Options include cardioversion, drugs and overdrive pacing.

Cardioversion

If sustained ventricular tachycardia causes cardiac arrest or shock, immediate cardioversion is necessary (see Chapter 21). Cardioversion should also be undertaken if antiarrhythmic drugs are ineffective, contraindicated or cause haemodynamic deterioration without restoring normal rhythm.

Antiarrhythmic drugs

Lignocaine is the first-line drug to stop ventricular tachycardia. Other drugs that are commonly used are sotalol, disopyramide and flecainide. These are markedly negatively inotropic (i.e. they can reduce the force of myocardial contraction) and are best avoided in patients with heart failure or in those known to have extensive myocardial damage. In general, no more than two drugs should be given before considering alternative methods of arrhythmia termination.

Amiodarone is a very useful second-line drug. It does not have a significant negative inotropic action and is extremely effective. However, it seldom works 'at the end of a needle' and can take up to 24 hours to act. If ventricular tachycardia keeps recurring it may be worth using amiodarone despite its delayed action rather than risking the complications associated with other less effective drugs, even if cardioversion or pacing is required while amiodarone is taking effect.

Though verapamil is effective in controlling supraventricular tachycardia it is, except for fascicular and right ventricular outflow tract tachycardia, useless in ventricular tachycardia and may cause severe hypotension. It cannot be emphasized too strongly that it is dangerous practice to use the drug as a therapeutic test to ascertain the origin of a tachycardia with broad QRS complexes.

In contrast to most ventricular tachycardias, both fascicular and right ventricular outflow tract tachycardia may be terminated by verapamil and the latter arrhythmia may also respond to adenosine.

Pacing

Pacing can sometimes be successful in terminating ventricular tachycardia (Figure 12.14). It should be considered when drugs are ineffective, when frequently recurrent tachycardia necessitates multiple cardioversions or when a temporary pacing wire is already in place for treatment of a bradycardia.

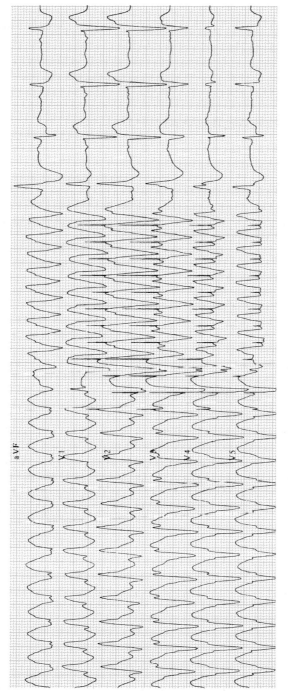

Figure 12.14 Monomorphic ventricular tachycardia terminated by burst of rapid ventricular pacing.

The usual method is overdrive right ventricular pacing. A burst for a couple of seconds at a rate 10–30 per cent in excess of that of the tachycardia will often terminate the arrhythmia. However, there is a significant risk of accelerating the tachycardia or precipitating ventricular fibrillation, in which case immediate cardioversion will be necessary.

In patients where there is a high risk that ventricular tachycardia might recur, or in whom antiarrhythmic drugs are ineffective, an automatic implantable cardiovertor defibrillator may be indicated (see Chapter 25).

PREVENTION OF RECURRENCE OF VENTRICULAR TACHYCARDIA

Intravenous drugs

Blood levels of most antiarrhythmic drugs fall rapidly after a single bolus. After a bolus has restored sinus rhythm it is usual to give a continuous infusion of the drug. This makes sense if ventricular tachycardia is expected to recur within a short period (e.g. after acute myocardial infarction). However, it is pointless to set up an infusion if either the bolus has failed or the tachycardia is known to occur infrequently.

Oral drugs

Unless ventricular tachycardia occurs during acute myocardial infarction or other acute events, recurrence is likely and long-term therapy is indicated. Therapy is particularly important if the arrhythmia is associated with significant structural heart disease or has caused marked hypotension or shock, since the prognosis without treatment is poor.

Several drugs may be useful: sotalol, disopyramide, flecainide and amiodarone. When ventricular tachycardia has occurred on exertion beta-blockers should be tried first.

Disopyramide, flecainide and beta-blockers may precipitate heart failure in patients with extensive myocardial damage. Amiodarone is by far the most effective drug and can be given to patients with poor ventricular function, but it can cause a number of unwanted effects. In patients who are at high risk from further arrhythmias it would seem reasonable to use amiodarone and consider alternatives if major side-effects occur.

Ambulatory electrocardiography has been compared with programmed electrical stimulation in patients presenting with ventricular tachycardia who had ten or more ventricular extrasystoles per hour to see which method best predicts antiarrhythmic efficacy. Suppression of extrasystoles was found to be as predictive of antiarrhythmic efficacy as prevention of inducibility of ventricular tachycardia by programmed electrical stimulation. However, neither method was found to be very reliable. Notably, sotalol was found to be a more effective antiarrhythmic drug than mexiletine, pirmenol, procainamide and propafenone.

The author's 'first-line' drugs to prevent ventricular tachycardia are sotalol and amiodarone.

Most antiarrhythmic drugs can be proarrhythmic. Class Ic drugs (see Chapter 19) are the main culprits and patients with extensive myocardial damage will be the most susceptible. If no progress is being made in maintaining normal rhythm or there are new arrhythmias, a proarrhythmic effect should be considered.

Pacing

Sometimes ventricular tachycardia arises during bradycardia. If the heart rate is low (e.g. less than 50 beats/min), the rate should be increased by pacing before drugs are given: often pacing alone will prevent ventricular tachycardia. Pacing at a rate of 80–90 per minute together with drugs may prevent ventricular tachycardia when the rate during sinus rhythm is relatively slow (e.g. 50–70 beats/min).

Catheter ablation

Delivery of radiofrequency energy via a catheter electrode to the site of origin of tachycardia is very effective in right ventricular outflow tract and fascicular tachy-cardias: it should be considered when troublesome symptoms occur, particularly since oral antiarrhythmic drugs are rarely effective.

Only modest rates of success have been achieved in patients with ventricular tachycardia caused by arrhythmogenic right ventricular dysplasia and coronary heart disease.

Surgery

There are several surgical techniques that involve the excision or isolation of the arrhythmia focus. However potential candidates for surgery often have impaired myocardial function. Cardiopulmonary bypass surgery carries a substantial risk when myocardial function is poor since ventriculotomy may worsen function. Only a few cardiac centres routinely perform surgery for ventricular tachycardia.

There are reports that myocardial revascularization alone may reduce the inci-dence of ventricular arrhythmias in some patients with coronary heart disease.

Occasionally, life-threatening, resistant ventricular arrhythmias are an indication for cardiac transplantation.

ASSESSMENT OF EFFICACY

Whatever treatment is chosen, it is important to ensure it is effective in preventing a recurrence of ventricular tachycardia. If the tachycardia has been frequent then monitoring the ECG at the bedside or using ambulatory electrocardiography is the best method of assessing efficacy. If ventricular tachycardia has been infrequent then it is unlikely that ECG monitoring will reflect antiarrhythmic control. Exercise ECG testing and electrophysiological testing should be considered.

Main points

- Monomorphic ventricular tachycardia consists of a rapid, regular succession of ventricular extrasystoles each with the same configuration. The duration exceeds 0.12 s and is usually greater than 0.14 s.

- The presence of P waves dissociated from ventricular activity or of fusion or capture beats indicates independent atrial activity and confirms ventricular tachycardia.

- The common causes of ventricular tachycardia are myocardial damage from coronary artery disease or from cardiomyopathy.

- Right ventricular outflow tract and fascicular tachycardia arise in patients with structurally normal hearts and are amenable to radiofrequency ablation.

- If ventricular tachycardia causes shock, prompt cardioversion is indicated.

- Lignocaine is the first-line drug for intravenous use. Generally, no more than two drugs should be tried before resorting to amiodarone or non-pharmacological methods of treatment. Verapamil should not be given except for right ventricular outflow tract and fascicular tachycardias.

- Ventricular tachycardia is often a recurrent problem and may lead to sudden death. An implantable defibrillator may be indicated, particularly in patients with poor ventricular function.

- Accelerated idioventricular rhythm is ventricular tachycardia at a rate less than 120 beats/min. Treatment is not required.

- Wherever possible, obtain and save a 12-lead ECG during tachycardia.

CHAPTER 13

Polymorphic ventricular tachycardia and ventricular fibrillation

POLYMORPHIC VENTRICULAR TACHYCARDIA

Whereas monomorphic ventricular tachycardia consists of a rapid succession of ventricular ectopic beats, each with the same configuration, polymorphic tachycardia is characterized by repeated progressive changes in the QRS complex so the complexes 'twist' about the baseline (Figure 13.1). It may result from acute myocardial infarction and from other causes of myocardial damage (Figure 13.2). In these situations the QT

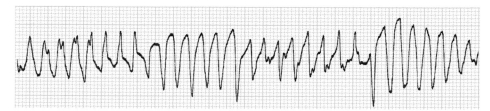

Figure 13.1 Polymorphic ventricular tachycardia.

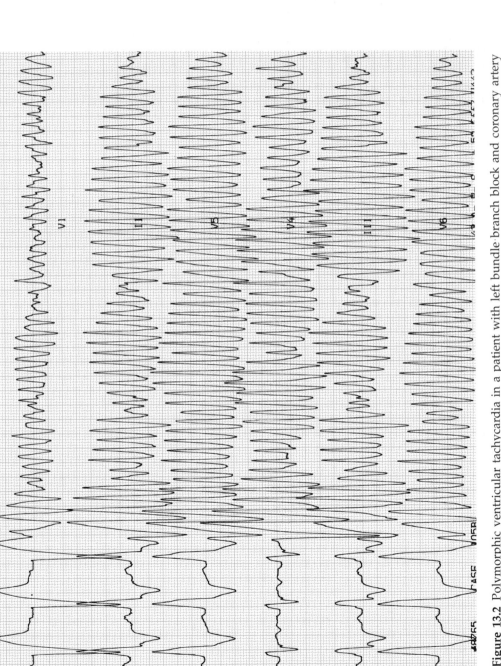

Figure 13.2 Polymorphic ventricular tachycardia in a patient with left bundle-branch block and coronary artery disease.

interval during sinus rhythm is normal and the management of the arrhythmia is the same as for monomorphic ventricular tachycardia.

TORSADE DE POINTES TACHYCARDIA

'Torsade de pointes' is the term applied to polymorphic ventricular tachycardia when the QT interval is prolonged in between episodes of the arrhythmia (Figure 13.3). Recognition is important because antiarrhythmic drugs may aggravate the tachycardia and because correction of or treatment aimed at its cause should prevent it.

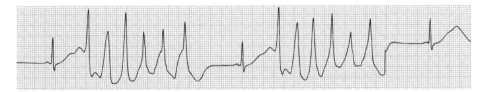

Figure 13.3 Two episodes of torsade de pointes tachycardia during sinus bradycardia; there is marked QT prolongation.

The arrhythmia is caused by bradycardia (Figure 13.4a,b) or by drugs (Figure 13.5a,b) or disorders that lead to abnormal ventricular repolarization (Table 13.1).

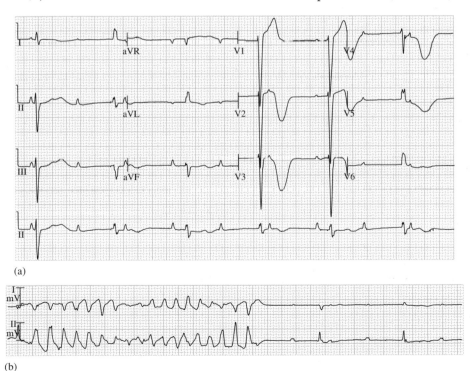

Figure 13.4 Complete atrioventricular block leading to a very long QT interval (a), with episodes of torsade de pointes tachycardia (b).

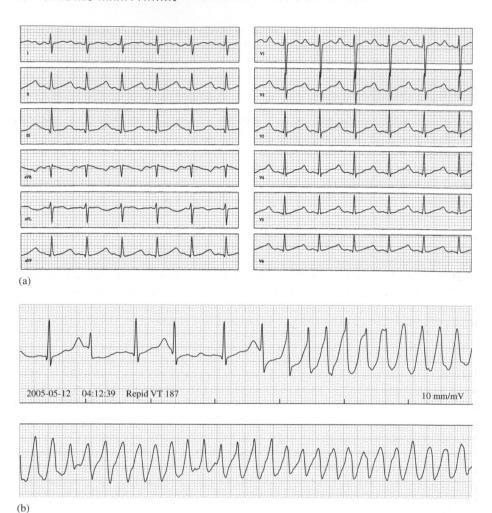

(a)

(b)

Figure 13.5 Overdose of the antipsychotic amisulpride leading to QT prolongation (a) and torsade de pointes tachycardia (b). (T wave alternans precedes the arrhythmia.)

Table 13.1 Causes of torsade de pointes tachycardia

Bradycardia due to sick sinus syndrome or atrioventricular block
Hereditary prolongation of the QT interval
Hypokalaemia, hypomagnesaemia
Antiarrhythmic drugs (e.g. quinidine, disopyramide, sotalol, amiodarone, ibutilide, dofetilide)
Non-antiarrhythmic drugs (e.g. erythromycin, clarithromycin, thioridazine, chlorpromazine, haloperidol, tricyclic antidepressants, prenylamine, bepridil, cisapride, domperidone, terfenadine, probucol, chloroquine, pentamidine)
Anorexia nervosa

Usually torsade de pointes tachycardia is non-sustained and repetitive but it can deteriorate to ventricular fibrillation. Onset usually follows a pause in rhythm caused by bradycardia or following an ectopic beat.

Drug interactions

Risk of torsade de pointes may be increased if an interaction between drugs leads to a higher blood level of a potentially proarrhythmic drug. For example, the erythromycins are metabolized by the liver's cytochrome P450 3A enzyme system. Commonly used drugs such as diltiazem and verapamil, as well as a number of antifungal agents, inhibit the enzyme system and have been shown to increase the risk of sudden death when administered together with erythromycin and clarithromycin.

QT INTERVAL

The QT interval is a measure of the duration of ventricular repolarization. It is measured from the onset of the QRS complex to the end of the T wave. Precise measurement is difficult because the timing of these events varies from ECG lead to lead and because it can be difficult to define the point at which the T wave ends and the U wave starts.

The QT interval normally shortens with increasing heart rate, partly due to the increase in rate itself and partly due to the increase in sympathetic nervous system activity associated with sinus tachycardia. When measuring the QT interval it is necessary to correct the measured interval for heart rate. The corrected QT interval (QTc) is usually calculated by selecting the ECG lead showing the longest QT interval, and then dividing the square root of the cycle length into the measured QT interval. For example, a patient with a measured QT interval of 0.38 s at a heart rate of 60 beats/min has a cycle length of 1.0 s and therefore also has a QTc of 0.38 s. A patient with a QT interval of 0.38 s at a heart rate of 120 beats/min has a QTc of 0.54 s. The normal QTc does not exceed 0.42 s in males and 0.44 s in females.

Prolongation of the QT interval may be due to either uniform prolongation of the process of repolarization throughout the myocardium, or variation in the rates of repolarization in disparate regions of myocardium. The latter situation is the one likely to cause ventricular arrhythmias.

Causes of QT prolongation include hereditary prolongation (i.e. the long QT syndromes; see below), hypocalcaemia, hypothyroidism, myocardial ischaemia (Figure 13.6) and subarachnoid haemorrhage.

MANAGEMENT OF TORSADE DE POINTES TACHYCARDIA

Treatment consists of reversal of the cause where possible, and cardiac pacing. Intravenous magnesium sulphate may be effective, even when serum magnesium is normal (8 mmol stat; 2.5 mmol/hour infusion).

Antiarrhythmic drugs should be stopped. Increasing the heart rate to 100 beats/min by pacing will often prevent the tachycardia while the drug(s) are being excreted or metabolized.

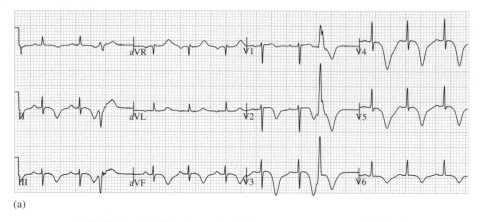

(a)

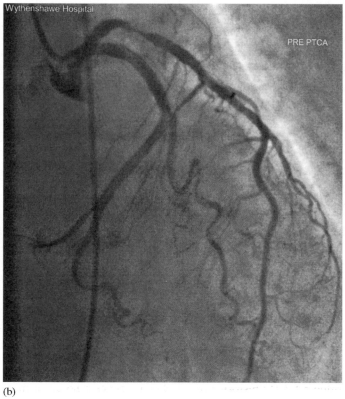

(b)

Figure 13.6 Marked QT prolongation (a) due to a severe stenosis in the proximal left anterior descending coronary artery (b). (There are two 'R on T' ventricular ectopic beats.)

HEREDITARY LONG QT SYNDROMES

The hereditary long QT syndromes are fairly rare disorders, with an estimated incidence of 1:5000, which can cause collapse, brief episodes of unconsciousness and sudden death due to torsade de pointes tachycardia and ventricular fibrillation (Figure 13.7). They are caused by abnormalities in the genes that control the functions of the cardiac cells' potassium and sodium ion channels. The common forms of long QT syndrome (at least five types have been described: LQT1–5) are caused by dominant genes and are also known as the Romano–Ward syndrome. There is no structural cardiac defect.

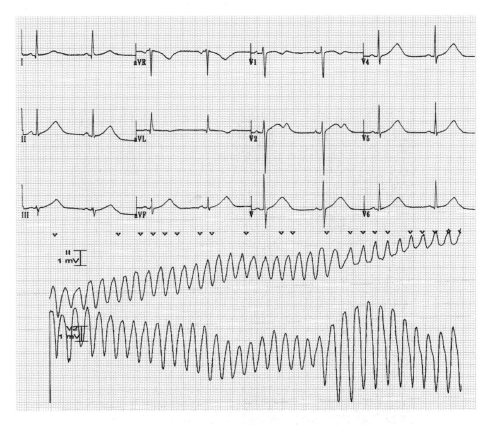

Figure 13.7 Hereditary QT prolongation and resultant torsade de pointes tachycardia. The QT interval is prolonged and the T wave is notched (LQT2 syndrome).

There is often a family history, but cases can arise as a result of mutation. Some patients can be severely affected and yet others with the same genetic defect can have little or no symptoms and a normal ECG (Figure 13.8a,b,c). Symptoms are most common in childhood and adolescence.

The clinical diagnosis is based on the ECG, which demonstrates a prolonged QT interval and an abnormally shaped T wave. There may be day to day variation in QT duration; it may be normal at times in some patients. Typically, the T wave is broad in LQT1 syndrome, of low amplitude and notched in LQT2 (Figure 13.7) and has a long isoelectric ST segment in LQT3 syndrome. Some patients are prone to marked sinus bradycardia.

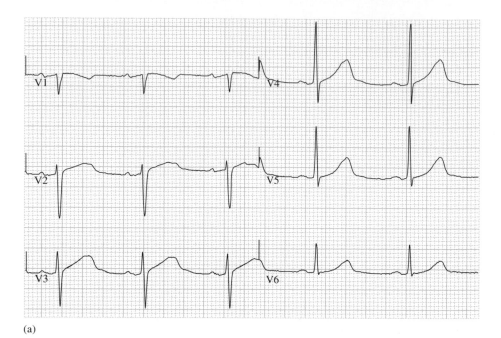

(a)

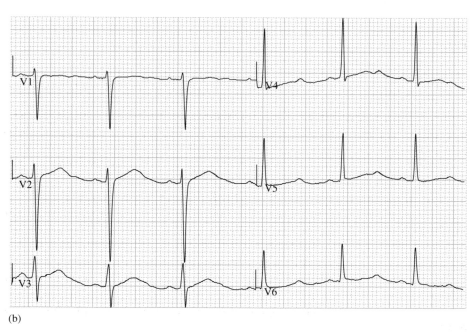

(b)

Figure 13.8 Hereditary QT prolongation: ECGs from asymptomatic father (a) and his two highly symptomatic daughters (b and c).

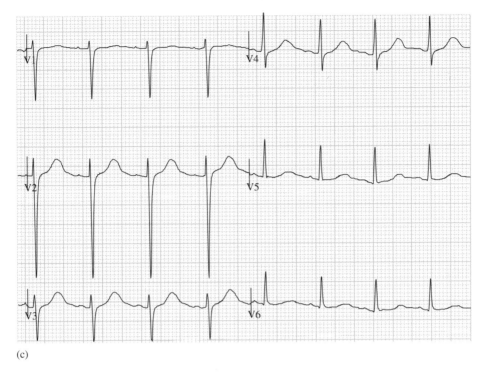

(c)

Figure 13.8 (Continued).

Thirty to forty per cent of patients with hereditary long QT syndrome will experience syncope, cardiac arrest or sudden death before the age of 40 years. In the more common forms of the syndrome, heart rhythm disturbances are initiated by exertion, excitement or fear. Sudden loud auditory stimuli, such as the ringing of a telephone, are also recognized as a common trigger for heart rhythm disturbances (typically in LQT2 but also in LQT1). In the LQT3 syndrome arrhythmias typically occur during sleep. Males who reach adulthood without an arrhythmia are unlikely to do so thereafter, whereas females are at risk at least into their fourth decade.

Very marked QT prolongation (QTc > 500 ms) and female gender (except for LQT3 syndrome) are associated with a higher risk of death. Arrhythmias are more common at the time of menstruation. T wave alternans (i.e. beat-to-beat alteration in T wave direction or amplitude) is also associated with a high risk of arrhythmia (see Figure 13.5). It is reported that a family history of sudden cardiac death is not a good guide to a patient's prognosis.

Genetic testing for the long QT syndromes is now becoming increasingly widely available.

It is likely that patients who develop torsade de pointes tachycardia as a result of a drug or bradycardia have the same genetic abnormalities of cardiac ion channels that cause the congenital long QT syndromes but in a subclinical form. Females are more susceptible.

The very rare Jervell and Lange–Nielsen long QT syndrome is due to a recessive gene and is associated with nerve deafness.

Treatment

Full beta-blockade is often effective. Ideally long-acting drugs should be used: nadolol (80–160 mg daily) has a very long half-life. Cardiac pacing in addition to beta-blockers should be considered in those patients with marked bradycardia prior to or because of beta-blockers. Asymptomatic patients who are young should receive a beta-blocker.

Left cervical sympathectomy has been performed where beta-blockade has failed. An implantable cardiovertor defibrillator should be considered in symptomatic patients, especially survivors of cardiac arrest.

Patients should be advised to avoid highly strenuous activities and, if possible, drugs that may enhance sympathetic nervous system activity, such as decongestants, midodrine, medications for asthma and fenfluramine.

It is very important that they avoid drugs that are recognized to prolong the QT interval, such as those listed in Table 13.1.

LQT3 is due to a defect in sodium rather than potassium ion transport and there are reports that flecainide will normalize the ECG and may prevent arrhythmias.

HEREDITARY SHORT QT SYNDROME

A hereditary short QT syndrome has recently been described. It appears to be very rare. The QTc interval is less than 300 ms. Sudden cardiac death due to ventricular arrhythmias and also atrial fibrillation can occur. It has been suggested that quinidine is effective in prolonging the QT interval and preventing arrhythmias, but implantation of an automatic cardiovertor defibrillator may be necessary.

VENTRICULAR FIBRILLATION

ECG CHARACTERISTICS

Ventricular fibrillation is the rapid, totally incoordinate contraction of ventricular myocardial fibres. This is reflected in the ECG by irregular, chaotic electrical activity (Figure 13.9).

Ventricular fibrillation causes circulatory arrest. Unconsciousness develops within 10–20 s.

CAUSES

Ninety per cent of deaths caused by acute myocardial infarction are due to ventricular fibrillation. The incidence of fibrillation is highest in the first hour. Ventricular fibrillation can also occur late after infarction and, in patients with severe coronary artery disease, without myocardial infarction. It may be the first clinical manifestation of the disease.

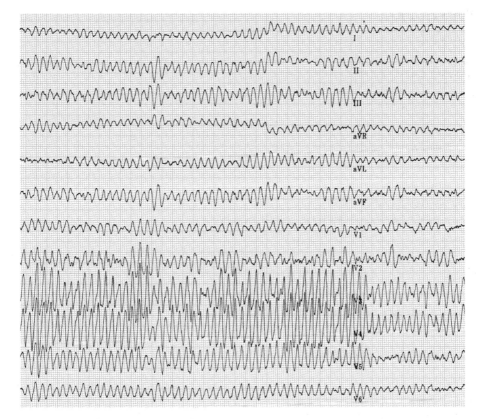

Figure 13.9 Ventricular fibrillation. Unusually, a full 12-lead ECG was obtained during ventricular fibrillation.

The arrhythmia can result from many other cardiac disorders, such as myocarditis and the cardiomyopathies. It may result from a primary electrical disorder (see Brugada syndrome, below).

It is usually initiated by a ventricular ectopic beat but can arise during a pause in cardiac rhythm or result from monomorphic or polymorphic ventricular tachycardia.

PRIMARY AND SECONDARY VENTRICULAR FIBRILLATION

If ventricular fibrillation develops in a heart that was functioning satisfactorily during normal rhythm it is termed 'primary' fibrillation, whereas if it occurs in the context of cardiac failure or cardiogenic shock, it is termed 'secondary'. Successful defibrillation is less likely in secondary ventricular fibrillation.

TREATMENT

Rarely, ventricular fibrillation is a brief event, spontaneously reverting to normal rhythm. Otherwise, without prompt treatment, irreversible cerebral and myocardial damage will quickly ensue.

Occasionally a praecordial blow is effective. Usually defibrillation is necessary (see Chapter 21).

Recurrent ventricular fibrillation

Acutely, intravenous lignocaine or amiodarone as well as correction of the pause, if possible, may be required. Addition of a beta-blocker can often be effective.

Longer term management is discussed in Chapters 21 and 25.

BRUGADA SYNDROME

Electrocardiographic appearance

The syndrome is characterized by a typical ECG pattern of ST elevation in leads V1, V2 and sometimes V3, usually together with partial right bundle branch block, a structurally normal heart and a risk of ventricular fibrillation.

The ventricular complex in lead V1 usually shows the most typical features: it ends with a positive component (akin to the J wave seen in hypothermia), followed by an elevated, *down-sloping* ST segment and negative T wave (Figure 13.10). Varying patterns of ST segment elevation may be seen in an individual patient: sometimes the ST segment elevation will have a concave or 'saddle-back' morphology. However, this appearance alone is not diagnostic of the Brugada syndrome.

There may be prolongation of the PR interval and paroxysmal atrial fibrillation is not uncommon.

The typical ECG abnormalities may be intermittent. Intravenous flecainide (2mg/kg over 10 minutes) or ajmaline (1mg/kg over 5 minutes) may induce the typical pattern: the latter is more effective at unmasking the syndrome but is not available in the United Kingdom. A high body temperature can also induce the abnormal pattern.

Aetiology

The Brugada syndrome is a genetically determined abnormality of a cardiac sodium ion channel. It is due to an autosomal dominant gene. Not all patients give a family history of sudden cardiac death because commonly the condition arises by mutation. Though due to an autosomal dominant gene, arrhythmias are more prevalent in males.

Ventricular fibrillation

Ventricular fibrillation can develop at any age but is most common in middle life. It is rare in the first two decades of life. It often occurs during sleep. No antiarrhythmic drugs have been shown to be effective but quinidine has been reported to be effective in patients with an 'arrhythmic storm'. The only treatment is implantation of an automatic defibrillator. Patients who have experienced syncope or have been resuscitated from ventricular fibrillation should receive such a device.

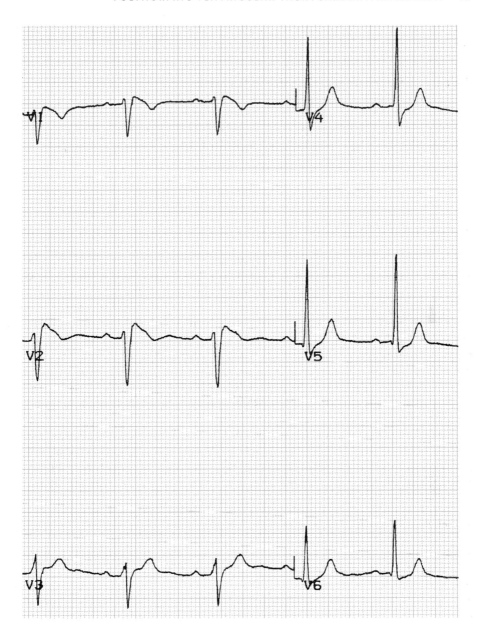

Figure 13.10 Chest leads from a patient with Brugada syndrome who developed ventricular fibrillation while driving.

Asymptomatic patients

The management of asymptomatic patients is controversial. Some studies have reported a fairly high incidence of ventricular fibrillation in previously asymptomatic patients (e.g. 8 per cent incidence over a three-year period). Other studies have demonstrated a much lower risk. It is generally agreed that patients who do not have

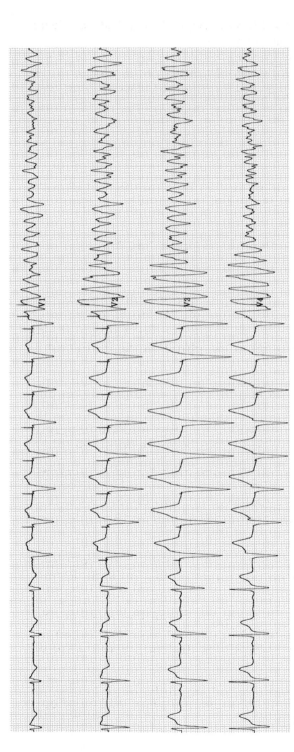

Figure 13.11 Asymptomatic patient with Brugada syndrome (leads V1–V4) who developed ventricular fibrillation during ventricular stimulation study: after eight paced beats at 120 beats/min a couplet of premature stimuli initiated ventricular fibrillation.

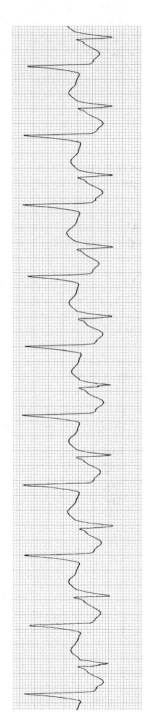

Figure 13.12 Bidirectional ventricular tachycardia.

a persistently abnormal ECG are at low risk. Surprisingly, it seems that a family history of sudden cardiac death is not a risk factor.

Some but not all authorities advocate a ventricular stimulation study in patients with a consistently abnormal ECG and recommend implantation of a defibrillator if ventricular fibrillation is initiated by programmed premature stimulation (Figure 13.11).

BIDIRECTIONAL VENTRICULAR TACHYCARDIA

This is a rare arrhythmia with two alternating ventricular complex morphologies (Figure 13.12). It cannot be described as either monomorphic or polymorphic!

CATECHOLAMINERGIC POLYMORPHIC VENTRICULAR TACHYCARDIA

This is a rare, genetically determined condition where polymorphic or bidirectional (Figure 13.12) ventricular tachycardia is induced by exercise. The QT interval is normal. It is mainly seen in children. It has a poor prognosis. Beta-blockers are indicated but are not always effective. An implantable defibrillator may be required.

Main points

- Polymorphic tachycardia is characterized by repeated progressive changes in the QRS complex so the complexes appear to 'twist' about the baseline.

- Torsade de pointes tachycardia refers to polymorphic tachycardia when there is QT prolongation in between tachycardias. Causes include bradycardia, a large number of drugs and the hereditary QT prolongation syndromes. Antiarrhythmic therapy may aggravate the arrhythmia and pacing is often effective.

- The hereditary long QT syndromes are an important cause of syncope and sudden cardiac death. Beta-blockers, pacing and/or an implantable defibrillator may be required.

- Ventricular fibrillation is the rapid, totally incoordinate contraction of ventricular myocardial fibres. It causes circulatory arrest. The commonest cause is myocardial ischaemia. Rarely it will stop spontaneously, otherwise immediate defibrillation is necessary.

- The Brugada syndrome is a genetic disorder characterized by a specific pattern of ST elevation in the right praecordial leads and may result in sudden death from ventricular fibrillation.

CHAPTER 14

Tachycardias with broad ventricular complexes

Tachycardias of supraventricular origin sometimes have broad ventricular complexes. Thus, they may mimic ventricular tachycardia. Now that this is widely appreciated, the tendency is to misinterpret ventricular tachycardia as supraventricular, rather than the reverse.

CAUSES OF A BROAD COMPLEX TACHYCARDIA

Tachycardias with broad ventricular complexes may be due to:

1. ventricular tachycardia;
2. supraventricular tachycardia when bundle branch block has already been present during sinus rhythm;
3. supraventricular tachycardia with rate-related bundle branch block (i.e. bundle branch block develops during tachycardia);
4. the Wolff–Parkinson–White syndrome, when atrial impulses during atrial flutter or fibrillation are conducted to the ventricles by the accessory AV pathway, or in the uncommon 'antidromic' form of AV junctional re-entrant tachycardia, when AV conduction is over the accessory pathway.

Several pointers are used to distinguish a supraventricular tachycardia with broad ventricular complexes from ventricular tachycardia.

USELESS GUIDELINES

It is often said that whereas ventricular tachycardia leads to major haemodynamic disturbance, supraventricular tachycardia does not. This is wrong. Sometimes ventricular tachycardia causes few or even no symptoms, whereas supraventricular tachycardia, if very fast or in the presence of underlying heart disease, can cause shock or heart failure (Figure 14.1).

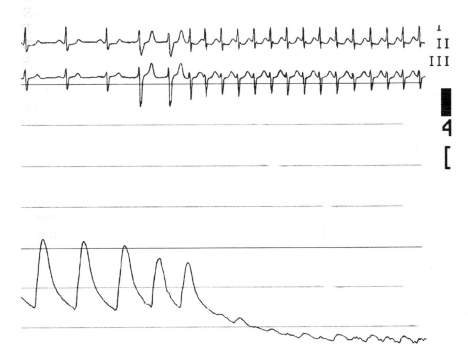

Figure 14.1 Dramatic drop in arterial pressure with onset of atrioventricular re-entrant tachycardia.

Another widely quoted but incorrect rule is that whereas supraventricular tachycardia is regular, ventricular tachycardia is slightly irregular.

Verapamil may terminate supraventricular tachycardia or slow the ventricular response to atrial fibrillation or flutter. It has been used as a 'therapeutic' test of the origin of tachycardia. However, dangerous hypotension may result when the drug is given during ventricular tachycardia. Never use verapamil to try to establish the origin of a broad complex tachycardia.

USEFUL GUIDELINES

CLINICAL CIRCUMSTANCES

Myocardial damage caused by coronary artery disease, by cardiomyopathy or by other diseases may cause ventricular tachycardia. On the other hand, myocardial damage is not going to create the additional electrical connection between atria and ventricles that is necessary to facilitate an AV junctional re-entrant tachycardia. Thus, a broad QRS tachycardia in a patient known to have myocardial damage is likely to be ventricular in origin.

Atrial flutter and tachycardia may occur in patients with myocardial damage and may lead to a regular ventricular rhythm with bundle branch block, but there are characteristic features which should lead to their identification. The ventricular rhythm during atrial fibrillation is totally irregular and should never be confused with ventricular tachycardia.

INDEPENDENT ATRIAL ACTIVITY

If there is direct or indirect (Figures 12.2, 12.4, 12.10, 14.2 and 14.3) evidence of independent atrial activity then supraventricular tachycardia is excluded. As discussed in Chapter 12, scrutiny of several ECG leads may be necessary to identify evidence of atrial activity (Figure 14.4). Wherever possible, a 12-lead ECG during tachycardia should be acquired (Figure 14.5).

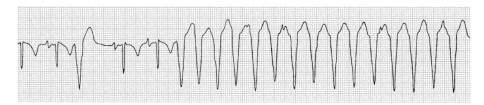

Figure 14.2 The second ventricular ectopic beat initiates ventricular tachycardia. Independent atrial activity can be seen.

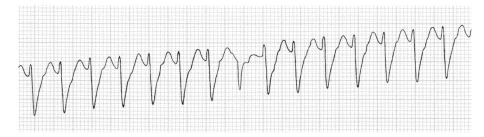

Figure 14.3 Ventricular tachycardia (lead II). The eighth complex is a capture beat.

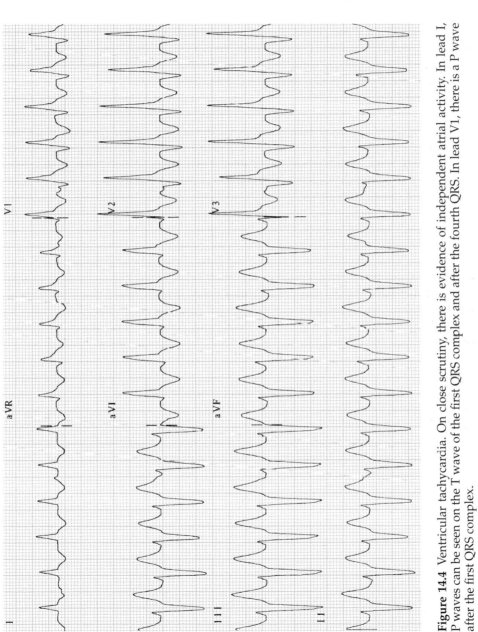

Figure 14.4 Ventricular tachycardia. On close scrutiny, there is evidence of independent atrial activity. In lead I, P waves can be seen on the T wave of the first QRS complex and after the fourth QRS. In lead V1, there is a P wave after the first QRS complex.

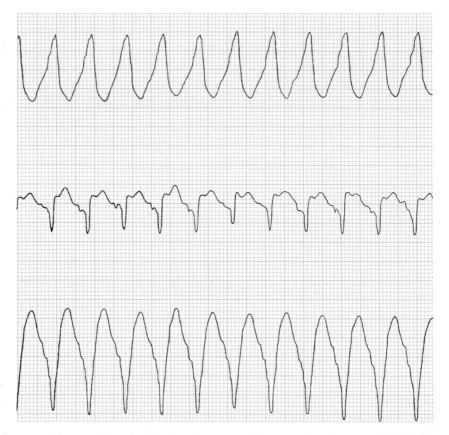

Figure 14.5 Advantage of simultaneous recording of ECG leads (I, II, III). Lead II suggests that there may be a P wave before each QRS complex and thus that the tachycardia is supraventricular in origin rather than ventricular. However, comparison with other leads indicates that the 'P' wave is in fact the initial vector of the ventricular complex.

Occasionally, independent atrial activity can only be demonstrated by recording an atrial ECG simultaneously with a surface ECG (Figure 14.6). An atrial ECG can be obtained by passing a transvenous electrode to the right atrium or by using an oesophageal electrode positioned behind the left atrium.

CAROTID SINUS MASSAGE

Carotid sinus massage can transiently slow AV node conduction and may thus terminate an AV re-entrant tachycardia. If a reduction in ventricular rate occurs during massage but sinus rhythm does not return, it is likely that the patient has atrial flutter or fibrillation. During the higher degree of AV block, flutter and fibrillation waves are more easily identifiable.

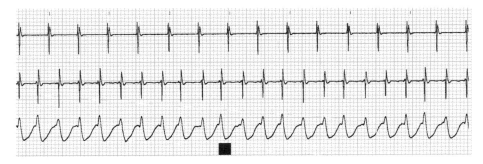

Figure 14.6 Right atrial (upper trace), right ventricular (middle trace) and surface (lower trace) electrograms. Atrial activity is slower than and independent of ventricular activity, confirming ventricular tachycardia.

Carotid sinus massage is not always effective in supraventricular tachycardia and its failure does not indicate ventricular tachycardia.

CONFIGURATION OF VENTRICULAR COMPLEX

The broader the ventricular complex the more likely is a ventricular origin. In ventricular tachycardia, the duration of the ventricular complex is usually 0.14 s or greater.

Marked axis deviation, left or right, also suggests ventricular tachycardia. Another pointer towards this arrhythmia is a 'concordant' pattern in the chest leads (i.e. the complexes are either all positive or all negative) (Figures 14.7 and 14.8).

When supraventricular tachycardias are associated with bundle branch block the morphology of the ventricular complexes is usually that of typical left or right bundle branch block (Figure 14.9).

RETROGRADE CONCEALED CONDUCTION

As discussed in Chapter 2, partial penetration of the AV node by a ventricular ectopic impulse may lead to prolongation of the PR interval during the following sinus beat. Prolongation of the PR interval in the first sinus beat after a tachycardia indicates a ventricular origin.

ECTOPIC BEATS

If the configuration of the ventricular complex during tachycardia is similar to that of an ectopic beat recorded during normal rhythm, a common origin is probable.

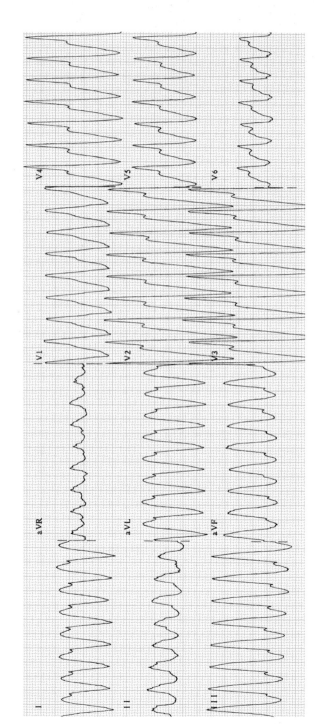

Figure 14.7 Ventricular tachycardia. QRS complex duration = 0.18 s. Positive concordant pattern in chest leads.

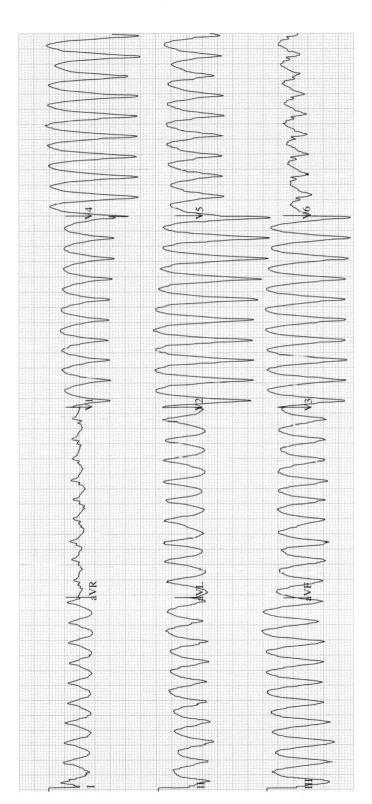

Figure 14.8 Ventricular tachycardia. QRS complex duration = 0.18 s. Negative concordant pattern in chest leads.

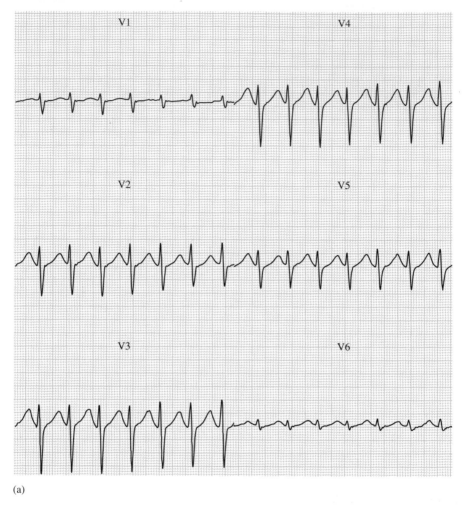

(a)

Figure 14.9 Atrioventricular nodal re-entrant tachycardia recorded during an electro-physiological study. Intraventricular conduction varied from normal (a), to right bundle branch block (b) and left bundle branch block (c).

It is relatively easy to ascertain the origin of single ectopic beats, especially if a full ECG is available (see Figure 14.2).

ADENOSINE

Adenosine is very effective at terminating supraventricular tachycardia due to an AV junctional re-entrant mechanism, and will transiently slow the ventricular response to atrial fibrillation and flutter, making the respective atrial 'f' or 'F' waves easily identifiable for diagnostic purposes. A positive response to adenosine points

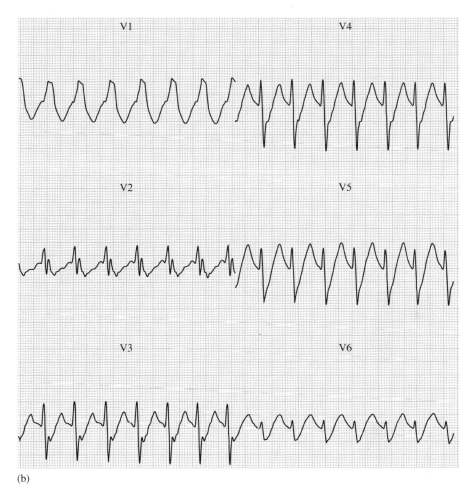

(b)

Figure 14.9 (Continued).

strongly towards a supraventricular origin to the tachycardia. Because its duration of action is very brief it is a safe drug to give (with the possible exception of patients with asthma).

However, a minority of supraventricular tachycardias will not respond to adenosine and the drug will terminate right ventricular outflow tract tachycardia. Thus response or lack of response to adenosine is a pointer towards the origin of the tachycardia but is not an absolutely reliable guide.

Adenosine is often used in a 'knee-jerk' response to a broad complex tachycardia in patients with known myocardial infarction or cardiomyopathy. Ventricular tachycardia is highly likely and it is pointless to use adenosine in these situations unless there is a very strong suspicion that the rhythm is atrial flutter or tachycardia with aberration.

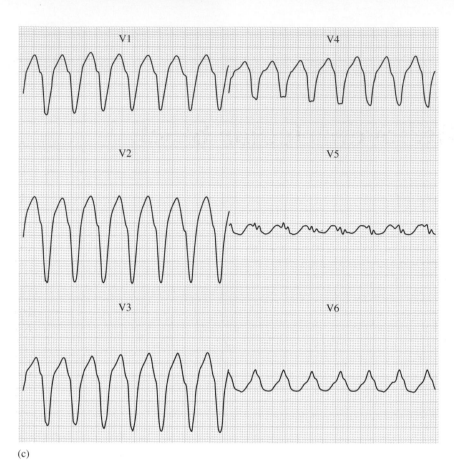

(c)

Figure 14.9 (Continued).

Main points

- Wherever possible, record a 12-lead ECG during tachycardia.

- Though bundle branch block can sometimes occur during supraventricular tachycardias, most wide complex tachycardias are ventricular in origin.

- Pointers towards ventricular tachycardia include the presence of myocardial damage, direct or indirect evidence of independent atrial activity, QRS duration greater than 0.14 s, a concordant pattern in the chest leads and marked axis deviation.

- Neither minor irregularities during tachycardia nor the haemodynamic effect of the arrhythmia are useful in ascertaining its origin.

- When supraventricular tachycardias are associated with bundle branch block the morphology of the ventricular complexes is usually that of typical left or right bundle branch block.

- Never use verapamil for a diagnostic test.

Atrioventricular block

CLASSIFICATION

Atrioventricular (AV) block is classified as first, second or third degree depending on whether conduction of atrial impulses to the ventricles is delayed, intermittently blocked or completely blocked.

FIRST-DEGREE ATRIOVENTRICULAR BLOCK

Delay in conduction of the atrial impulse to the ventricles results in prolongation of the PR interval (Figures 15.1–15.3). The PR interval is measured from the onset of the P wave to the onset of the ventricular complex – whether this is a Q or an R wave – and is prolonged if it is greater than 0.21 s. Since conduction of the atrial impulse is only delayed, the term first-degree AV block is, in fact, a misnomer.

First-degree AV block does not cause symptoms but may sometimes progress to higher degrees of block. In young people it is usually due to high vagal tone and is benign.

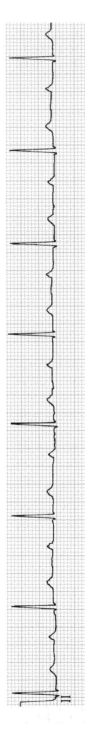

Figure 15.1 First-degree atrioventricular block (lead II). PR interval = 0.32 s.

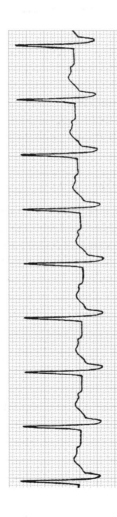

Figure 15.2 First-degree atrioventricular block and sinus tachycardia (lead I). PR interval = 0.24 s.

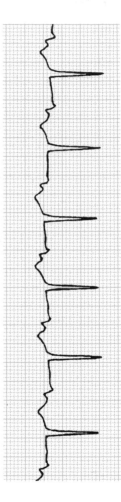

Figure 15.3 First-degree atrioventricular block (lead V1). The P wave is superimposed on the terminal portion of the preceding T wave. PR interval = 0.38 s.

SECOND-DEGREE ATRIOVENTRICULAR BLOCK

In second-degree AV block there is intermittent failure of conduction of atrial impulses to the ventricles (i.e. some P waves are not followed by QRS complexes).

Second-degree block is subdivided into Mobitz type I (which is also termed 'Wenckebach') and Mobitz type II block.

Mobitz type I or Wenckebach atrioventricular block

In this form of second-degree block, delay in AV conduction increases with each successive atrial impulse until an atrial impulse fails to be conducted to the ventricles. After the dropped beat, AV conduction recovers and the sequence starts again (Figures 15.4 and 15.5).

Wenckebach AV block is usually due to impaired conduction in the AV node. Like first AV block, it can be benign (particularly during sleep) and is due to high vagal tone. Wenckebach block that cannot be attributed to high vagal tone has a prognosis similar to that of Mobitz II block.

Mobitz type II atrioventricular block

In Mobitz type II block there is intermittent failure of conduction of atrial impulses to the ventricles without preceding progressive lengthening of the PR interval, and thus the PR interval of conducted beats is constant (Figure 15.6).

In contrast to first-degree and Wenckebach AV block, Mobitz type II block is usually due to impaired conduction in the bundle of His or bundle branches i.e. infranodal. Thus, because there is bundle branch disease, the QRS complexes are usually broad (Figure 15.7). Block below the AV node is more likely to be associated with Stokes–Adams attacks, slow ventricular rates and sudden death.

The ratio of conducted to non-conducted atrial impulses varies. Commonly 2:1 AV conduction occurs. A similar pattern may be caused by an extreme form of Wenckebach block so it is difficult to make prognostic inferences from 2:1 AV block with narrow QRS complexes (Figure 15.8).

Usually, during Mobitz type II block, the atrial rate is regular. Sometimes, however, the P–P interval encompassing a ventricular complex is shorter than a P–P interval that does not. This is known as ventriculophasic sinus arrhythmia.

THIRD-DEGREE ATRIOVENTRICULAR BLOCK

Third-degree or complete AV block occurs when there is total interruption of transmission of atrial impulses to the ventricles. Third-degree block may be due to interrupted conduction at either AV nodal or infranodal level. When the block is within the AV node, subsidiary pacemakers arise within the bundle of His and, unless there is additional bundle branch block, will lead to narrow QRS complexes (Figure 15.9). Often, pacemakers within the bundle of His discharge reliably at a fairly rapid rate. In contrast, in infranodal block subsidiary pacemakers usually arise in the left or right bundle branches. These pacemakers will produce broad QRS complexes and

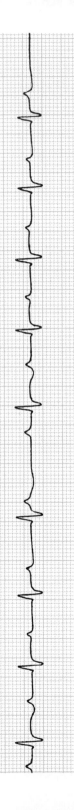

Figure 15.4 Wenckebach atrioventricular block.

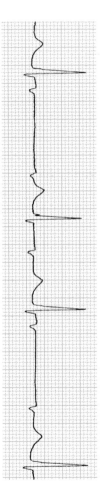

Figure 15.5 Wenckebach atrioventricular block. Unlike many textbook examples, but as often occurs in practice, the trace does not start with the shortest PR interval.

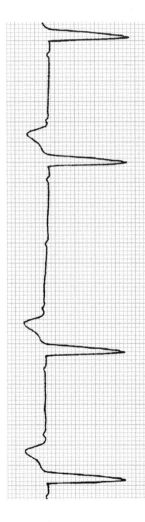

Figure 15.6 Mobitz type II atrioventricular block. In this example the ratio between conducted and non-conducted atrial impulses varies.

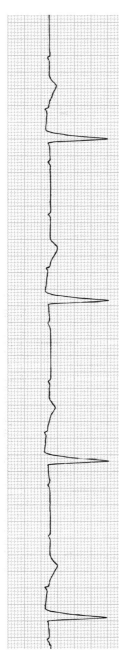

Figure 15.7 Mobitz type II atrioventricular block. The QRS complex is broad.

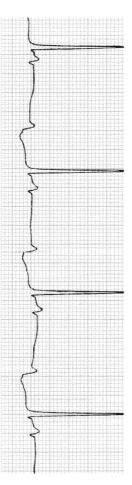

Figure 15.8 2:1 atrioventricular block with narrow QRS complexes (lead V1). The non-conducted atrial beats are superimposed on preceding T waves.

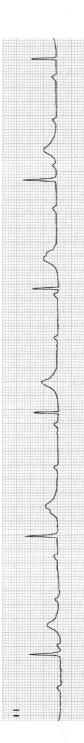

Figure 15.9 Complete atrioventricular block with narrow QRS complexes.

slower ventricular rates (Figures 15.10 and 15.13). They are less reliable and thus Stokes–Adams attacks are more likely.

Complete AV block can occur during atrial fibrillation and flutter (Figures 6.4, 15.11 and 15.12).

Occasionally, heart block only occurs during exercise and can be the cause of exertional syncope or weakness.

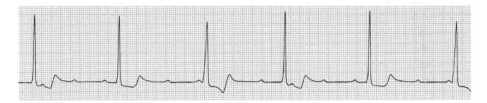

Figure 15.10 Complete atrioventricular block with broad QRS complexes.

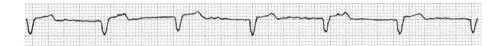

Figure 15.11 Complete atrioventricular block with atrial fibrillation.

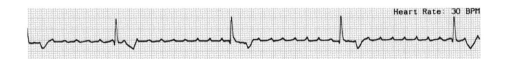

Figure 15.12 Complete atrioventricular block with atrial flutter.

Supernormal conduction

Rarely, even during third-degree AV block, atrial impulses may be conducted to the ventricles. There is a short period immediately after recovery from excitation when AV conduction may transiently improve. This period usually coincides with inscription of the latter portion of the T wave (Figure 15.13). As a result, atrial impulses falling on this part of the T wave will be followed by a premature QRS complex.

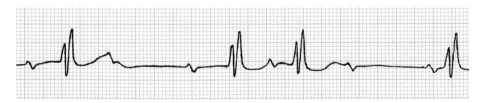

Figure 15.13 Complete atrioventricular block. There is supernormal conduction of the atrial impulse that falls on the T wave of the second ventricular complex (lead V1).

CAUSES OF ATRIOVENTRICULAR BLOCK

Idiopathic fibrosis of the AV junction and/or bundle branches is the most common cause. The causes of AV block are listed in Table 15.1.

Table 15.1 Causes of atrioventricular block

Idiopathic fibrosis of conduction tissues
Myocardial infarction
Aortic valve disease
Congenital isolated lesion
Congenital heart disease (e.g. corrected transposition)
Cardiac surgery
Infiltration (e.g. tumour, sarcoidosis, haemochromatosis, syphilis)
Inflammation (e.g. endocarditis, ankylosing spondylitis, Reiter's syndrome)
Rheumatic fever
Diphtheria
Dystrophia myotonica
Chagas' disease (South America)
Lyme carditis (tick-borne spirochaetal infection, *Borrelia burgdorferi*, mainly North America)
Rarely, familial

ATRIOVENTRICULAR DISSOCIATION

During third-degree AV block, atrial activity is *faster* than and dissociated from ventricular activity. Dissociation between atrial and ventricular activity also occurs when, often during sinus bradycardia, an escape rhythm faster than the sinus rate arises from the AV junction or ventricles (Figure 15.14). The term 'AV dissociation' should be reserved for this latter situation, in which the atrial rate is *slower* than the ventricular rate. If AV dissociation is not distinguished from complete AV block, inappropriate action can result. For example, AV dissociation often occurs in acute myocardial infarction and, if not recognized as such, a pacemaker may be inserted unnecessarily.

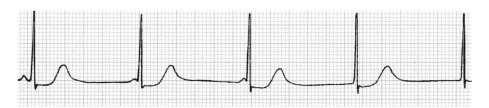

Figure 15.14 Atrioventricular dissociation. Atrial and ventricular rates are 49 and 51 beats/min, respectively. The fourth and fifth P waves are concealed by superimposed QRS complexes.

BILATERAL BUNDLE BRANCH DISEASE

Infranodal AV block is most often caused by disease in both left and right bundle branches.

Although the anatomical situation may be more complex, functionally the bundle of His can be considered to divide into three: the right bundle branch and the anterior and posterior fascicles of the left bundle branch (see Chapter 4).

If conduction is blocked in only two of the three fascicles (bifascicular block), the functioning fascicle will conduct atrial impulses to the ventricles and maintain sinus rhythm. Block in the third fascicle will lead to complete AV block.

BIFASCICULAR BLOCK

The most common pattern of bifascicular block is right bundle branch plus left anterior fascicular block (Figure 15.15). The posterior fascicle of the left bundle branch is a stouter structure than the anterior fascicle and is therefore less vulnerable. As a result, right bundle branch plus left posterior fascicular block is a less common occurrence (Figure 15.16).

PR interval prolongation is usually due to impaired AV node conduction, but in the context of bifascicular block it is more likely to reflect abnormal conduction in the functioning fascicle (Figure 15.17, see page 151). The combination of bifascicular block and a long PR interval is sometimes referred to as 'trifascicular block'. This is incorrect. Trifascicular block indicates that there is complete block of AV conduction; 'trifascicular disease' would be a better term.

TRIFASCICULAR BLOCK

Interrupted conduction in all three fascicles results in complete AV block. In many patients one of the three fascicles is capable of intermittent conduction so that, for part of the time, there will be sinus rhythm with evidence of bifascicular block.

The risk of bifascicular block progressing to trifascicular block is low. In patients with right bundle and left anterior fascicular block, it is a few per cent per year. There is little evidence to suggest that prophylactic implantation of a permanent pacemaker in asymptomatic patients with bifascicular block improves prognosis. The major determinants of prognosis are the states of the myocardium and coronary arteries.

The risk is increased when there is right bundle and left posterior fascicular block and when there is alternating complete right and left bundle branch block.

CLINICAL FEATURES OF ATRIOVENTRICULAR BLOCK

First-degree and Mobitz type I second-degree AV block do not usually cause symptoms but may progress to higher grades of block. Very rarely, the resultant delay

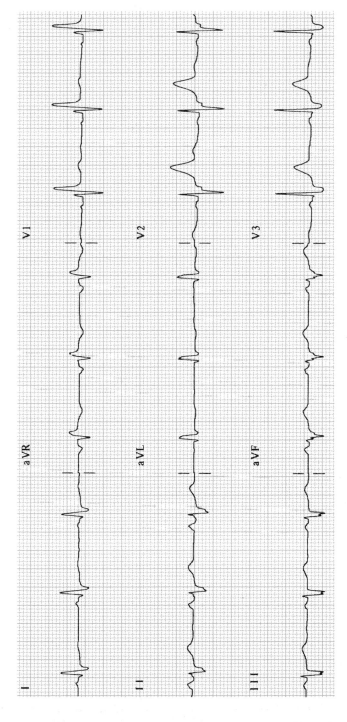

Figure 15.15 Left anterior fascicular and right bundle branch block.

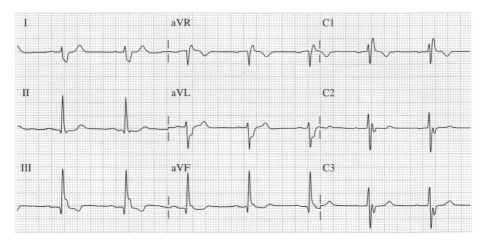

Figure 15.16 Left posterior fascicular and right bundle branch block.

between atrial and ventricular activation can significantly reduce cardiac output and thereby cause symptoms.

In Mobitz type II and complete AV block, a low ventricular rate may cause tiredness, dyspnoea or heart failure.

In some patients the ventricular pacemaker may at times discharge very slowly or actually stops, leading to syncope or, if ventricular activity does not quickly return, sudden death (Figure 15.18). Not uncommonly, syncope is due to torsade de pointes tachycardia which has resulted from the low ventricular rate during heart block.

STOKES–ADAMS ATTACKS

Syncope due to transient asystole (or ventricular tachyarrhythmia) – a Stokes–Adams attack – has characteristic features. These features are of great diagnostic importance. On the one hand, abnormalities of AV conduction and/or sinus node function may be intermittent and therefore routine electrocardiography will be normal. The typical features of a Stokes–Adams attack will point to the likelihood that collapse is due to an arrhythmia and the need for ambulatory electrocardiography. On the other hand, it is possible that a patient who does have evidence of disease of the specialized conducting tissues syncope may collapse from an unrelated cause such as epilepsy: if the symptoms are not typical of a Stokes–Adams attack a non-arrhythmic cause should be suspected.

In a Stokes–Adams attack, loss of consciousness is sudden. There is virtually no warning, though the patient will sometimes feel that he or she is going to faint, just before loss of consciousness. The patient collapses, lying motionless, pale and pulseless, and looks as though he or she is dead. Usually, within a minute or two, consciousness returns, and as cardiac action resumes there may be a vivid flushes to the skin. Incontinence does occur occasionally but is not a regular feature as it is in epilepsy. Unlike epilepsy, recovery is quick, and confusion and headache after the attack are unusual.

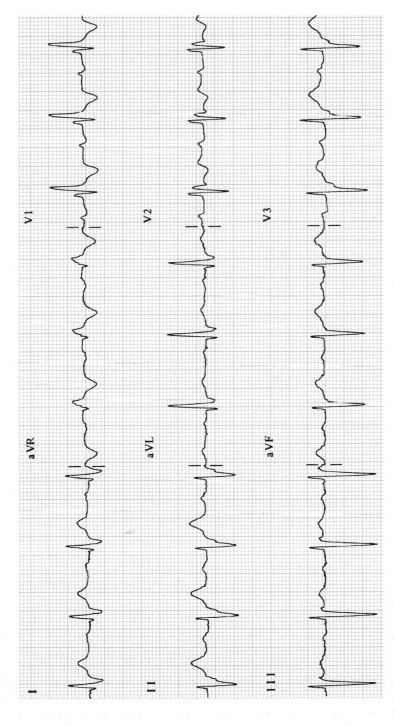

Figure 15.17 Bifascicular and first-degree atrioventricular block.

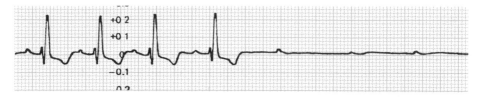

Figure 15.18 Sudden onset of complete atrioventricular block with no escape rhythm in a patient with bifascicular block.

NEAR-SYNCOPE

In some patients the rhythm disturbance does not last long enough to cause syncope but the patient feels as though he or she is going to faint and then recovers. The patient may complain of 'dizziness' but does not experience true vertigo.

CONGENITAL HEART BLOCK

In congenital heart block AV conduction is interrupted at the AV nodal level. Consequently, the subsidiary ventricular pacemaker is situated in the proximal part of the bundle of His (producing narrow QRS complexes) and discharges reliably at a moderately fast rate (40–80 beats/min), which may accelerate on exercise. Often, there are no symptoms and exercise tolerance is good. However, syncope and sudden death do occur in a minority of patients (see Chapter 24).

There is a high incidence of congenital AV block in babies whose mothers have systemic lupus erythematosus.

ACQUIRED HEART BLOCK

Heart block complicating myocardial infarction is discussed in Chapter 18.

As discussed above, the commonest cause of heart block is idiopathic fibrosis of the AV junction or bundle branches. This mainly affects the elderly but – as with the other causes of AV block – can affect the young and middle aged as well.

The bradycardia associated with Mobitz type II and third-degree AV block may reduce cardiac output and lead to symptoms such as shortness of breath, tiredness and heart failure. Stokes–Adams attacks will sooner or later occur in about two-thirds of patients with these higher grades of AV block.

TREATMENT

Artificial cardiac pacing has greatly improved symptoms and prognosis. The indications are discussed in Chapters 23 and 24.

Main points

- AV block is classified as first, second or third degree depending on whether conduction of atrial impulses to the ventricles is delayed, intermittently blocked or completely blocked.

- Second-degree AV block is subdivided into Mobitz I (Wenckebach) and Mobitz II types. In the former, there is progressive lengthening of the PR interval prior to non-conduction of an atrial impulse, whereas the PR interval of conducted atrial impulses is constant in Mobitz II. The QRS complex in Mobitz II block is usually broad.

- During AV dissociation (in contrast to complete AV block), the atrial rate is slower than the ventricular rate.

- First-degree block, Wenckebach block and third-degree block with narrow QRS complexes are usually due to disease within the AV node, whereas Mobitz II and complete AV block with broad QRS complexes are likely to be due to infranodal block.

- Bifascicular block may deteriorate intermittently or permanently to complete (trifascicular) AV block.

- Stokes–Adams attacks are characterized by an abrupt, brief loss of consciousness following which recovery is usually rapid. Patients with conduction tissue disease often experience 'near syncope' as well as episodes of complete loss of consciousness.

Sick sinus syndrome

The sick sinus syndrome, also referred to as sinoatrial disease, is caused by impairment either of sinus node automaticity (automaticity is defined as the ability of a cell to initiate an electrical impulse) or of conduction of impulses from the sinus node to the atria. It can lead to sinus bradycardia, sinoatrial block or sinus arrest.

In some patients, atrial fibrillation, flutter or tachycardia may also occur. The term 'bradycardia–tachycardia' (often shortened to 'brady–tachy') syndrome applies to these patients.

Sick sinus syndrome is a common cause of syncope, dizzy attacks and palpitation. Though found most often in the elderly, it can occur at any age.

CAUSES

The cause is usually idiopathic fibrosis of the sinus node. Cardiomyopathy, myocarditis, cardiac surgery, antiarrhythmic drugs and lithium toxicity can also cause the syndrome.

ECG CHARACTERISTICS

Any of the following can occur. They are often intermittent, normal sinus rhythm being present for most of the time.

SINUS BRADYCARDIA

Sinus bradycardia is a common finding (Figure 16.1).

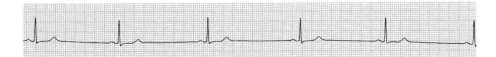

Figure 16.1 Sinus bradycardia. Rate 33 beats/min.

SINUS ARREST

Sinus arrest occurs due to failure of the sinus node to activate the atria. The result is absence of normal P waves (Figures 16.2 and 16.3).

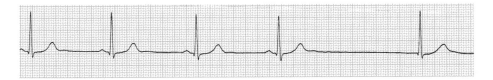

Figure 16.2 Sinus arrest leading to a junctional escape beat.

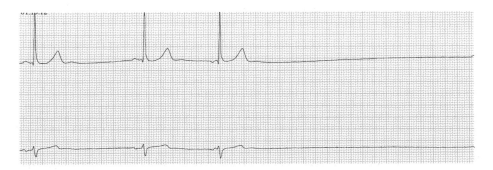

Figure 16.3 Sinus arrest after a junctional beat leading to a prolonged period of ventricular standstill.

Sinoatrial block

Sinoatrial block occurs when sinus node impulses fail to traverse the junction between the node and surrounding atrial myocardium. Like atrioventricular block, sinoatrial block can be classified into first, second or third degrees. However, the ECG allows only recognition of second-degree sinoatrial block. Third-degree or complete block is indistinguishable from sinus arrest.

In second-degree sinoatrial block, intermittent failure of atrial activation results in intervals between P waves that are multiples of (often twice) the cycle length during sinus rhythm (Figure 16.4).

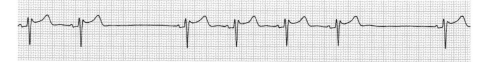

Figure 16.4 Two pauses due to second-degree sinoatrial block during which both the P waves and QRS complexes are dropped for one cycle.

Escape beats and rhythms

When sinus bradycardia or arrest occurs, subsidiary pacemaker tissue may give rise to an escape beat or rhythm (Figures 16.2 and 16.5). A junctional or idioventricular rhythm suggests impaired sinus node function.

Atrial ectopic beats

These are common. Long pauses often follow because sinus node automaticity is depressed by the ectopic beat (Figure 16.6).

BRADYCARDIA–TACHYCARDIA SYNDROME

Atrial fibrillation, flutter or tachycardia may occur in patients with the sick sinus syndrome (Figure 16.7). However, AV re-entrant tachycardia is not part of this syndrome.

Sinus node automaticity is often depressed by these tachycardias, so sinus bradycardia or arrest follows the tachycardia (Figure 16.7). Conversely, tachycardias often arise as an escape rhythm during bradycardia (Figures 16.8 and 16.9). Thus, tachycardia often alternates with bradycardia.

ATRIOVENTRICULAR BLOCK

AV block sometimes coexists with the sick sinus syndrome.

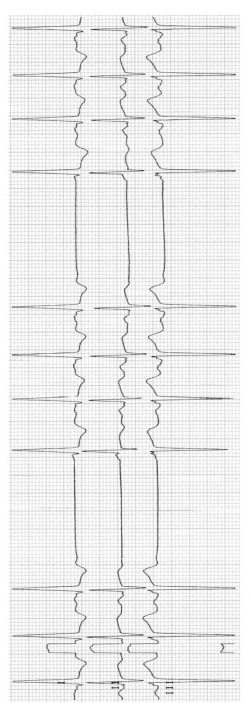

Figure 16.5 Junctional escape beats following sinus arrest.

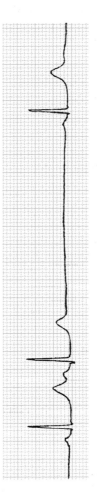

Figure 16.6 Atrial ectopic beat leads to depression of sinus node automaticity.

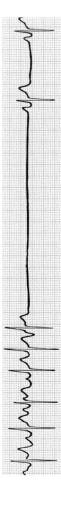

Figure 16.7 Termination of atrial fibrillation followed by sinus arrest.

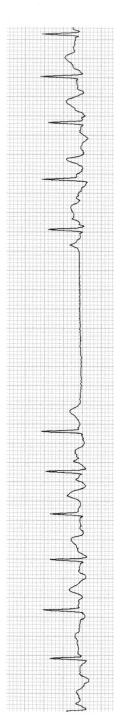

Figure 16.8 Sinus arrest after termination of atrial fibrillation. After a single sinus beat atrial fibrillation recurs.

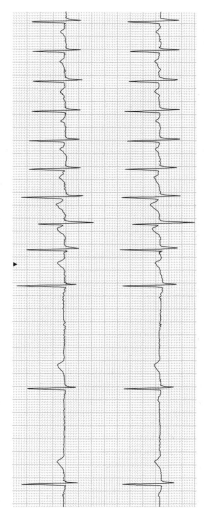

Figure 16.9 Bradycardia–tachycardia syndrome. Atrial tachycardia arises during sinus bradycardia.

In patients with the sick sinus syndrome who develop atrial fibrillation there is often a slow ventricular response without AV nodal-blocking drugs, suggesting coexistent impaired AV nodal function.

CLINICAL FEATURES

Sinus arrest without an adequate escape rhythm may cause syncope or dizzy attacks, depending on its duration. Tachycardias often produce palpitation, and resultant sinus node depression may lead to syncope or near-syncope after palpitation.

Some patients will experience symptoms several times each day, whereas in others symptoms will be infrequent.

Systemic embolism is common in the bradycardia–tachycardia syndrome.

CHRONOTROPIC INCOMPETENCE

Impaired sinus node function may result in an inadequate increase in heart rate during exertion, resulting in an impaired ability to exercise. Chronotropic incompetence is defined as the inability to achieve a heart rate of 100 beats/min in response to maximal exertion.

DIAGNOSIS

Suspect the sick sinus syndrome when there is syncope, near-syncope or palpitation in the presence of sinus bradycardia or an escape rhythm. Prolonged sinus arrest or sinoatrial block confirms the diagnosis.

Sometimes the standard ECG will provide diagnostic information but often ambulatory electrocardiography will be necessary.

Sinus bradycardia and short pauses during sleep are normal and are not evidence for the sick sinus syndrome. Furthermore, pauses in sinus node activity of up to 2.0 s during the daytime due to high vagal tone may be found in fit, young people.

A 24-hour tape recording in a normal subject will inevitably show sinus bradycardia during sleep and sinus tachycardia during exercise. Sometimes these are wrongly taken as evidence of the bradycardia–tachycardia syndrome!

TREATMENT

SINUS BRADYCARDIA OR ARREST

Cardiac pacing is necessary to control symptoms (see Chapter 24).

Atrial pacing, which preserves the normal sequence of cardiac chamber activation, is preferable to ventricular pacing for two reasons: ventricular pacing may result in the pacemaker syndrome and atrial systole lessens the risk of systemic embolism.

An AV sequential pacemaker is required if there is AV or bundle branch block or if at implantation, atrial pacing at 120 beats/min causes AV block.

A pacemaker that has the facility to increase heart rate in response to exercise (see Chapter 24) can markedly improve the ability to exercise in patients with chronotropic incompetence.

BRADYCARDIA–TACHYCARDIA SYNDROME

Antiarrhythmic drugs often worsen sinus node function. A pacemaker is usually necessary if drugs are needed to control tachycardias.

Tachycardias often arise during sinus bradycardia or pauses. Atrial pacing may well prevent tachyarrhythmias.

The risk of systemic embolism is high. Anticoagulation is indicated unless tachyarrhythmias can be prevented.

Main points

- The sick sinus syndrome is due to impaired sinus node function or sinoatrial conduction and may cause sinus bradycardia, sinoatrial block or sinus arrest.

- A long pause in sinus node activity without an adequate junctional or ventricular escape rhythm will cause near-syncope or syncope.

- The bradycardia–tachycardia syndrome is the association of sinus node dysfunction with episodes of atrial fibrillation, flutter or tachycardia (but not AV re-entrant tachycardia). There is a high risk of systemic embolism.

- Artificial cardiac pacing is required for control of symptoms and to prevent bradycardia if antiarrhythmic drugs are to be prescribed for the bradycardia–tachycardia syndrome.

Neurally mediated syncope

This term refers to the carotid sinus syndrome, malignant vasovagal syncope and less common syndromes such as micturition syncope, in which triggering of an autonomic nervous system reflex results in syncope due to inappropriate bradycardia and/or hypotension due to vasodilatation.

Neurally mediated syncope should be considered in patients with unexplained syncope without electrocardiographic evidence of the sick sinus syndrome or AV block.

CAROTID SINUS SYNDROME

The diagnosis of carotid sinus syndrome is made in patients who suffer from near-syncope or syncope in whom unilateral carotid sinus massage for 5–10 s causes sinus arrest or complete AV block for 3 s or more (Figure 17.1). In some patients, severe hypotension due to vasodilation (vasodepression) occurs as well as bradycardia (cardioinhibition).

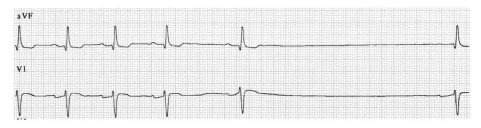

Figure 17.1 Carotid sinus syndrome. Carotid sinus massage causes 3 s sinus arrest.

In contrast to syncope caused by the sick sinus syndrome or AV block, loss of consciousness may be prolonged due to persistent hypotension; and fitting and incontinence can occur.

Cardiac pacing (see Chapter 24) will improve or abolish symptoms. However, in some patients, the vasodepressor element continues to cause symptoms in spite of pacing.

Some asymptomatic subjects, particularly among the elderly, may develop a marked bradycardia on carotid massage. Carotid sinus syndrome should only be diagnosed in patients with typical spontaneous symptoms.

MALIGNANT VASOVAGAL SYNDROME

The term 'malignant' is used to distinguish this syndrome from vasovagal syncope or faint commonly seen in young people. With the former, there are no prodromal symptoms or triggering factors, such as pain or the sight of blood.

The syndrome is characterized by recurrent, abrupt syncope, when standing or sitting (including car driving), and a positive tilt table test. Results from other usual tests performed to investigate syncope are negative. Even though asystole may occur, the syndrome is not a cause of sudden death. Frequency of recurrence of attacks is variable and unpredictable. It occurs in both young and elderly people.

Syncope is thought to result from pooling of blood in the lower extremities during standing or sitting. Reduced venous return leads to hypotension. This is detected by baroreceptors in the aortic arch and carotid arteries and leads to reflex-enhanced sympathetic nervous system activity and thus increased force of myocardial contraction. Because of reduced venous return, the left ventricle is relatively empty. Systole results in excessive stimulation of ventricular mechanoreceptors, which trigger inappropriate reflex vasodilatation and bradycardia. Reflex control of venous tone has also been shown to be abnormal. In some patients 'cardioinhibition' (i.e. bradycardia, either sinus arrest or AV block) predominates, while in others it is the 'vasodepressor' element (i.e. vasodilatation) that is the main problem.

Tilt table test

The patient is gently secured on a tilt table and rapidly tilted from the supine position to a 60 degree angle. They stay in this position, standing on a footplate, for up to 45 min. The ECG and blood pressure are continuously monitored. The test is positive if syncope results from profound bradycardia (often asystole) and/or hypotension (Figures 17.2–17.4, see pages 163–5). A positive result rarely occurs in normal subjects. Blood pressure and heart rate are rapidly restored on returning to a horizontal position (Figure 17.5, see page 166).

Isoprenaline or glyceryl trinitrate are sometimes used to increase the sensitivity of the test (i.e. more positive results are obtained) but the drugs also reduce the test's sensitivity (i.e. a positive test may occur in a person who has not experienced spontaneous reflex syncope).

It should also be appreciated that sometimes a predominantly vasodepressor response will be observed during tilt table testing and yet a cardioinhibitory response is responsible for spontaneous symptoms.

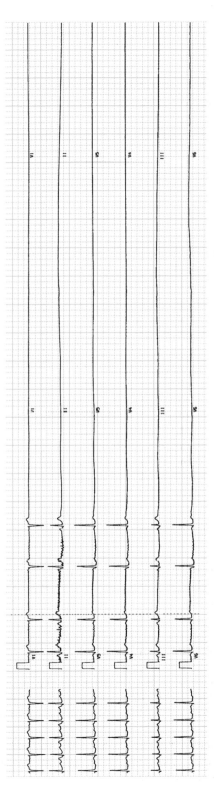

Figure 17.2 Malignant vasovagal syndrome. Asystole and then fitting developed after 3 min on a tilt table.

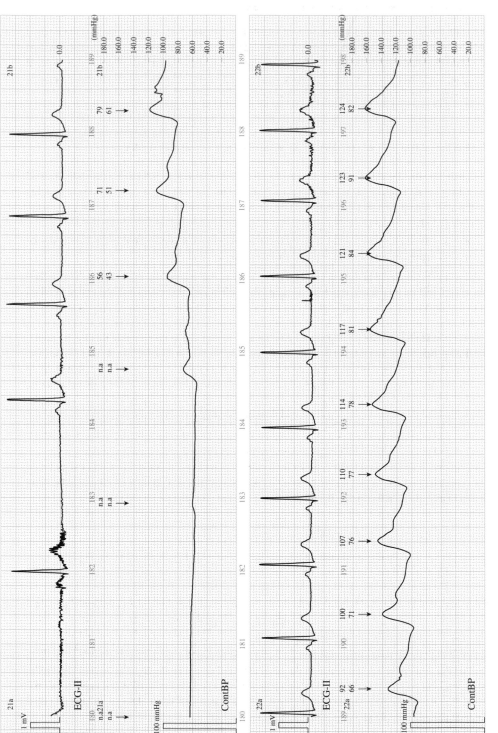

Figure 17.5 Blood pressure and heart rate rapidly restored to normal on returning to a horizontal position after profound bradycardia and hypotension during tilt table testing.

Postural orthostatic tachycardia syndrome

Tilt table testing can also be used to demonstrate another condition: the postural orthostatic tachycardia syndrome. This syndrome is characterized by an intolerance to standing due to symptoms such as palpitation, light-headedness, near-syncope and fatigue, together with a rise in heart rate by 30 beats/min or to a rate in excess of 120 beats/min without significant hypotension.

Treatment of malignant vasovagal syndrome

Patients should be advised measures to prevent venous pooling. They should avoid standing or sitting for prolonged periods and should regularly contract the muscles in their legs to aid venous return. Dehydration should also be avoided. A generous salt intake should be encouraged.

One study has shown that a programme of progressively prolonged periods of 'enforced upright posture' or 'tilt-training' can be effective.

Isometric arm muscle contraction at the first signs of an impending vasovagal attack has been shown to elevate blood pressure and to avoid syncope: the patient should extend both arms and then very forcefully push one hand against the other.

Dual-chamber cardiac pacing is indicated to treat the cardioinhibitory element of the syndrome in patients who have experienced frequent blackouts. Because pacing will not prevent the vasodepressor element of the syndrome, symptoms may continue. In general, pacing will reduce the frequency and severity of symptoms but only a minority will be rendered symptom free. A rate-drop algorithm is probably the best method of pacing for patients with the malignant vasovagal syndrome: a sudden reduction in heart rate will trigger pacing at a high rate: 90–130 beats/min. The high rate may compensate for the vasodepressor effect.

Treatment of the vasodepressor component is difficult. A number of drugs have been tried: beta-blockers, disopyramide, scopolamine skin patches, midodrine and fludrocortisone. None have been shown to be very effective.

SIMPLE FAINT

Syncope due to the malignant vasovagal syndrome must be distinguished from the 'simple' faint that is common in young people. This is triggered by a variety of 'situational factors' such as unpleasant sights (e.g. sight of blood or needles), pain, extreme emotion or stuffy rooms. Common places for fainting are churches, hospitals and restaurants. In contrast to the malignant vasovagal syndrome, where syncope is of abrupt onset, there is a history of preceding dizziness, sweating and nausea prior to loss of consciousness. Witnesses often report marked pallor. Weakness and nausea usually occur during recovery.

CAUSES OF SYNCOPE

When a patient presents with syncope it is important to bear in mind the many possible causes as listed in Table 17.1.

Table 17.1 Causes of syncope

Cardiac arrhythmias:
  sinus node disease
  atrioventricular block
  paroxysmal supraventricular tachycardia
  paroxysmal ventricular tachycardia or fibrillation,
      including hereditary long QT syndromes and the
      Brugada syndrome
Neurally mediated syncope:
  simple, common faint
  carotid sinus syndrome
  malignant vasovagal syndrome
Structural heart disease:
  aortic stenosis
  hypertrophic cardiomyopathy
  atrial myxoma
  acute myocardial ischaemia
  pulmonary embolism
Orthostatic hypotension:
  disorders of autonomic nervous syndrome: primary
      and caused by diabetes, amyloidosis
  haemorrhage
  diarrhoea
  Addison's disease
Postural orthostatic tachycardia syndrome

Main points

- Carotid sinus and malignant vasovagal syndromes are caused by abnormal autonomic nervous system reflexes and can cause syncope due to bradycardia and/or hypotension.

- The malignant vasovagal syndrome is characterized by recurrent, abrupt syncope, when sitting or standing, and a positive tilt table test.

- Tilt table testing can be used to demonstrate the cardioinhibitory and/or vasodepressor elements of the malignant vasovagal syndrome. Pacing may prevent or reduce syncope when caused by the former but will not influence symptoms due to the latter.

Arrhythmias due to myocardial infarction

Myocardial infarction causes a wide variety of arrhythmias, some of which require immediate action, whereas for others no treatment is necessary. Arrhythmias are most frequent in the early hours after infarction (Table 18.1).

Table 18.1 Incidence of arrhythmias in a series of patients within 4 hours of myocardial infarction

Ventricular fibrillation	16%
Ventricular tachycardia	4%
Ventricular ectopic beats	93%
Supraventricular arrhythmias	6%
Sinus or junctional bradycardia	34%
Second- or third-degree atrioventricular block	7%

The main sustained arrhythmias caused by myocardial infarction are ventricular fibrillation, atrial fibrillation and ventricular tachycardia. In recent years, serious cardiac arrhythmias due to acute myocardial infarction seem to be less prevalent: presumably due to the reduction in infarct size resulting from the widespread use of thrombolytic therapy and primary angioplasty.

VENTRICULAR FIBRILLATION

Ninety per cent of deaths caused by myocardial infarction are due to ventricular fibrillation. The incidence of fibrillation is highest in the first hour after the onset of chest pain and decreases progressively thereafter. Forty per cent of deaths occur within the first hour. Thus, many patients die before they can receive medical aid.

In those patients who reach hospital, however, ventricular fibrillation and other arrhythmias are sufficiently common to necessitate continuous ECG monitoring for 24–48 hours in an area where facilities for resuscitation are immediately available (i.e. a coronary care unit). Between 3 and 10 per cent of patients with acute myocardial infarction develop ventricular fibrillation while in a coronary care unit. The shorter the delay before admission, the greater the incidence of ventricular fibrillation.

Ventricular fibrillation is most often initiated by an 'R on T' ventricular ectopic beat (Figure 18.1).

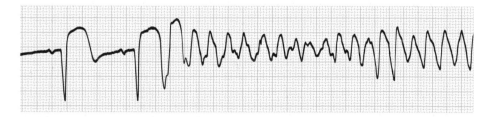

Figure 18.1 Ventricular ectopic beat initiating ventricular fibrillation.

Ventricular fibrillation can also occur late after infarction and, in patients with severe coronary artery disease without myocardial infarction it may be the first clinical manifestation of the disease.

PRIMARY AND SECONDARY VENTRICULAR FIBRILLATION

If ventricular fibrillation develops in a heart that was functioning satisfactorily during normal rhythm it is termed 'primary' fibrillation, whereas if it occurs in the context of cardiac failure or cardiogenic shock it is termed 'secondary'. Successful defibrillation is less likely in secondary ventricular fibrillation.

TREATMENT

Rarely, ventricular fibrillation is a brief event, spontaneously reverting to normal rhythm. Otherwise, without prompt treatment, irreversible cerebral and myocardial damage will quickly ensue.

Occasionally a praecordial blow is effective but usually defibrillation is necessary (see Chapter 21). On a coronary care unit, a defibrillator should be immediately available so little or no time need be spent on cardiopulmonary resuscitation.

A 200 J shock will successfully defibrillate 90 per cent of cases. If unsuccessful, a second shock at the same energy level may be effective. The energy of a further shock should be increased to 360 J. Sequential shocks, delivered by means of two defibrillators with separate pairs of electrodes, should be considered in any patient who does not defibrillate with repeated 360 J shocks. With a biphasic defibrillator the initial energy level should be 150 J.

Following restoration of normal rhythm, an infusion of lignocaine may be given to prevent further ventricular fibrillation, though there is little evidence to show that lignocaine or other antiarrhythmic drugs are effective in this situation. Lignocaine is best reserved for the few patients with recurrent fibrillation. If lignocaine fails, alternative drugs including beta-blockers and amiodarone may be effective.

VENTRICULAR FLUTTER

Ventricular flutter is a very rapid ventricular rhythm in which there are continuous changes in waveform, distinction between QRS complexes and T waves being impossible (Figure 18.2). For practical purposes, it is the same as ventricular fibrillation.

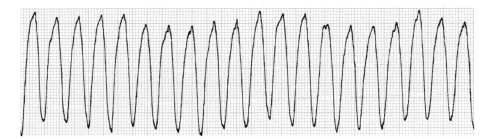

Figure 18.2 Ventricular flutter.

PREVENTION OF VENTRICULAR FIBRILLATION IN ACUTE INFARCTION

Conventional teaching used to be that ventricular ectopic beats that were frequent, multifocal, 'R on T' or repetitive – the 'warning arrhythmias' – heralded ventricular fibrillation or tachycardia (Figures 18.3–18.6). It was common practice to suppress these ectopic beats with antiarrhythmic agents.

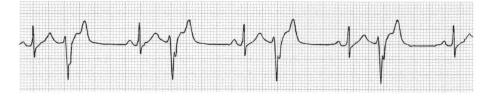

Figure 18.3 Frequent unifocal ventricular ectopic beats.

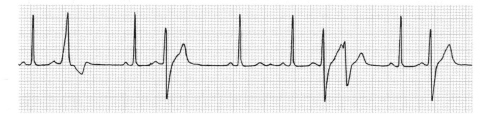

Figure 18.4 Frequent multifocal ventricular ectopic beats. The first ectopic beat arises from a different focus from that of subsequent ectopic beats. There is a couplet of ectopic beats after the fourth sinus beat.

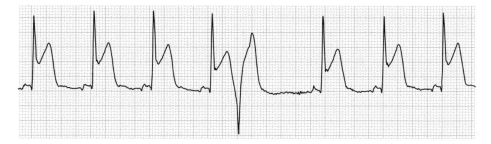

Figure 18.5 'R on T' ventricular ectopic beat.

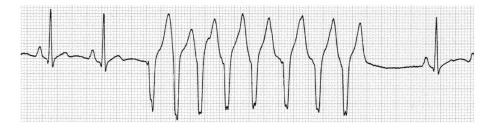

Figure 18.6 Salvo of ventricular ectopic beats.

However, analysis of continuous ECG recordings has shown that ventricular ectopic beats occur in almost all cases of acute infarction and warning arrhythmias are as common in patients who do not develop ventricular fibrillation as in those who do. Furthermore, warning arrhythmias may not precede ventricular fibrillation and when these do occur, staff in even the best coronary care units often fail to detect them.

Since 'warning arrhythmias' do not in fact warn, it has been advocated that all patients should receive lignocaine. Several recent studies in the 'thrombolytic era' have shown that lignocaine does reduce the incidence of ventricular fibrillation but mortality from acute infarction is not reduced: in fact, a trend to increased mortality has been shown. Furthermore, these studies have shown that even though thrombolysis may sometimes cause ventricular fibrillation (a reperfusion arrhythmia) the overall incidence of ventricular fibrillation is low. The current consensus is that prophylactic lignocaine is not advisable.

Oral mexiletine, a drug similar to lignocaine, has been shown to increase mortality in acute infarction.

VENTRICULAR TACHYCARDIA

Ventricular tachycardia may be self-terminating (Figure 18.6) or sustained (Figure 18.7). Ventricular tachycardia may be initiated by either 'R on T' or later ventricular ectopic beats (Figure 18.8). It may be monomorphic or polymorphic.

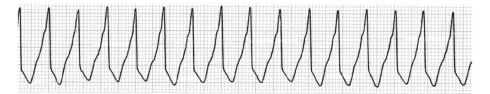

Figure 18.7 Monomorphic ventricular tachycardia.

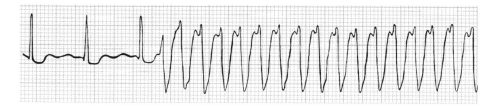

Figure 18.8 Ventricular tachycardia initiated by 'R on T' ectopic beat.

Sometimes ventricular tachycardia will result in shock or circulatory arrest. On the other hand, ventricular tachycardia may cause few or no symptoms. In myocardial infarction a regular tachycardia with broad ventricular complexes is usually ventricular in origin, even in the absence of haemodynamic deterioration.

Non-sustained ventricular tachycardia is very common in the first 24 hours following acute infarction. Only sustained ventricular tachycardia requires treatment. If cardiac arrest or shock occurs, immediate synchronized cardioversion (see Chapter 21) is necessary. Otherwise intravenous lignocaine should be given. If lignocaine fails, second-line drugs include sotalol and amiodarone. Cardioversion may be necessary if a second-line drug fails. Overdrive ventricular pacing may help in recurrent ventricular tachycardia.

REPERFUSION ARRHYTHMIAS

Reperfusion of an occluded coronary artery by thrombolysis or by balloon angioplasty can lead to a reperfusion arrhythmia: ventricular fibrillation, accelerated idioventricular rhythm (see below) or ventricular tachycardia.

LONG-TERM SIGNIFICANCE OF VENTRICULAR ARRHYTHMIAS

Ventricular tachycardia and fibrillation within the first 24 hours of myocardial infarction are unlikely to recur after that period. While most studies suggest that early ventricular arrhythmias are not related to the amount of myocardial damage and are not of long-term prognostic significance, there are studies that suggest that early primary ventricular fibrillation is associated with an impaired prognosis and may be a mark of extensive infarction (Table 18.2).

Table 18.2 Relation of ventricular tachycardia/fibrillation to infarct size and long-term treatment

	Related to infarct size	Long-term treatment
Early	Probably not	Not indicated
Late	Yes	Indicated

In contrast to early arrhythmias, ventricular tachycardia or fibrillation occurring more than 24–48 hours after infarction is likely to recur days, weeks or even months later. Long-term antiarrhythmic therapy such as sotalol or amiodarone should be prescribed. Most patients with late arrhythmias will have poor ventricular function and should therefore benefit from an angiotensin-converting enzyme inhibitor and beta-blockade.

The more extensive the myocardial damage the worse the prognosis. The incidence of late ventricular arrhythmias is related to the size of the infarct. However, ventricular arrhythmias are also an independent predictor of prognosis. That is, a patient with both extensive myocardial damage and late ventricular arrhythmias has a poorer prognosis than a patient with the same degree of myocardial damage but no arrhythmia (Table 18.2).

Frequent ventricular ectopic beats at the time of hospital discharge have been shown to indicate extensive myocardial damage and hence a poor prognosis but not an increased risk of arrhythmic death. There is no evidence that suppression of ventricular ectopic beats or non-sustained ventricular tachycardia improves prognosis. Studies have shown that class I antiarrhythmic drugs actually worsen prognosis. A study in which defibrillators were implanted within six weeks after myocardial infarction which had resulted in an ejection fraction ≤35 per cent showed no reduction in mortality.

ASSESSMENT OF EFFICACY OF LONG-TERM ANTIARRHYTHMIC THERAPY

It is important to ensure that the treatment that is chosen is effective in preventing a recurrence of the arrhythmia. It should not be assumed that an oral preparation of a drug that had restored normal rhythm when given intravenously will be effective in preventing a recurrence of arrhythmia.

If the tachyarrhythmia has been frequent then monitoring the ECG at the bedside or ambulatory electrocardiography are the best methods of assessing the efficacy of antiarrhythmic therapy. Sometimes, where control has been difficult to achieve it may be necessary to accept ventricular extrasystoles and even short runs of ventricular tachycardia, provided the rate during tachycardia is significantly slower than before treatment.

If the arrhythmia has been an infrequent event then it is unlikely that ECG monitoring will reflect antiarrhythmic control. Exercise ECG testing and electrophysiological testing may be helpful.

ACCELERATED IDIOVENTRICULAR RHYTHM

This is also referred to as idioventricular tachycardia or 'slow' ventricular tachycardia. It is benign and treatment is not necessary (Figure 18.9).

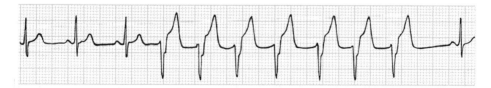

Figure 18.9 Accelerated idioventricular rhythm.

SUPRAVENTRICULAR TACHYCARDIAS

AV junctional re-entrant tachycardia can only occur if there is an additional AV connection, either bypassing or within the AV node (see Chapter 5). Thus, it is highly unlikely to occur for the first time during acute myocardial infarction. When supraventricular tachycardia is diagnosed in a patient with acute infarction, the correct diagnosis is usually atrial fibrillation, atrial flutter or erroneously ventricular tachycardia.

ATRIAL FIBRILLATION

In atrial fibrillation, the resultant rapid ventricular rate and reduction in cardiac output from loss of atrial systole can sometimes cause severe hypotension (Figure 18.10). If shock occurs, immediate cardioversion may be necessary. Otherwise, the ventricular rate should be lowered by intravenous verapamil. If contraindicated, a beta-blocker or amiodarone are alternatives. Spontaneous reversion to sinus rhythm is common.

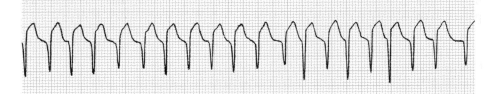

Figure 18.10 Atrial fibrillation with rapid ventricular rate in anterior infarction (lead V3).

Atrial fibrillation is usually associated with extensive myocardial damage or older patients and hence a poor prognosis. Frequent atrial ectopic beats often herald atrial fibrillation.

SINUS AND JUNCTIONAL BRADYCARDIAS

Sinus and junctional bradycardias are common, particularly in inferior infarction (Figures 18.11 and 18.12). If uncomplicated, no treatment is required.

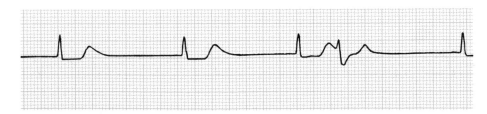

Figure 18.11 Junctional bradycardia. The fourth beat is an 'R on T' ventricular ectopic.

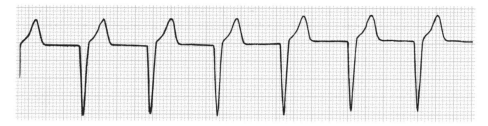

Figure 18.12 Junctional escape rhythm as a result of sinus bradycardia in anterior infarction (lead V4).

Bradycardia may be beneficial in acute infarction, in that myocardial oxygen consumption is related to heart rate and low oxygen consumption might limit infarct size.

However, if bradycardia causes hypotension (systolic blood pressure less than 90 mmHg), mental confusion, oliguria, cold peripheries or ventricular arrhythmias, intravenous atropine (initially 0.3–0.6 mg) should be given. Temporary cardiac pacing is occasionally necessary and is preferable to frequent doses of atropine.

ATRIOVENTRICULAR BLOCK

The management and prognosis of AV block in inferior and anterior infarction differ markedly.

INFERIOR INFARCTION

In inferior infarction, AV block is common and is often due to ischaemia of the AV node. Recovery of AV node function usually occurs within a few hours or days, although sometimes it takes up to three weeks. Permanent AV node damage is exceptional. The prognosis for inferior infarction is widely accepted as good, but some studies do indicate increased in-hospital mortality.

First-degree and Mobitz type I second-degree (Wenckebach) AV block require no action other than stopping drugs that may worsen AV nodal conduction (e.g. verapamil, diltiazem, beta-blockers) (Figures 18.13 and 18.14).

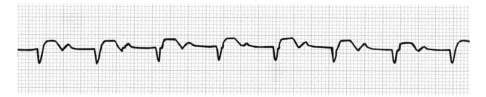

Figure 18.13 First-degree atrioventricular block (lead aVF).

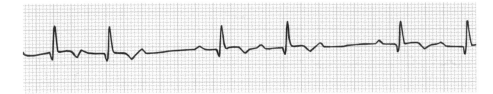

Figure 18.14 Wenckebach atrioventricular block in inferior infarction (lead aVF).

If complete AV block develops, subsidiary pacemakers in the bundle of His will control the ventricular rate (Figure 18.15). These pacemakers usually discharge at an adequate rate. However, sometimes the ventricular rate does fall very low (less than 40 beats/min), when syncope, hypotension, mental confusion, oliguria or ventricular arrhythmia may occur. In these circumstances, temporary pacing is necessary. There is no place for steroids or catecholamines although in the first 6 hours atropine may be effective.

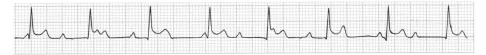

Figure 18.15 Inferior infarction complicated by complete atrioventricular block (lead II).

AV block will almost always resolve within three weeks of infarction, and it is highly unlikely that long-term cardiac pacing will be necessary.

ANTERIOR INFARCTION

In anterior infarction, it is the bundle branches rather than the AV node which are usually the site of ischaemic damage. AV block is more serious than in inferior infarction for two reasons. First, subsidiary pacemakers that arise below the level of the block in the distal specialized conducting system tend to be slower and less reliable. Thus circulatory disturbances due to a low ventricular rate are common and ventricular standstill often occurs. Second, an extensive area of infarction is necessary to affect both bundle branches. Prognosis after myocardial infarction is related to the extent of infarction. Hence it is poor in patients with anterior infarction complicated by AV block.

Evidence of bilateral bundle branch damage (alternating right and left bundle branch block, or right bundle branch block with left anterior or posterior hemiblock) usually precedes the onset of second-degree (Mobitz type II) or complete AV block (Figures 18.16–18.19). The chance of bilateral bundle branch damage progressing to second-degree or complete heart block is approximately 30 per cent. The first manifestation of these higher degrees of block may be ventricular standstill (Figure 18.20). Temporary transvenous pacing should be considered if there is evidence of

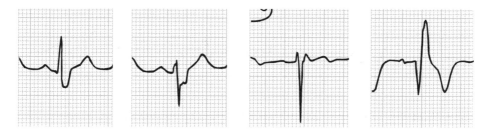

Figure 18.16 Left anterior fascicular and right bundle branch block in anterior infarction (leads I, II, III and V1).

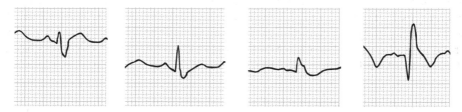

Figure 18.17 Left posterior fascicular and right bundle branch block in anterior infarction (leads I, II, III and V1).

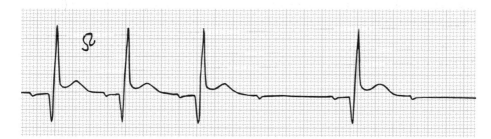

Figure 18.18 Intermittent Mobitz type II atrioventricular block in a patient with bifascicular block due to anterior infarction (lead V2).

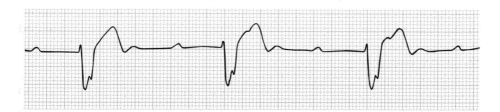

Figure 18.19 Complete atrioventricular block in anterior infarction.

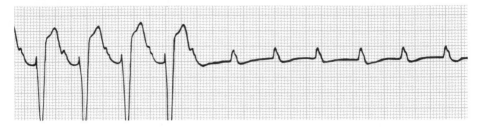

Figure 18.20 Ventricular asystole due to complete atrioventricular block in a patient with bifascicular block due to anterior infarction.

bilateral bundle branch damage, provided an experienced operator is available, otherwise the risks of temporary pacing will outweigh the advantages of pacing.

Second- and third-degree AV block due to anterior infarction are always indications for temporary pacing. Sinus rhythm often returns after a few days, but in some patients AV block will persist and may necessitate long-term pacing.

Mortality is high in the first three weeks after anterior infarction complicated by AV block, and long-term pacing should not be undertaken until the patient has survived this period.

If sinus rhythm does return, bifascicular block often persists. Complete AV block may recur in the weeks and months after acute infarction, but there is no conclusive evidence to show that implantation of a pacemaker will improve prognosis. This is because the extensive myocardial damage associated with this situation will often lead to ventricular fibrillation or heart failure.

ATRIOVENTRICULAR DISSOCIATION

In contrast to complete AV block, in AV dissociation the atrial rate is lower than the ventricular rate and no treatment is necessary.

TREATMENTS TO IMPROVE PROGNOSIS

A number of treatments have been shown to improve prognosis following myocardial infarction whether by arrhythmia reduction or other means and all should be instituted unless there is a contraindication (Table 18.3).

Table 18.3 Treatments to improve prognosis after myocardial infarction

Beta-blocker
Angiotensin-converting enzyme inhibitor or angiotensin II receptor blocker
Aspirin and clopidogrel
Statins
Eplerenone (in patients with poor ventricular function)
Smoking cessation

Main points

- Ventricular fibrillation occurs during the first hour of acute myocardial infarction in more than 30 per cent of patients; the incidence falls progressively thereafter.

- Frequent, 'R on T' and other 'warning arrhythmias' are common in acute infarction and are not predictive of ventricular fibrillation. Antiarrhythmic drugs are not indicated.

- Immediate defibrillation should be carried out if ventricular fibrillation occurs.

- Ventricular fibrillation or other major ventricular arrhythmia during the first 24 hours of infarction is not an indication for long-term antiarrhythmic therapy, whereas therapy should be given if these arrhythmias occur after 24 hours.

- Atrial fibrillation, and ventricular arrhythmias arising 24 hours or more after acute infarction, are usually associated with extensive myocardial damage and hence an impaired prognosis.

- Sinus and junctional bradycardia and complete AV block due to inferior infarction do not require treatment unless there are symptoms, marked hypotension, other signs of shock or ventricular arrhythmias. AV block due to acute inferior infarction may persist for up to three weeks and is not an indication for permanent pacemaker implantation.

- Bilateral bundle branch damage or higher degrees of AV block in anterior infarction imply extensive myocardial damage and a poor prognosis.

Antiarrhythmic drugs

LIMITATIONS

Drugs are widely used in the treatment of arrhythmias but their limitations, as summarized in Table 19.1, should be appreciated.

Antiarrhythmic drugs are of limited effectiveness. In other words, a drug prescribed in the correct dose for an appropriate indication may fail to work.

With many antiarrhythmic drugs it is difficult to maintain consistently therapeutic drug levels.

Table 19.1 Limitations of antiarrhythmic drugs

Limited efficacy
Difficulty in maintaining therapeutic drug levels
Selection of an effective drug is often based on trial and error
Unwanted effects are common

Considerable insight into the mode of action of antiarrhythmic drugs has been gained, but selection for an individual patient of a drug that is both effective and well tolerated is often a process of trial and error.

Unwanted effects often occur. The most common are hypotension, heart failure, impairment of the specialized cardiac conducting tissues and symptoms from the gastrointestinal and central nervous systems.

PROARRHYTHMIC EFFECT

Many antiarrhythmic drugs, particularly those in class IC (see below), can sometimes worsen or cause arrhythmias, sometimes with fatal consequences. Patients with poor ventricular function are at greatest risk, while the risk is low in those with structurally normal hearts.

CHOICE OF TREATMENT

Drugs are only one form of treatment and in some situations other approaches such as vagal stimulation, cardioversion, artificial pacing, catheter ablation or surgery may be more appropriate.

A number of factors influence the choice of treatment: the type of arrhythmia, the urgency of the situation, the need for short- or long-term therapy, and the presence of impaired myocardial performance, sinus node dysfunction or abnormal AV conduction.

It is important to consider whether an antiarrhythmic drug is being given to terminate an arrhythmia, to prevent its recurrence or to slow the heart rate during the arrhythmia. In some situations drugs are given to control symptoms, whereas in others the purpose may be to prevent dangerous arrhythmias.

MODES OF ACTION

The modes of action of antiarrhythmic drugs can be classified according to their effects in the intact heart (clinical classification) or according to their effects at cellular level as established by *in vitro* studies (action potential classification). The latter classification is widely referred to though it is of limited practical value.

CLINICAL CLASSIFICATION

In this classification drugs are divided, according to their main site or sites of action in the intact heart, into three groups: those that act on the AV node, those that act on the ventricles, and those that act on the atria, ventricles and accessory AV pathways (Table 19.2).

Table 19.2 Classification of antiarrhythmic drugs according to principal site(s) of action in intact heart

Site of action	Examples
AV node	Verapamil, diltiazem, adenosine, digoxin, beta-blockers
Ventricles	Lignocaine, mexiletine
Atria, ventricles and accessory atrioventricular pathways	Quinidine, disopyramide, amiodarone, flecainide, procainamide, sotalol, propafenone

The first group consists of drugs whose chief action is to slow conduction in the AV node. These drugs are therefore useful in the treatment of arrhythmias of supraventricular origin but are of little use in the treatment of ventricular arrhythmias. In the second group, there are drugs that work mainly in ventricular arrhythmias. The third group comprises drugs that act on the atria, ventricles and, in cases of the Wolff–Parkinson–White syndrome, accessory AV pathways. Thus, they may be effective in both supraventricular and ventricular arrhythmias.

ACTION POTENTIAL CLASSIFICATION

In this classification, drugs are divided into four main classes depending upon their electrophysiological effects at cellular level (Table 19.3).

Table 19.3 Classification of antiarrhythmic drugs according to electrophysiological effects

I	II	III	IV
A. Quinidine Procainamide Disopyramide	Beta-blockers Bretylium	Amiodarone Sotalol Dofetilide Bretylium	Verapamil Diltiazem
B. Lignocaine Mexiletine			
C. Flecainide Propafenone			

Class I drugs impede the transport of sodium across the cell membrane during the initiation of cellular activation and thereby reduce the rate of rise of the action potential (phase 0). They are subdivided into classes A, B and C according to their effect on the duration of the action potential (which is reflected in the surface ECG by the QT interval).

IA drugs increase the duration of the action potential, IB drugs shorten it and IC drugs have little effect. The antiarrhythmic action of IB drugs is confined to the ventricles, whereas IA and IC drugs affect both atria and ventricles. IA and particularly IC drugs slow intraventricular conduction.

Class II drugs interfere with the effects of the sympathetic nervous system on the heart. They do not affect the action potential of most myocardial cells but do reduce the slope of spontaneous depolarization (phase 4) of cells with pacemaker activity and thus the rate of pacemaker discharge.

Class III drugs prolong the duration of the action potential and hence the length of the refractory period and the QT interval, but do not slow phase 0.

Class IV drugs antagonize the transport of calcium across the cell membrane which follows the inward flux of sodium during cellular activation. Cells in the AV and sinus nodes are particularly susceptible. It should be noted that the dihydropyridine calcium channel blockers (e.g. nifedipine and amlodipine) do not have an antiarrhythmic action.

As can be seen from Table 19.3, the majority of drugs are in class I: drugs within this class differ significantly in their clinical effects. Some drugs have more than one class of action; amiodarone has class I, II and IV actions as well as its main class III effect! Furthermore, some drugs (e.g. digoxin and adenosine) cannot be classified.

NOTES ON INDIVIDUAL DRUGS

LIGNOCAINE

Lignocaine is the first-line drug for ventricular arrhythmias but is ineffective in supraventricular arrhythmias. The drug is a vasoconstrictor and, unlike many drugs, rarely causes hypotension or heart failure.

A 100 mg bolus given intravenously over 2 min will often be successful. If not, a further bolus (50–75 mg) should be given after 5 min.

Several concentrations of lignocaine are available. Disasters have occurred because the wrong concentration has been used. Remember that 10 mL 1 per cent lignocaine contains 100 mg.

Lignocaine is often used for short-term prevention of ventricular arrhythmias. The therapeutic effect of lignocaine is closely related to plasma levels, which fall rapidly after a bolus injection. Thus it is necessary to give a continuous infusion immediately after the bolus. There is, however, no point in giving a continuous infusion if the bolus has failed to work or, since lignocaine cannot be administered by mouth, if long-term prophylaxis is required.

It can be difficult to maintain therapeutic levels of lignocaine. With subtherapeutic levels, the patient is at risk from arrhythmias while toxic levels may cause symptoms related to the central nervous system, including light-headedness, confusion, twitching, paraesthesiae and epileptic fits. With conventional infusion rates (1–4 mg/min) subtherapeutic levels commonly occur in the first hour or two after the infusion is commenced.

Lignocaine is metabolized by the liver: where there is liver disease or where hepatic blood flow is reduced by heart failure or by shock, dosages should be halved to avoid toxicity. Hypokalaemia may impair lignocaine's efficacy.

MEXILETINE

Mexiletine is similar to lignocaine in its therapeutic and haemodynamic actions but it can be given by mouth as well as intravenously. There is a narrow margin between therapeutic and toxic effects; and symptoms such as nausea, vomiting, confusion, tremor, ataxia, as well as bradycardia and hypotension, are not uncommon.

Intravenously, the drug is given in a dose of 100–250 mg over 5–10 min, followed by 250 mg over 1hour and a further 250 mg over 2hours. The infusion can then be continued at 0.5–1.0 mg/min or oral therapy started. The oral dose is 200–300 mg 8-hourly. If the patient has not received a prior infusion, a loading dose of 400 mg can be given. Up to one-third of patients experience unwanted effects with long-term administration. The drug is mainly metabolized by the liver and doses should be reduced if there is hepatic disease or heart failure. Approximately 10 per cent is excreted unchanged in the urine. Renal excretion is inhibited by alkaline urine but this is not a problem in practice.

The author does not recall the oral preparation ever having been effective when given alone! Occasionally, it has been found to be effective in combination with amiodarone when the latter has not achieved control of ventricular tachycardia.

QUINIDINE

Quinidine can cause torsade de pointes tachycardia. Several surveys have shown that it increases mortality, even in patients with non-dangerous arrhythmias. There are safer alternative drugs for many arrhythmias.

However, recently there have been reports about the value of this drug in treating the 'arrhythmia storms' that may occur in the Brugada syndrome and in the treatment of the rare short QT syndrome.

DISOPYRAMIDE

Disopyramide has been widely used for both supraventricular and ventricular arrhythmias. However, it is only moderately effective and does have significant unwanted effects.

The intravenous dose is 1.5–2.0 mg/kg up to a maximum of 150 mg, given over no less than 5 min. The injection should be stopped if the arrhythmia is terminated. Therapy can be continued by intravenous infusion at 20–30 mg/h up to a maximum of 800 mg daily or the patient can be transferred to oral therapy. The oral dose is 300–800 mg daily in three or four divided doses. If necessary, a loading dose of 300 mg can be given.

Given intravenously, the drug is more likely to cause hypotension and heart failure than lignocaine and related drugs and its use can be disastrous if the recommended minimum period of administration is ignored.

Orally, the drug's side-effects are mainly related to its anticholinergic (atropine-like) action, which often causes a dry mouth, blurred vision, urinary hesitancy or retention and, by enhancing AV nodal conduction, an increase in the ventricular response to atrial flutter and fibrillation. The drug may precipitate heart failure in patients with impaired myocardial function. It may occasionally induce torsade de pointes tachycardia and should not be given to patients with QT interval prolongation. Disopyramide may worsen impaired sinus node function and is contraindicated in the sick sinus syndrome. The drug is partially excreted by the kidneys and dosage should be reduced in renal disease.

PROCAINAMIDE

Procainamide has similar antiarrhythmic properties to quinidine. It is not widely used and is now never used by the author. It has a short half-life, necessitating very frequent dosage when given by mouth. Even with a slow-release preparation, 8-hourly administration is necessary. Furthermore, unwanted effects such as systemic lupus syndrome, gastrointestinal symptoms, hypotension and agranulocytosis make it unsuitable for long-term use. Impaired renal function and a slow acetylator status both reduce procainamide requirements. N-Acetyl-procainamide, a metabolite of procainamide, has been shown to have a longer duration of action and not to cause systemic lupus.

FLECAINIDE

Flecainide is a potent drug which can be given both orally and parenterally. Its indications include paroxysmal atrial fibrillation, ventricular arrhythmias and pre-excitation syndromes. It is very effective at suppressing ventricular ectopic beats but somewhat less so in the treatment of ventricular tachycardia.

It has a long half-life of approximately 16 hours which facilitates twice daily oral administration. The usual dosage is 100 mg twice daily. If side-effects occur then reduction of the daily dosage by as little as 50 mg can help. Occasionally, daily dosages up to 300 mg are required.

The intravenous dose is 1–2 mg/kg body weight over not less than 10 min; it should be given more slowly in patients with impaired ventricular function. Flecainide is both metabolized by the liver and excreted by the kidney.

The drug has a narrow therapeutic range (i.e. it can be difficult to achieve a therapeutic action without unwanted effects). High levels can cause visual disturbance, particularly on rotating the head, and light-headedness and nausea. Marked prolongation of the QRS complex indicates the blood level may be too high. The drug has been shown to increase the threshold of pacemaker stimuli.

The drug does have an important negative inotropic action and should be avoided in patients in heart failure or with extensive myocardial damage. It can be proarrhythmic, particularly in patients with a history of sustained ventricular tachycardia and/or poor ventricular function.

In a major study of patients with ventricular extrasystoles following myocardial infarction, flecainide was found to increase mortality. It is now generally agreed that the drug should not be given to patients known to have coronary artery disease.

Flecainide causes slight prolongation of the QRS complex and hence the QT interval: it does not prolong the JT component of the QT interval as does quinidine and disopyramide.

Flecainide is effective and safe when used to prevent atrial fibrillation and AV re-entrant tachycardias in patients with structurally normal hearts. It is also indicated in patients with highly symptomatic idiopathic ventricular extrasystoles. It should be avoided in patients with myocardial damage.

Occasionally, like other class I drugs, flecainide can worsen atrial arrhythmias: either converting atrial fibrillation to flutter, or increasing the ventricular rate during atrial flutter (Figure 19.1).

PROPAFENONE

This drug has both IC and mild beta-blocking properties and has been shown to be effective in both supraventricular and ventricular arrhythmias. It can be proarrhythmic and should not be given to patients with impaired ventricular function. In the author's experience, non-cardiac unwanted effects are common.

AMIODARONE

Amiodarone has several advantages over other drugs. It is highly effective in both supraventricular and ventricular rhythm disorders: even in arrhythmias refractory to other drugs there is a 70 per cent success rate. It has a remarkably long half-life (20–100 days), so that the drug need only be given once daily or even less frequently. It does not significantly impair ventricular performance and can be given to patients in heart failure.

Though it is effective in the treatment of ventricular arrhythmias, recent studies have clearly shown that it has no role in 'primary prevention' in patients with poor ventricular function (i.e. it does not reduce the incidence of fatal ventricular arrhythmias in these patients).

Amiodarone has important unwanted effects that dictate the long-term use of amiodarone being confined to patients with arrhythmias that are dangerous or resistant to other drugs, or where the risk of side-effects is not a major consideration because the patient's prognosis is poor (e.g. in the elderly and those with severe myocardial damage).

Administration

The drug has a delayed onset of action. When given by mouth, it usually takes 3–7 days before it takes effect and it may take 50 days to achieve its maximal action.

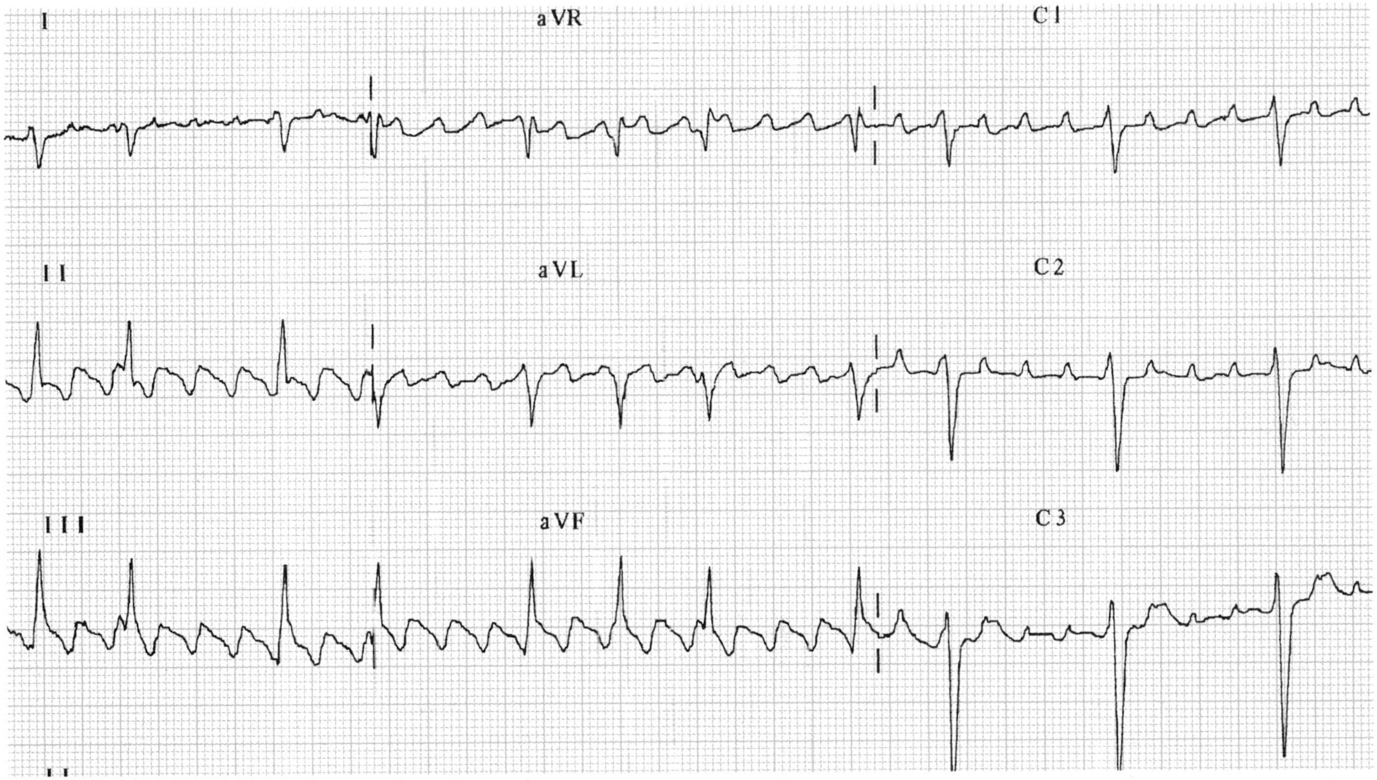

Figure 19.1 (a) Patient with atrial futter with 2:1 atrioventricular conduction.

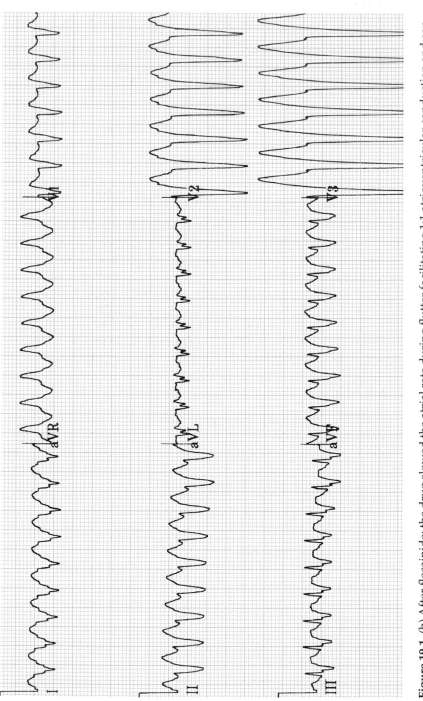

Figure 19.1 (b) After flecainide: the drug slowed the atrial rate during flutter facilitating 1:1 atrioventricular conduction and consequently a marked increase in ventricular rate.

If necessary, delay can be minimized by giving large doses (e.g. 1200 mg) daily for one or two weeks. The dose can then be reduced to 400 mg daily.

Once the arrhythmia is controlled, it is recommended that the dose be progressively reduced until the lowest effective dose is found. The usual maintenance dose is 200–400 mg daily. In a few patients, a dose as small as 200 mg on alternate days will suffice. In the author's experience, arrhythmias often recur if the dose in adults is reduced below 300 mg daily. With dangerous arrhythmias where a recurrence cannot be risked, it is best not to reduce the dose below 400 mg daily: above 400 mg daily there is a marked increase in unwanted effects.

The drug is metabolized by the liver. It is not excreted by the kidneys. The main metabolite is desethylamiodarone, which may itself have an antiarrhythmic action. Very high concentrations of amiodarone and its metabolite are achieved in the lungs, heart, liver and adipose tissue.

Intravenous administration will lead to an earlier effect than oral therapy, but unlike most drugs, an immediate antiarrhythmic effect does not often occur: an effect is usually seen within 1–24 hours. When an arrhythmia has been difficult to control, it is often worth resorting to intravenous amiodarone in spite of possible delay in action rather than to try further drugs which are less potent and which often cause unwanted effects.

The recommended intravenous dosage is 5 mg/kg body weight over 30 min to 1 hour followed by 15 mg/kg over 24 hours. In an emergency, the initial infusion can be given more rapidly but its vasodilator action may cause marked hypotension. It is important to give the drug via a central venous line to avoid phlebitis. If this is not possible, frequent changes of peripheral infusion site will often suffice.

Unwanted effects

Short-term treatment with intravenous amiodarone is unlikely to cause side-effects although a few cases of hepatitis associated with the drug have been described.

Longer term oral therapy is associated with a high incidence of side-effects (Table 19.4).

Table 19.4 Amiodarone: main unwanted effects

Dermatological: photosensitivity and blue–grey pigmentation
Corneal microdeposits
Thyroid dysfunction: hyperthyroidism and hypothyroidism
Pulmonary alveolitis
Hepatitis
Neuropathy
Myopathy
Sleep disturbance: insomnia, vivid dreams, and nightmares
Tremor
Alopecia
Torsade de pointes tachycardia
Warfarin potentiation

Skin photosensitivity to UVA radiation affects two-thirds of patients. Though only a minority experience severe photosensitivity, all patients should be warned about the possibility. If necessary, protective clothing, avoidance of prolonged sunlight and barrier creams containing zinc oxide may be recommended. Severe photosensitivity is the commonest reason for stopping the drug. Symptoms may persist for over a year afterwards. There appears to be no relation between skin type or dosage and this unwanted effect.

After prolonged usage a minority develop marked blue–grey pigmentation of the skin, particularly the nose and forehead. This pigmentation will persist for many years after amiodarone is stopped.

Corneal microdeposits occur in virtually all patients but permanent damage does not occur. The microdeposits disappear if the drug is stopped and are a useful sign of compliance. There have been a few reports of a possible association between the drug and optic neuropathy.

Amiodarone contains large amounts of iodine and causes moderate elevation of both serum thyroxine and reverse tri-iodothyronine, and depression of serum tri-iodothyronine. Thyroid stimulating hormone (TSH) can be depressed. These changes are compatible with normal thyroid function when on amiodarone. However, amiodarone can cause both hypothyroidism and hyperthyroidism. Up to 15 per cent of patients can be affected.

Hyperthyroidism can result from activation of pre-existing subclinical thyroid disease which results in increased thyroid hormone synthesis, or from thyroiditis developing in a previously normal thyroid gland and thus increased hormone release. If hyperthyroidism occurs, the patient will often become unwell with weight loss and other signs of thyroid overactivity. Previously controlled arrhythmia may recur. *Both* serum thyroxine and tri-iodothyronine will be increased. Hyperthyroidism may be very severe and sudden in its onset. It *may develop many months after amiodarone has been stopped.* There should always be a high index of suspicion of hyperthyroidism in a patient who is taking or who has taken amiodarone. Amiodarone should, if possible, be stopped. Large doses of carbimazole may be required. In severe cases short-term steroid therapy should be given. Referral to an endocrinologist is advisable. Thyroiditis may be self-limiting and there are reports of reintroduction of amiodarone without further hyperthyroidism.

If hypothyroidism occurs, serum thyroxine will be low and TSH will be elevated. Sometimes there will be no clinical signs of hypothyroidism. Thyroid hormone replacement is indicated. It is not essential to stop amiodarone.

Patients receiving long-term amiodarone should have thyroid tests 6–12 monthly.

Testicular dysfunction is another endocrine problem that may occasionally occur.

Other serious side-effects include pulmonary alveolitis, hepatitis, neuropathy and myopathy. Pulmonary alveolitis is the most common of these problems. It usually presents with dyspnoea, which may be severe, and widespread shadowing in the lung fields which can be mistaken for pulmonary oedema. Amiodarone should be stopped and short-term therapy with steroids given. Sometimes several major unwanted effects occur together. A reduction in total diffusing capacity without clinical manifestations is common.

Usually, but not invariably, serious side-effects are associated with higher dosages of amiodarone.

Other unwanted effects include nausea, rash, alopecia, tremor, insomnia and nightmares, which can be very vivid.

The drug's class III action results in QT prolongation, often with prominent U waves. There are a few reports of the drug causing torsade de pointes tachycardia. The drug commonly causes sinus bradycardia.

It is important to note that the drug potentiates oral anticoagulants: usually halving the required dosage. Amiodarone increases blood levels of digoxin, quinidine, verapamil, flecainide and ciclosporin.

With many arrhythmias, the major advantages of amiodarone – its efficacy, absence of important negative inotropic action and long duration of action – are outweighed by the formidable list of side-effects. However, most of the side-effects are reversible and the risk of them should not be a contraindication in patients with life-threatening arrhythmias, a short life expectancy or in whom other antiarrhythmic measures have failed.

DRONEDARONE

Dronedarone is a derivative of amiodarone that is currently being evaluated. It has similar electrophysiological actions to amiodarone, including its class III effect. Unlike amiodarone, there is no iodine radical and it appears to be free of amiodarone's thyroid, pulmonary, hepatic and dermatological unwanted effects. It has a shorter duration of action than amiodarone with a half-life of 1–2 days. Typical dosage is 400 mg twice daily. It does not have a significant proarrhythmic effect.

It has been shown to be moderately effective in preventing recurrences of atrial fibrillation. It can also slow the ventricular rate during atrial fibrillation. Its role in treating other arrhythmias has not yet been explored nor has its efficacy been compared with amiodarone.

DOFETILIDE

Dofetilide is new class III antiarrhythmic drug that has been shown to be moderately successful in terminating and preventing atrial fibrillation and flutter. It does not have a negative inotropic effect.

Like amiodarone, it prolongs the QT interval. It causes torsade de pointes tachycardia in approximately 3 per cent of patients. In spite of its proarrhythmic action, the drug was shown not to increase mortality in a large group of patients with heart failure. Torsade de pointes usually (but not always) occurs within the first few days of therapy and in-hospital ECG monitoring and serial QTc measurements for at least three days are essential.

Orally, the usual dose is 500 mg twice daily but dosage should be reduced if there is renal impairment. If the QT interval prolongs by more than 15 per cent after the first dose, subsequent doses should be halved. The drug should be stopped if the QTc exceeds 500 ms.

The drug should not be given to patients who have a prolonged QT interval or who are receiving verapamil, cimetidine, ketaconazole, timethoprim or prochlorperazine. A number of drugs, including amiodarone, diltiazem, metformin and amiloride, and grapefruit juice may increase blood levels.

ADENOSINE

Adenosine is a potent blocker of AV nodal conduction. It has an extremely short duration of action: 20–30 s. It is very effective in terminating supraventricular tachycardia due to an AV re-entrant mechanism (Figure 19.2) and will transiently slow or interrupt the ventricular response to atrial fibrillation and flutter, making the respective 'f' or 'F' waves more easily identifiable (Figure 19.3). It will terminate some atrial tachycardias (Figure 19.4). Because of its very short duration of action and its safety, it is the drug of choice for the termination of AV and AV nodal re-entrant tachycardias.

A positive response to adenosine points strongly towards a supraventricular origin to the tachycardia. However, a minority of supraventricular tachycardias will not respond to adenosine, perhaps because a dose in excess of the recommended upper limit is required, and the drug will terminate right ventricular outflow tract tachycardia. Thus response or lack of response to adenosine is a useful pointer towards the origin of a tachycardia but cannot be taken as an absolutely reliable guide.

Most patients will experience chest tightness, dyspnoea and flushing but the symptoms last less than 60 s. There may be complete AV block for a few seconds following termination of the tachycardia. The drug does not have a negative inotropic action. It is a safe drug to give except perhaps to patients with asthma, in whom there is a possibility of bronchospasm. The drug is antagonized by aminophylline and potentiated by dipyridamole. Adenosine does cause sinus bradycardia and may briefly worsen sinus node function in patients with the sick sinus syndrome.

It should be given as a rapid (2.0 s) intravenous bolus, followed by a flush of saline. The initial dose in adults and in children is 3 mg and 0.05 mg/kg, respectively. If ineffective, further dosages of 6 mg (0.10 mg/kg) and, if necessary, 12 mg (0.25 mg/kg) can be given after 1.0 min intervals.

Adenosine abuse

Adenosine is often used in a 'knee-jerk' response to a broad complex tachycardia in patients with known myocardial infarction or cardiomyopathy. Ventricular tachycardia is highly likely and it is pointless to use adenosine in these situations unless there is a very strong suspicion that the rhythm is atrial flutter or tachycardia with aberration, in which case the drug is being used for diagnostic purposes.

The drug is also commonly given to patients who present with atrial fibrillation. Even if the QRS complexes are broad, the diagnosis will be clear from the totally irregular ventricular rhythm. All adenosine will achieve is slowing of the ventricular response for a few seconds which is clearly futile! (Figure 19.5).

VERAPAMIL

Intravenous verapamil (5–10 mg over 30–60 s) quickly and effectively slows AV nodal conduction. It will terminate AV re-entrant junctional tachycardia and will promptly slow the ventricular response to atrial fibrillation and flutter.

Orally, verapamil is less effective in the treatment of AV junctional re-entrant tachycardias but will often control the ventricular response to atrial fibrillation.

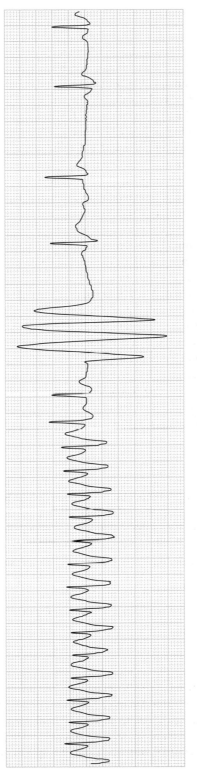

Figure 19.2 Atrioventricular junctional re-entrant tachycardia with rate-related right bundle branch block. Adenosine slows the rate slightly, facilitating normal intraventricular conduction for two cycles and then terminates the arrhythmia. After termination, as often occurs, there is a triplet of ventricular ectopic beats and a brief period of atrioventricular block.

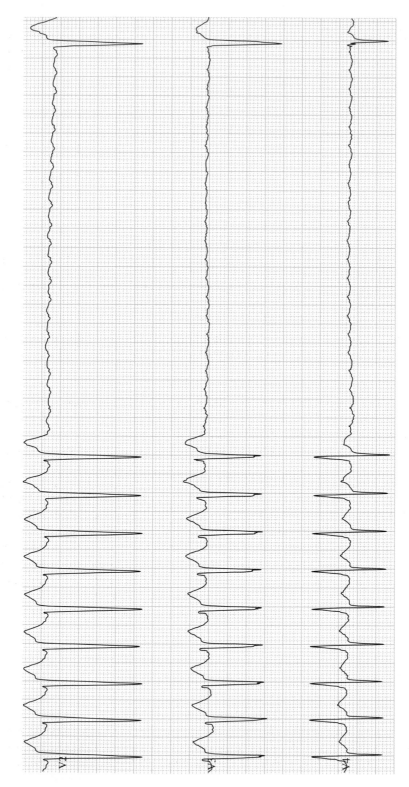

Figure 19.3 Adenosine briefly interrupts atrioventricular nodal conduction, demonstrating atrial flutter.

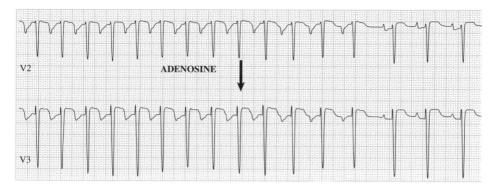

Figure 19.4 Adenosine terminates atrial tachycardia with 1:1 atrioventricular conduction.

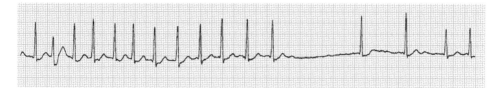

Figure 19.5 Adenosine abuse. The rhythm is totally irregular and clearly due to atrial fibrillation. The drug leads to a short pause in ventricular activity. So what!

Because much of each dose is metabolized by the liver, large doses (120–360 mg daily), preferably given in a controlled release preparation, are required.

The drug is recognized to be able to terminate right ventricular outflow tract tachycardia and fascicular tachycardia. However, when given orally it does not appear to be effective in preventing the onset of these arrhythmias.

Intravenous verapamil is contraindicated if the patient has received an intravenous or oral beta-blocker. Profound bradycardia or hypotension can result and may be fatal. Sometimes, the combination of oral verapamil and an oral beta-blocker will cause profound sinus or junctional bradycardia. Verapamil is contraindicated in patients with impaired sinus or AV node function or digoxin toxicity unless a ventricular pacing wire is *in situ* because of its depressant effects on the sinus and AV nodes.

Verapamil does have a significant negative inotropic effect and may cause hypotension in patients with very poor myocardial function. Two studies report that administration of intravenous calcium chloride immediately prior to intravenous verapamil prevents hypotension.

DILTIAZEM

The actions of diltiazem are similar to those of verapamil.

Orally, a controlled release preparation should be used; the dosage being 200–300 mg daily. Intravenously, the dosage is 20 mg as a bolus, repeated after 15 min if necessary. A maintenance infusion of 5–15 mg hourly can be given if required.

BETA-ADRENOCEPTOR ANTAGONISTS

Beta-blockers have antiarrhythmic properties by virtue of their principal action – antagonizing the effects of catecholamines on the heart. They are most effective in arrhythmias caused by increased sympathetic nervous system activity (e.g. those caused by exertion, emotion, thyrotoxicosis, acute myocardial infarction and the hereditary QT prolongation syndromes).

Beta-blocking drugs slow AV nodal conduction and thus, like verapamil, are useful in arrhythmias of supraventricular origin and in particular, reduction of the ventricular rate during atrial fibrillation. Unwanted bradycardia caused by beta-blockade can usually quickly be reversed by atropine.

Intravenous esmolol has an extremely short half-life of only 2 min. Its beta-adrenoceptor antagonist action and any associated unwanted effects will therefore be brief.

SOTALOL

Sotalol, in addition to its beta-blocking property, prolongs the duration of the action potential and hence QT interval: it has a significant class III or amiodarone-like action. Unlike other beta-blockers, sotalol has a marked effect upon the recovery periods of atrial and ventricular myocardium and accessory AV pathways.

It has a long half-life and can be given once daily. The oral dosage is 160–320 mg daily. The drug is excreted by the kidneys: dosage should be reduced if renal function is impaired. Intravenously, it should be given slowly up to a dosage of 1.5 mg/kg.

There are reports of the drug – usually in association with other drugs or hypokalaemia – of causing torsade de pointes tachycardia. It should not be given to patients whose QT interval is already prolonged or if there is a family history of hereditary QT prolongation.

Several but not all studies show that sotalol is considerably more effective than other beta-blockers for prevention of atrial fibrillation and other supraventricular arrhythmias. It has been shown to be effective in the treatment of ventricular tachycardia, including patients with implantable defibrillators.

DIGOXIN

Digoxin is widely used as an AV nodal-blocking drug in the control of the ventricular rate during atrial fibrillation. However, it is often ineffective at rate control when the patient is active.

The usual dose is 0.25–0.375 mg daily. A number of factors, such as hypokalaemia, renal impairment, dehydration (often caused by diuretics) and therapy with quinidine, verapamil or amiodarone, predispose to digoxin toxicity and are an indication for dosage reduction.

Digoxin toxicity(c)

Digoxin toxicity is a common problem. Over 10 per cent of patients receiving the drug who are admitted to hospital have been found to have evidence of digoxin toxicity.

A number of symptoms suggest digoxin toxicity. These include anorexia, nausea, vomiting, diarrhoea, mental confusion, xanthopsia and visual blurring. However, none of these symptoms is specific to digoxin toxicity; in patients with severe congestive heart failure in particular, gastrointestinal symptoms are often caused by heart failure rather than digoxin.

Digoxin toxicity can cause a number of disorders of cardiac rhythm. These include atrial tachycardia with AV block (Figure 19.6), junctional tachycardia (Figure 19.7), ventricular ectopic beats (often bigeminy) (Figure 19.8), ventricular tachycardia, first-, second- and third-degree AV block, a slow ventricular response to atrial fibrillation (Figure 19.9) and sinoatrial block (Figure 19.10).

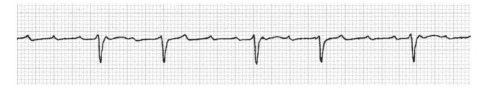

Figure 19.6 Atrial tachycardia with varying degrees of atrioventricular block.

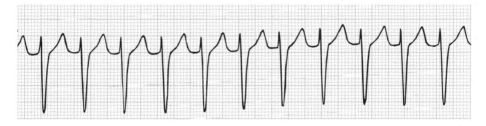

Figure 19.7 Junctional tachycardia.

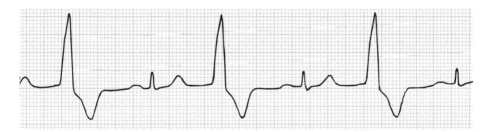

Figure 19.8 First-degree atrioventricular block with ventricular bigeminy.

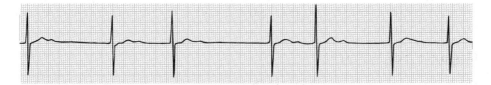

Figure 19.9 Slow ventricular response to atrial fibrillation.

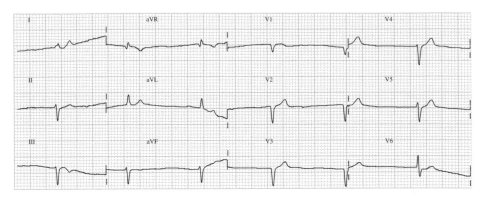

Figure 19.10 Junctional rhythm in a patient receiving digoxin for atrial fibrillation. Digoxin level 5.9 nmol/L.

The main use of digoxin is to control the ventricular rate during atrial fibrillation. When a patient receiving digoxin for this purpose develops a regular pulse a number of possibilities should be considered. First, sinus rhythm may have returned. Second, an arrhythmia due to digoxin toxicity may have developed (e.g. atrial tachycardia with AV block, junctional tachycardia or atrial fibrillation with complete AV block). Without an ECG it may be difficult to ascertain whether the regular rhythm is due to an arrhythmia or not.

Plasma digoxin levels can be measured but must be interpreted in conjunction with clinical features. Levels less than 1.5 ng/mL, in the absence of hypokalaemia, indicate that digoxin toxicity is unlikely. Levels in excess of 3.0 ng/mL indicate that toxicity is probable. With levels between 1.5 and 3.0 ng/mL digoxin toxicity should be considered a possibility, particularly if there are symptoms or arrhythmias attributable to digoxin toxicity or if there is renal impairment, or if the patient appears to be on an inappropriately large dose of digoxin. Blood for digoxin concentration estimation must be taken at least 6 hours after the last dose.

Usually, temporary discontinuation of the drug and correction of hypokalaemia, if present, are all that is required. Serious toxicity can be treated with specific digoxin binding antibodies raised in sheep.

If high degrees of AV block occur, temporary cardiac pacing may be necessary. Cardioversion is dangerous in the presence of digoxin toxicity. If cardioversion is essential, low energy levels (e.g. 5–10 J), increasing gradually as necessary, should be used and lignocaine 75–100 mg should be given.

GRAPEFRUIT

Grapefruit juice and fresh segments have been shown to inactivate the hepatic cytochrome P450 system and can lead to increased levels of a wide variety of cardiac medications: antiarrhythmic drugs including verapamil, amiodarone, quinidine, disopyramide and propafenone and other cardiac medications, including carvedilol, atorvastatin, simvastatin and nifedipine.

Grapefruit juice alone has been shown to slightly prolong the QT interval.

ANTIARRHYTHMIC DRUGS DURING PREGNANCY

No antiarrhythmic drug is completely safe during pregnancy. Where possible, drugs should be avoided in patients with well-tolerated arrhythmias, particularly in the first trimester.

Of the commonly used drugs, beta-blockers and flecainide have been used quite widely and appear relatively safe. Amiodarone has been reported to cause congenital abnormalities.

Main points

- Antiarrhythmic drugs are of limited efficacy and often cause unwanted effects.

- Choice of antiarrhythmic therapy should be tailored to the individual patient and depends on the arrhythmia, the degree of associated circulatory disturbance, the presence of impaired myocardial, sinus node or AV node function, need for short- or long-term treatment and concurrent administration of other drugs.

- Drugs are better at terminating arrhythmias than at preventing their recurrence.

- Disopyramide, flecainide and beta-blockers may precipitate heart failure in patients with extensive myocardial damage.

- Many drugs can have a proarrhythmic action, particularly if ventricular function is impaired.

- Adenosine is the treatment of choice for termination of AV junctional re-entrant tachycardias.

- Intravenous verapamil will quickly control the ventricular response to atrial fibrillation and flutter. It should not be given to a patient who has received a beta-blocker.

- Lignocaine is the first-line drug for termination of ventricular tachycardia.

- Sotalol is effective in a wide variety of arrhythmias.

- Amiodarone is the most effective antiarrhythmic agent currently available but because of its many unwanted effects its long-term use should generally be confined to the treatment of patients with arrhythmias that are dangerous or are refractory to other forms of treatment, or who have a poor prognosis.

Sudden cardiac death

Sudden death due to cardiac disease is common. The annual incidence in the United Kingdom is estimated to be 100 000.

DEFINITION

Many sudden deaths are unwitnessed and few occur during ECG monitoring. Thus, it cannot be assumed that sudden death is synonymous with arrhythmic death because there are other possible causes such as valvular heart disease, congenital heart disease, cardiac tumours, electromechanical dissociation (EMD), cerebrovascular accident, pulmonary embolism and massive haemorrhage (e.g. from a ruptured aortic aneurysm). Furthermore, even a documented episode of ventricular fibrillation might be a terminal event resulting from a cardiovascular catastrophe such as massive myocardial infarction or pulmonary embolism, or cerebrovascular accident. Nevertheless, most sudden cardiac deaths are caused by an arrhythmia, usually ventricular tachycardia or fibrillation.

Ventricular fibrillation often results from degeneration from ventricular tachycardia rather than being the primary arrhythmia (Figure 20.1).

A minority of arrhythmic deaths are caused by bradycardias.

CAUSES

Coronary heart disease is by far the most common cause of sudden cardiac death. Though acute myocardial infarction commonly leads to ventricular fibrillation, it accounts for less than one-third of patients presenting with sudden death. The majority have been found to have extensive coronary disease and poor left ventricular function but not acute infarction.

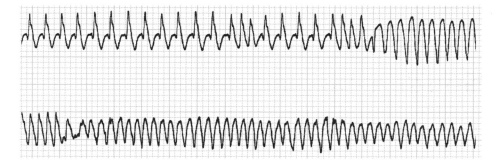

Figure 20.1 Continuous recording as monomorphic ventricular tachycardia deteriorates into ventricular fibrillation.

The main causes are listed in Table 20.1. They are discussed elsewhere in this book, except for commotio cordis which is described below.

Table 20.1 Causes of arrhythmic sudden cardiac death

Acute myocardial infarction
Acute myocardial ischaemia
Myocardial damage due to coronary heart disease
Congenital coronary artery abnormalities
Dilated cardiomyopathy
Hypertrophic cardiomyopathy
Arrhythmogenic right ventricular cardiomyopathy
Myocarditis
Atrioventricular block
Hereditary and acquired long QT syndromes
Brugada syndrome
Wolff–Parkinson–White syndrome
Idiopathic ventricular fibrillation
Catecholaminergic ventricular tachycardia
Short QT syndrome
Electrolyte abnormalities
Proarrhythmic drugs (including cocaine)
Commotio cordis

COMMOTIO CORDIS

Commotio cordis is sudden death caused by a blunt, non-penetrating blow to the praecordium that coincides with the upstroke of the ventricular T wave and initiates ventricular fibrillation. It typically occurs in young people during ball games and other contact sports.

The sooner defibrillation can be carried out, the greater the chance of survival.

EXERTION

Patients with a recognized cause of sudden cardiac death should be advised to avoid competitive sport and strenuous activities.

ABORTED SUDDEN CARDIAC DEATH

Several centres, mainly in North America, have shown that facilities for out-of-hospital cardiopulmonary resuscitation do save lives. As a result, information on the syndrome of 'aborted sudden cardiac death' is increasing. It is now clear that patients who are resuscitated and who have not sustained acute infarction remain at risk. There is a recurrence rate of up to 60 per cent within two years.

Patients resuscitated from cardiac arrest not caused by acute infarction or by a correctable cause must be investigated to assess the need for myocardial revascularization, antiarrhythmic drug therapy and/or implantation of an automatic defibrillator before discharge from hospital.

It should be noted that hypokalaemia is commonly found after resuscitation. It is usually the result of the stress of collapse and resuscitation and cannot be assumed to be the cause of a ventricular arrhythmia unless the patient was known to have a low potassium level prior to his or her arrest.

Management to prevent or deal with a recurrence will depend on the cause of the arrest. Treatment of specific conditions is discussed in other chapters.

IMPAIRED VENTRICULAR FUNCTION

In patients whose arrest was a consequence of poor ventricular function, the worse the ejection fraction the more likely is a recurrence. There are additional factors pointing to a poor prognosis, including left bundle branch block and non-sustained ventricular tachycardia.

Amiodarone has little or no effect on mortality and other antiarrhythmic drugs have been shown to increase mortality.

Beta-blockers, angiotensin-converting enzyme inhibitors, spironolactone or eplerenone, and statins have all been shown to improve prognosis whether by antiarrhythmic or by other actions. The most important treatment to consider is defibrillator implantation (see Chapter 25).

Main points

- Sudden cardiac death is common. It is most commonly due to ventricular tachycardia or fibrillation caused by poor ventricular function resulting from coronary artery disease or less commonly cardiomyopathy.

- Other causes of sudden cardiac death include the Brugada syndrome, the hereditary long QT syndromes, arrhythmogenic right ventricular dysplasia and hypertrophic cardiomyopathy.

- Patients resuscitated from sudden cardiac death not due to acute infarction or reversible cause are likely to experience a recurrence and investigation and treatment, which often includes an implantable defibrillator, must be undertaken.

Cardioversion

Electrical cardioversion is the use of an electric shock of brief duration and high energy to terminate a tachyarrhythmia (Figure 21.1). The shock depolarizes the myocardium, thus interrupting the tachycardia and allowing the sinus node to resume control of the heart rhythm.

Chemical cardioversion is the restoration of normal rhythm by antiarrhythmic drugs and is discussed elsewhere.

TRANSTHORACIC CARDIOVERSION

Cardioversion is usually carried out by delivering a shock between two electrodes placed on the chest.

PROCEDURE

Facilities for monitoring the ECG and for cardiopulmonary resuscitation must be available.

The rhythm should be checked immediately before cardioversion to ensure that spontaneous reversion has not occurred.

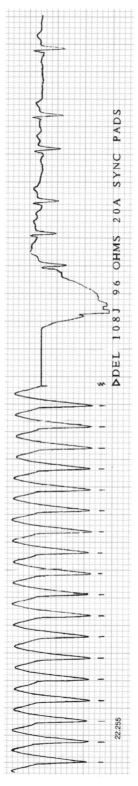

Figure 21.1 Termination of ventricular tachycardia by delivery of 100 J shock.

ANAESTHESIA

The patient should fast for 4 hours before elective cardioversion.

A conscious patient should receive a short-acting general anaesthetic or, in the absence of an anaesthetist, intravenous drugs to achieve deep but brief sedation. The author finds that small incremental doses of intravenous midazolam (total: 1–10 mg) in combination with fentanyl (50 µg) very effective. It is essential that the patient's airway and oxygen saturation are carefully monitored and that drugs to reverse fentanyl (i.e. naloxone) and midazolam (i.e. flumazenil) are immediately available in the unlikely event of respiratory depression.

DELIVERY OF SHOCK

The shock is delivered between two electrode paddles. Correct positioning is essential. Usually one electrode is placed at the level of the cardiac apex, close to the mid-axillary line, and the other is positioned to the right of the upper sternum.

Alternatively, a flat paddle, if available, can be placed beneath the patient's back, behind the heart, and a second paddle positioned over the praecordium. Standard paddles can be applied antero-posteriorly if the patient is turned onto his or her side: one paddle is placed over the praecordium and the other paddle below the left shoulder to the left of the spine.

To achieve good electrical contact and to avoid burning the skin, electrode jelly must be applied to the areas beneath the paddles. However, it is essential to avoid spreading jelly between the two paddles. Pads impregnated with electrode gel prevent jelly being spread over inappropriate areas, including the operator!

The defibrillator is charged to the desired energy level (see below) which takes a few seconds. The charge is usually delivered by pressing the button(s) on the defibrillator paddle(s). The paddles should be applied with firm pressure to reduce the electrical resistance of the thorax.

Before discharge it is essential to ensure that no one is in contact with the patient.

If cardioversion is unsuccessful, depending on the circumstances, further shocks with higher energy levels may be tried.

The heart rhythm should be monitored during and after cardioversion.

Synchronization

Ventricular fibrillation may be induced if a shock coincides with the ventricular T wave. Therefore, defibrillators have a mechanism whereby discharge is triggered to coincide with the R or S wave. This mechanism should be used during cardioversion for all arrhythmias except ventricular fibrillation. With ventricular fibrillation there will be no detectable R wave and thus, if the mechanism is in operation, the defibrillator will not discharge.

Before synchronized cardioversion, the operator should check that the synchronizing signal coincides with the onset of the QRS complex. Sometimes, the amplitude of the ECG has to be increased to enable synchronization.

BIPHASIC WAVEFORM

Modern defibrillators now deliver a biphasic rather than a monophasic shock. With biphasic shocks the direction of current flow is reversed approximately half way during the discharge. Biphasic defibrillation allows delivery of greater energy at lower voltage. A biphasic 150 J shock is roughly equivalent to a monophasic 200 J shock. It has been suggested that early recurrence of an arrhythmia is less likely following a biphasic shock.

Complications

Complications are rare.

Cardioversion often causes marked elevation in creatinine kinase but does not significantly elevate troponin levels. Thus, cardioversion may affect skeletal muscle but does not cause myocardial damage. Biphasic shocks are less likely to affect skeletal muscle. Skin burns can sometimes result from cardioversion. This complication has been shown to be less likely with biphasic shocks.

Transient arrhythmias occasionally occur but these are rarely a problem unless there is digoxin toxicity.

In patients with the bradycardia–tachycardia syndrome cardioversion may cause a major bradycardia: a temporary pacing wire should be inserted before cardioversion.

Systemic embolism may occur when cardioversion is carried out for atrial fibrillation (see below).

Digoxin toxicity

Cardioversion in the presence of digoxin toxicity can produce dangerous ventricular arrhythmias. For this reason cardioversion should be a last resort and should be preceded by lignocaine 75–100 mg. When digoxin toxicity is likely, very low levels should be used, starting at 5–10 J.

Because of the dangers of digoxin toxicity, it has become common practice to stop digoxin for 24–48 hours before cardioversion. However, cardioversion in the presence of therapeutic levels of digoxin is safe. There is no need to postpone cardioversion provided the patient is receiving standard doses of digoxin, renal function and plasma electrolytes are normal and there are no symptoms or ECG findings suggestive of digoxin toxicity (see Chapter 19).

IMPLANTED PACEMAKERS AND DEFIBRILLATORS

Cardioversion may cause pacemaker or defibrillator damage unless the paddles are at least 15 cm from the device and preferably are positioned so they are at right angles to the line between the device and the heart.

INDICATIONS

Ventricular fibrillation

Immediate cardioversion is necessary. The initial energy level should be 200 J (150 J biphasic). If unsuccessful, a further 200 J shock should be given. If ventricular fibrillation persists a 360 J shock should be delivered.

Sequential or simultaneous shocks, delivered by means of two defibrillators with separate pairs of electrodes, should be considered in any patient who does not defibrillate with repeated 360 J shocks.

Ventricular tachycardia

Cardioversion is indicated if the arrhythmia causes shock or cardiac arrest, or if drug therapy has failed. With very fast ventricular tachycardias it may be difficult to synchronize delivery of the shock and it may be necessary to deliver an unsynchronized shock. Energy levels as for ventricular fibrillation should be used.

Atrial fibrillation

Sinus rhythm can be restored by cardioversion in most patients with atrial fibrillation. However, not infrequently the arrhythmia returns.

High energy shocks are usually required. The first shock should be 200 J monophasic or 150 J biphasic. A 360 J monophasic or 200 J biphasic shock applied between anterior and posterior paddles may be successful in resistant cases and cardioversion should not be deemed to be unsuccessful unless these approaches have been tried.

Anticoagulation

Cardioversion can result in systemic embolism because of dislodgement of pre-existing thrombus. New atrial thrombus can develop after cardioversion because atrial mechanical activity often does not return for up to three weeks after the procedure and because cardioversion itself can increase blood hypercoagulability. Hence embolism can also occur in the following few weeks. It is therefore recommended that non-urgent cardioversion in patients who have been in atrial fibrillation for more than 24–48 hours is preceded by warfarin for at least three weeks and that anti-coagulation is continued for at least four weeks after restoration of normal rhythm. In patients who are at high risk of embolism long-term anticoagulation should be considered because there is a significant possibility of further atrial fibrillation: either paroxysmal or sustained.

If urgent cardioversion is required, transoesophageal echocardiography can be used to exclude left atrial thrombus or stasis. The echocardiographic signs of left atrial stasis are spontaneous echo contrast and reduced left atrial appendage flow velocity. If cardioversion has to be carried out urgently, heparin should be given until adequate anticoagulation is achieved with warfarin.

TRANSVENOUS CARDIOVERSION

Transvenous cardioversion is now an established technique for terminating atrial fibrillation. A low energy shock (15–30 J) is delivered between transvenous electrodes positioned in the right atrium and either the coronary sinus or pulmonary artery. Though energy levels are lower, sedative or anaesthetic requirements are the same as for transthoracic cardioversion.

A single-lead, balloon-guided system is available which also facilitates atrial and ventricular pacing, if required (Figure 21.2).

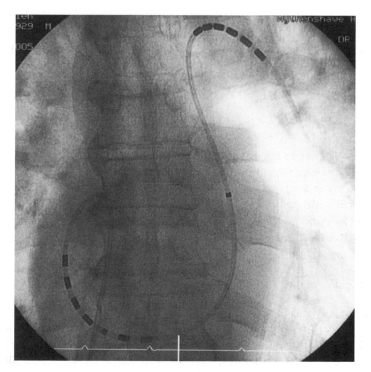

Figure 21.2 Transvenous cardioversion. There is a single lead with a multipolar cathode in the left pulmonary artery and a multipolar anode in the right atrium.

Success rates are higher than for transthoracic cardioversion, especially in very large patients.

This approach should be considered in patients where transthoracic cardioversion has failed but restoration of normal rhythm is thought to be of great importance, and as a first-line strategy in large patients.

Recurrence of atrial fibrillation

While cardioversion only leads to long-term sinus rhythm in a minority of patients, an attempt at restoring sinus rhythm should be considered in those patients with recent atrial fibrillation (less than 12 months) where no cause has been identified or in whom the disorder which has caused the arrhythmia has resolved or is self-limiting. Cardioversion should be considered in those patients with atrial fibrillation which has been present for more than 12 months if symptoms due to the arrhythmia are severe, even when there is only a small chance of long-term normal rhythm.

If there is a recurrence, a further attempt at cardioversion, after initiation of antiarrhythmic therapy, should only be undertaken in those with troublesome symptoms attributable to the arrhythmia. Several drugs such as disopyramide, flecainide, sotalol and especially amiodarone reduce the relapse rate after cardioversion.

ATRIAL FLUTTER

This arrhythmia, which is often difficult to treat with drugs, responds to low energy shocks (50 J). The need for anticoagulation is controversial. The risk of embolism is lower than with atrial fibrillation. However, flutter and fibrillation can sometimes coexist so some recommend the same anticoagulant regime as for atrial fibrillation. Anticoagulation is definitely indicated if there is myocardial or valve disease, or a history of embolism.

Though cardioversion is almost always successful, atrial flutter will recur in half of cases though there many be many months before the arrhythmia does recur.

ATRIOVENTRICULAR RE-ENTRANT TACHYCARDIA

Cardioversion is indicated on the very few occasions when other measures, such as vagal stimulation or intravenous adenosine or verapamil, have failed.

Main points

- The usual positions for the defibrillator paddles are the cardiac apex and to the right of the upper sternum.

- Firm paddle pressure should be applied prior to delivery of the DC shock.

- Except for ventricular fibrillation, delivery of the shock should be synchronized to the R or S wave of the ECG.

- Initial energy levels depend on the clinical circumstances: 50 J for atrial flutter, 200 J for ventricular fibrillation, 100 J for most other arrhythmias. A level of 300 J is often required to cardiovert atrial fibrillation. Lower energies are required if biphasic shocks are used.

- Digoxin toxicity is a contraindication to cardioversion.

- Temporary transvenous pacing should precede cardioversion if the bradycardia–tachycardia syndrome is suspected.

- In patients with atrial fibrillation or flutter due to conditions associated with a significant risk from systemic embolism, anticoagulation should precede cardioversion.

- Damage to an implanted pacemaker or defibrillator can be prevented if the paddles are placed at least 15 cm from the generator and preferably positioned so they are at right angles to the pacing system.

Ambulatory ECG monitoring

The standard resting ECG records the heart rhythm for no more than 30 s and is, therefore, not suitable for detecting intermittent disturbances in heart rhythm. Ambulatory ECG monitoring is an invaluable diagnostic tool. The ECG can be continuously or intermittently recorded for long periods.

CONTINUOUS ECG RECORDING

The ECG can be continuously recorded, usually for 24–120 hours, using a portable battery-operated recorder that is usually worn on a belt at the waist. The ECG is either recorded as an analogue signal on tape or, now more commonly, in digital form in solid state recording systems. If appropriate, the patient can be fully ambulant, carrying out his or her normal day-to-day activities.

The ECG is recorded by means of electrodes applied to areas of thoroughly cleaned skin. Usually one electrode is placed over the upper sternum and the other electrode over the V5 chest lead position. As an alternative, a modified V1 lead can be obtained by placing one electrode over the V1 chest lead position and the other electrode beneath the lateral part of the left clavicle.

Most systems allow simultaneous recording of two or more leads. This increases diagnostic accuracy and aids in the detection of artefacts, which are unlikely to appear on both leads at the same time (Figure 22.1). Furthermore, sometimes one lead does not reveal important diagnostic information while the other does (Figure 22.2).

The recording is analysed by replaying it at 60–100 times real-time. Playback systems have facilities for printing out selected portions of the recording on ECG paper at standard speed. Most recording systems can automatically detect bradycardias, tachycardias and ectopic beats, though in practice an operator has to supervise the analysis.

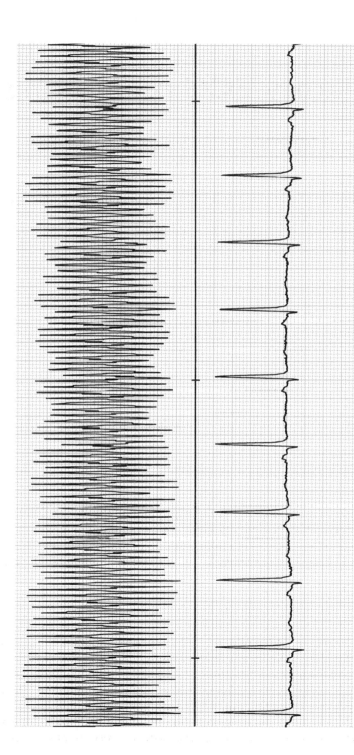

Figure 22.1 The artefact in the upper trace might have been misinterpreted as ventricular fibrillation had not the lower trace been recorded simultaneously.

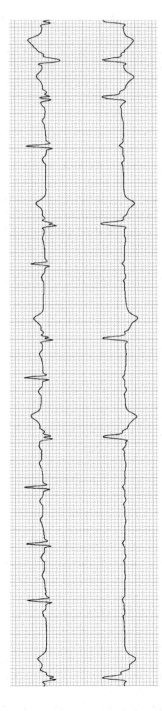

Figure 22.2 The lower trace suggests atrioventricular block but the simultaneous upper trace clearly shows that the small complexes in the lower trace are not P waves.

ARTEFACTS

Several technical problems during ambulatory electrocardiography can result in what appear to be arrhythmias to the unwary.

If the tape speed slows for any reason, complexes will appear closer together and mimic tachycardia. However, the duration of each ventricular complex will be shorter than normal and this should alert the observer to the likelihood of artefact. Conversely, if the tape runs too fast, apparent bradycardia with broader than normal complexes will result.

Not infrequently, a lead will become disconnected during a recording: because no activity is being recorded the ECG will appear as a straight line and mimic sinus arrest. Furthermore, sometimes an electrical connection can intermittently fail, resulting in repeated episodes of apparent sinus arrest. However, if a lead becomes disconnected it may do so at any point in the cardiac cycle, and it is unlikely the onset of 'asystole' will arise after the ventricular T wave as it would if sinus arrest were real. If the onset of sinus arrest occurs during the inscription of an atrial or ventricular complex, artefact can be assumed (Figure 22.3a).

Occasionally, an artefact can produce an apparent tachycardia, but close inspection will reveal that normal QRS complexes are 'walking through' the tachycardia (Figure 22.3b).

CLINICAL APPLICATIONS

Ambulatory ECG monitoring enables the detection and diagnosis of intermittent disorders of cardiac rhythm and may thus reveal the cause of symptoms such as syncope, near-syncope, palpitation and chest pain (Figures 22.4–22.8, pages 220–223).

The technique is most valuable when the patient experiences his or her usual symptoms during an ECG recording. The patient should be instructed to record the time of onset and nature of the symptoms so these can be correlated with the heart rhythm. With most recorders the patient can operate an event marker that indicates the time of symptoms on the tape.

Even when the patient does not experience symptoms during a recording, rhythm abnormalities of diagnostic significance may be detected. Obviously, if the patient does not experience symptoms during the recording and no rhythm abnormalities are found, an arrhythmic cause for the patient's symptoms is not excluded. Conversely, if a patient experiences typical symptoms during the recording and yet no arrhythmia is found then it can be concluded that symptoms are not due to a disturbance of heart rhythm. In the absence of typical symptoms, the finding of a minor abnormality of rhythm does not rule out a more major rhythm disturbance being responsible for the patient's complaints.

In patients with poor ventricular function or hypertrophic cardiomyopathy the technique can be useful in identifying patients who may be at risk from a ventricular arrhythmia (Figure 22.9, see page 224).

It is important to analyse the heart rate immediately prior to the onset of an arrhythmia. For example, sinus bradycardia prior to the onset of an atrial arrhythmia

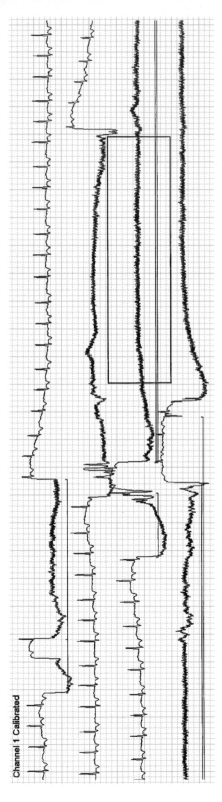

Figure 22.3 (a) Artefact due to intermittent lead disconnection.

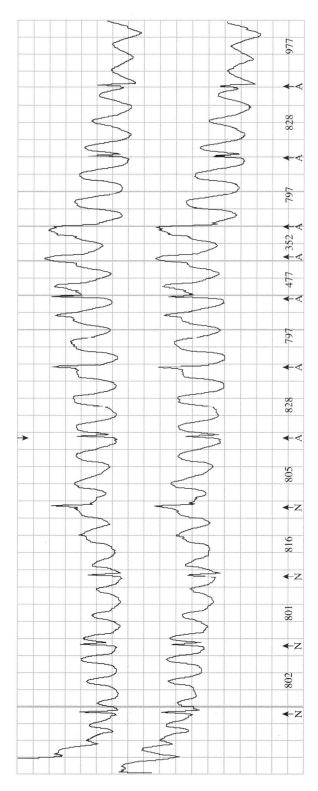

Figure 22.3 (b) On close inspection narrow QRS complexes (indicated by letters N and A at the bottom of the trace) can be seen walking through apparent ventricular arrhythmia.

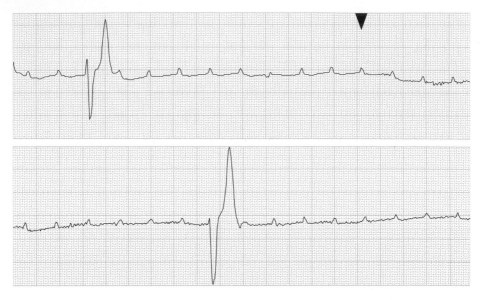

Figure 22.4 Stokes–Adams attack due to complete atrioventricular block with only two ventricular complexes during 24-hour tape recording. During the rest of the recording the patient was in sinus rhythm.

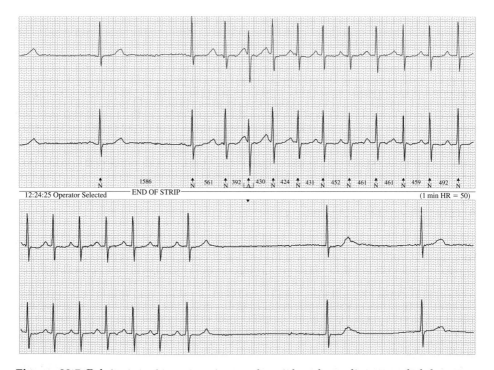

Figure 22.5 Palpitation due to paroxysmal atrial tachycardia, preceded by sinus bradycardia and succeeded by a junctional escape rhythm (i.e. bradycardia–tachycardia syndrome).

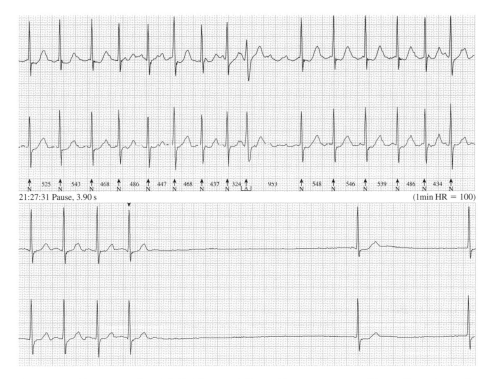

Figure 22.6 Paroxysmal atrial fibrillation followed by sinus arrest. (Recordings from the same patient as in Figure 22.5.)

points to the possibility that atrial pacing may prevent the tachyarrhythmia. Sinus tachycardia prior to the onset of a tachyarrhythmia points to the possibility that the rhythm disturbance was initiated by catecholamines and that beta-blockade may prevent it.

Ambulatory electrocardiography can also be useful in assessing pacemaker function.

Antiarrhythmic therapy

Ambulatory monitoring may be of value in assessing a patient's response to therapy. For example, not uncommonly ambulatory electrocardiography will reveal frequent ventricular arrhythmias despite the use of an antiarrhythmic agent. One problem in using ambulatory monitoring to assess therapy is there is a marked spontaneous variation in the frequency of arrhythmias and so based on one recording, absence or improvement in arrhythmia may not necessarily be a result of drug therapy.

More importantly, ambulatory electrocardiography may reveal a drug's proar-rhythmic effect.

Ambulatory electrocardiography is also useful for ensuring that AV nodal block-ing drugs prescribed for atrial arrhythmias are achieving control of the ventricular rate.

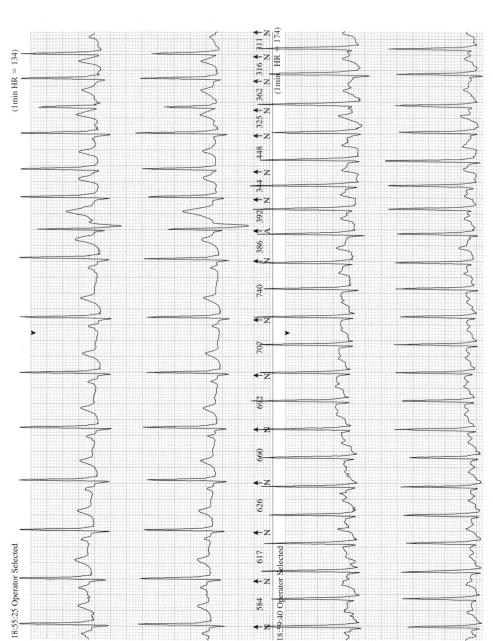

Figure 22.7 Palpitation due to paroxysmal atrial fibrillation.

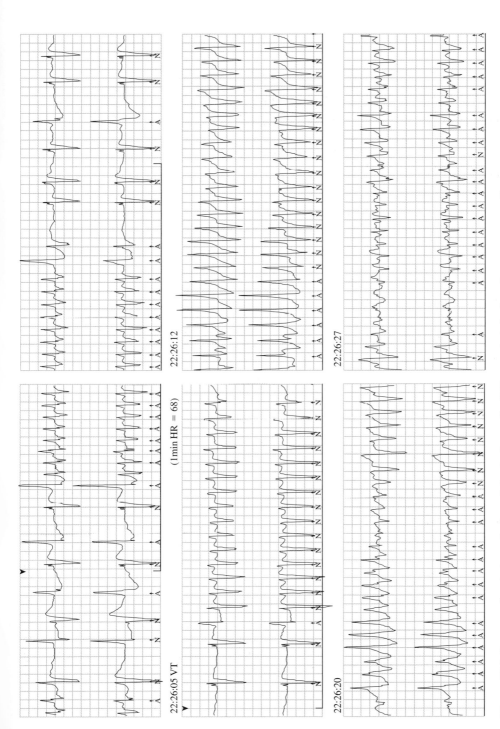

Figure 22.8 Syncope due to torsade de pointes tachycardia (NB recorded during slow paper speed).

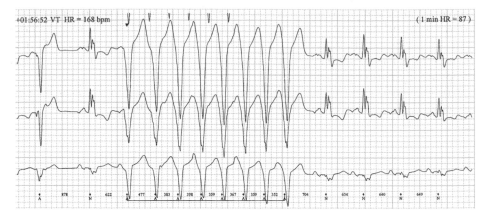

Figure 22.9 Non-sustained ventricular tachycardia in a patient with hypertrophic cardiomyopathy.

'NORMAL' FINDINGS

Sinus bradycardia; short pauses, up to 2 s, due to sinoatrial block; first-degree and AV Wenckebach block can occur in normal people during sleep and should not be regarded as evidence of conduction tissue disease (Figure 22.10). These rhythms may also occur during the day in young people with high vagal tone.

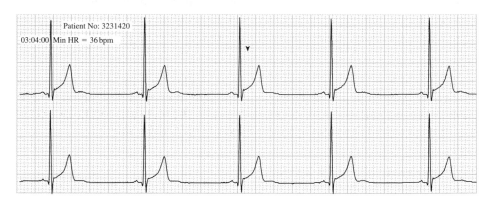

Figure 22.10 Sinus bradycardia during sleep.

Sinus tachycardia will of course also be seen in recordings from people with normal hearts at times of exertion.

Whereas a routine 12-lead ECG records approximately 60 heart beats, a normal 24-hour tape recording is likely to contain at least 90000 beats. Thus ambulatory electrocardiography is a much more sensitive tool than a standard recording. For example, the finding of a single ventricular ectopic beat on a routine ECG suggests a much higher frequency than a hundred ectopic beats on a 24-hour tape. In fact, studies of apparently normal people using ambulatory electrocardiography have shown that unifocal ventricular extrasystoles occur commonly, as do supraventricular ectopic beats. The frequency of ventricular ectopic beats increases with age. Some studies have also found short runs of relatively slow ventricular tachycardia in apparently normal young subjects.

Non-sustained ventricular tachycardia only rarely occurs in subjects without structural heart disease but if it does it is not associated with risk.

INTERMITTENT ECG RECORDING

EVENT RECORDERS

Patients with symptoms occurring at intervals of less than one week are unlikely to experience an episode during the 24–120 hours of continuous ambulatory electrocardiography. A hand-held event recorder is a very useful and inexpensive device that enables a patient to record his or her ECG for 30 s during symptoms. The patient can carry the device around until an attack occurs. He or she then applies the device to the chest wall and initiates the recording that is stored in a memory and can be replayed directly or transmitted via the telephone into an ECG machine. Some devices enable several recordings to be made.

It is very important to explain to the patient precisely when and how to use the recorder. Clearly, these devices are not suitable for the investigation of episodes that disable the patient to the extent that they cannot activate the recorder.

Sometimes patients will record sinus tachycardia. It may well be that this rhythm was responsible for the patient's symptoms. However, another possibility to be borne in mind is that sinus tachycardia resulted from a tachyarrhythmia which had stopped by the time the recorder was activated.

More recently, a small device has become available which can be worn for up to seven days. Arrhythmias that the device detects and rhythms when the patient activates an event marker can be stored in memory. Importantly, the heart rhythm immediately prior to a symptomatic or detected event is also saved.

IMPLANTABLE LOOP RECORDER

An implantable ECG loop recorder is now available. It is a very small device (only 17 g) that can easily be implanted subcutaneously, a few inches beneath the left clavicle. It facilitates ECG monitoring for up to 14 months and is therefore ideal for patients with infrequent symptoms. After the patient experiences typical symptoms, an external device can be held over the implanted recorder that triggers storage of the ECG before, during and after the event (Figure 22.11). Depending on how the implanted device is programmed, the patient may have up to 30 min after the event to initiate the recording. Thus, the ECG of an arrhythmia that has caused temporary incapacity can be recorded. Memory is sufficient to save ECGs relating to several events. The data can then be downloaded into a computer for analysis.

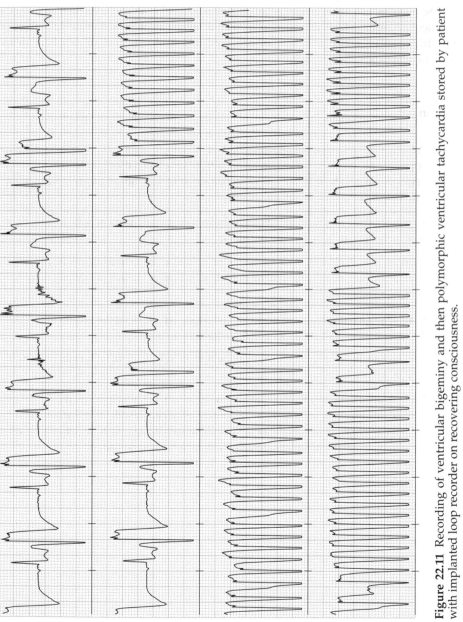

Figure 22.11 Recording of ventricular bigeminy and then polymorphic ventricular tachycardia stored by patient with implanted loop recorder on recovering consciousness.

The latest devices also automatically record the ECG below or above a predetermined heart rate. Though this facility will ensure that major arrhythmias are stored even if the patient fails to use the external activating device, there is the disadvantage that arrhythmias may be recorded which do not coincide with symptoms and may be of doubtful significance.

The manufacturer recommends patients should avoid magnetic resonance imaging, diathermy, high sources of radiation, electrosurgical cautery, external defibrillation, lithotripsy and radiofrequency ablation in order to avoid electrical reset of the device and/or inappropriate sensing.

Main points

- Ambulatory electrocardiography is very useful for the investigation of syncope, near-syncope, palpitation and other symptoms thought to be due to an arrhythmia when routine electrocardiography has not provided diagnostic information.

- Artefacts can produce apparent arrhythmias but can usually be recognized by careful inspection of the recording.

- Studies in apparently normal subjects have demonstrated that certain rhythms detected by ambulatory electrocardiography are not of pathological significance.

- For patients with infrequent, non-disabling palpitation, provision of an event recorder is the best method of investigation.

- An implantable loop recorder can facilitate ECG recording in patients with infrequent episodes.

- Useful information will be provided from an ambulatory recording if an arrhythmia is demonstrated or if a patient experiences his or her usual symptoms without a disturbance in rhythm. Clearly if there is no arrhythmia and no symptoms, an episodic arrhythmia has not been excluded.

Temporary cardiac pacing

The transvenous route is usually used for temporary pacing but, in emergencies, transcutaneous and oesophageal approaches are possible short-term alternatives.

Temporary transvenous pacing is a simple procedure. However complications are common because it is often carried out by inexperienced, unsupervised operators. The need for temporary pacing should be carefully considered before proceeding. In general, patients with infrequent bradycardias should not receive a temporary pacemaker while awaiting implantation of a long-term pacemaker.

INDICATIONS

MYOCARDIAL INFARCTION

1. Second- and third-degree AV block due to acute anterior myocardial infarction.
2. Second- and third-degree AV block caused by acute inferior infarction only when complicated by hypotension, ventricular tachyarrhythmia or a ventricular rate less than 40 beats/min.
3. Symptomatic sinus arrest or junctional bradycardia due to acute myocardial infarction.

CHRONIC CONDUCTION TISSUE DISEASE

Temporary pacing may be necessary as a first measure in patients with recent syncope caused by chronic disease of the sinus node or AV junction who are to be referred for long-term pacing. Patients with infrequent bradycardias should not receive a temporary pacemaker while awaiting implantation of a long-term pacemaker.

TACHYCARDIAS

Pacing is useful in terminating AV re-entrant tachycardia, atrial flutter and ventricular tachycardia. In the bradycardia–tachycardia syndrome temporary pacing should be used to cover cardioversion if required for the termination of supraventricular arrhythmias.

METHODS

TEMPORARY TRANSVENOUS PACING

Temporary ventricular pacing is carried out by introducing a transvenous pacing electrode under local anaesthesia into a systemic vein and advancing it, with the aid of X-ray screening, to the right ventricle. The electrode is connected to an external battery-powered pulse generator. During insertion, the heart rhythm must be monitored and equipment for resuscitation should be available.

Subclavian vein puncture

Puncture of the subclavian vein provides the most suitable route of access to the venous system. The vein runs behind the medial third of the clavicle and can be punctured using either supraventricular or infraclavicular approaches. Only the latter will be described.

The patient should lie flat or, if possible, in a slight head-down position. Alternatively, the legs should be raised to aid venous return and hence distension of the subclavian vein. If the patient is dehydrated an infusion of saline may aid puncture of the vein. A needle is introduced, through a 0.5 cm skin incision just below the inferior border of the clavicle and slightly medial to the mid-clavicular point, and is directed towards the sternoclavicular joint so it passes immediately behind the posterior surface of the clavicle. When first advancing the needle it is advisable to locate the clavicle with the needle tip to avoid going in too deeply, with consequent risk of pneumothorax or subclavian artery puncture.

As the needle punctures the vein, venous blood will be easily aspirated. If there is only a trickle of blood the needle tip is unlikely to be in the subclavian vein.

Cannulation of the vein is best achieved by introducing a guidewire through the needle into the vein. A guidewire with a flexible J-shaped tip is much easier to advance around the junction between the subclavian vein and superior vena cava. The needle is then withdrawn and a sheath within which there is a vessel dilator is passed over the wire into the vein. The guidewire and dilator are then removed, and the pacing lead is passed through the sheath.

The main advantages of subclavian vein puncture are that it is quick and infection and electrode displacement are unusual. Possible complications, which are rare in experienced hands, are pneumothorax, haemothorax, subclavian artery puncture and air embolism.

Antecubital vein cut-down

It is important to select a medially situated vein. It is unusual to be able to negotiate an electrode into the superior vena cava from a lateral vein.

The disadvantages of this approach are poor electrode stability, and infection and phlebitis are common. It may be safer to use this approach in patients who have received thrombolytic therapy.

Femoral vein puncture

This method is very easy and quick, provided that pulsation of the laterally adjacent femoral artery is easily palpable. However, it should be reserved for short-term emergency purposes because electrode stability is poor and there is a risk of venous thrombosis. The femoral vein is medial to the femoral artery. Pressure on the abdomen causes distension of the femoral vein and makes venipuncture much easier.

Positioning of the electrode

If there is resistance to the introduction of the electrode into the vein, the lumen has not been entered. Once in the venous system, it should be possible to advance the electrode without resistance. If an obstruction is encountered, the electrode should be withdrawn slightly, rotated and then advanced again. Nothing will be achieved by forcing the electrode.

Once the electrode has reached the right atrium, a loop should be formed by imping-ing the electrode tip on the atrial wall (Figure 23.1A) and then advancing the electrode a little further (Figure 23.1B). By twisting the electrode, the loop can be rotated so the electrode tip lies near the tricuspid valve (Figure 23.1C). Slight withdrawal of the elec-trode will allow the tip to 'flick' through the valve into the right ventricle.

Ventricular ectopic beats are invariably provoked as the valve is crossed. If these do not occur, the coronary sinus rather than the right ventricle may have been entered. An electrode lying in the coronary sinus assumes a characteristic shape (Figure 23.1F). (A lateral view will show the electrode is pointing posteriorly whereas an electrode in the right ventricular apex points anteriorly.) It can be con-firmed that the right ventricle has been entered by advancing the electrode into the pulmonary artery (Figure 23.1D).

Once in the right ventricle, the electrode tip is positioned in or near the apex of the ventricle by a process of advancement, withdrawal and rotation (Figure 23.1E).

Pacing

When a stable electrode position in or near the right ventricular apex has been achieved, the distal and proximal poles of the electrode should be connected to the

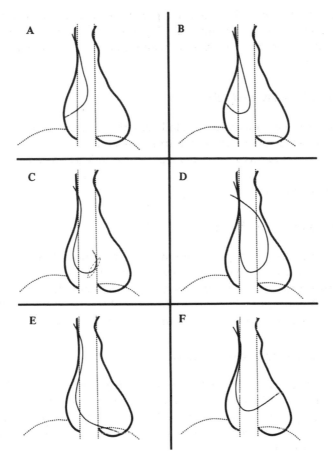

Figure 23.1 Insertion of a transvenous pacing lead. A loop is formed in the right atrium (A and B). The loop is positioned near the tricuspid valve, indicated by the oval of dashes (C). Entry into the right ventricle can be confirmed by passing the wire into the pulmonary artery (D). The pacing lead is then positioned in the apex of the right ventricle (E). (F) The characteristic appearance of a pacing lead in the coronary sinus.

pacemaker cathode (−) and anode (+), respectively. If the poles are reversed, the stimulation threshold will be substantially higher.

The pacing threshold, which is the minimum voltage necessary for pacing stimuli to capture the ventricles consistently, should then be measured (Figure 23.2). It should be less than 1.0 V, assuming the pulse generator delivers impulses whose duration is 1 or 2 ms. Some temporary pacemakers allow adjustment of the pulse width: shorter pulse durations lead to a higher threshold and are not indicated for temporary pacing. Sometimes, in an emergency, a pacing threshold or electrode position which is less than optimal has to be accepted. Occasionally a patient may become dependent on the pacemaker, making adjustment of the electrode position risky. In these circumstances it may be necessary to insert a second pacing electrode (e.g. via the femoral vein) to cover the period of repositioning.

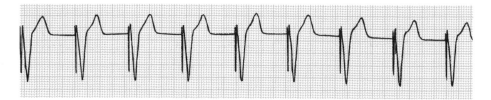

Figure 23.2 Ventricular pacing (lead II). Each pacing stimulus is followed by a ventricular complex. An electrode positioned in the apex of the right ventricle will produce left axis deviation of the paced beats.

The stability of the pacing lead should be tested by ensuring there is consistent pacing during coughing and deep inspiration. During the latter manoeuvre, if there is the correct number of slack in the lead, there will be a slight curve in its right atrial portion (Figure 23.1E).

To avoid lead displacement, it is essential to suture securely the electrode to the skin at its point of entry. The pacing threshold often rises to 2–3 V during the first few days after electrode insertion. The threshold should be checked daily and the output set at twice the measured threshold. Battery and electrical connections should also be checked daily.

It is surprising how often the connections between pacemaker and pacing lead, on which a patient's life may depend, are found to be loose or insecure!

Pacing complications

Causes of failure to pace (Figure 23.3) include electrode displacement, myocardial perforation, exit block and a break in either the electrical connections or in the pacing electrode.

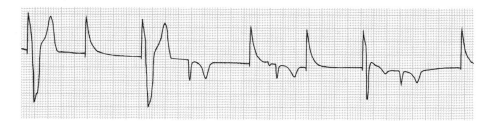

Figure 23.3 Intermittent failure to pace (lead II). Only the first and third pacing stimuli capture the ventricles.

Electrode displacement

Electrode displacement may cause intermittent or complete failure to pace. The electrode may fall back into the right atrial cavity and lead to atrial rather than ventricular pacing (Figure 23.4).

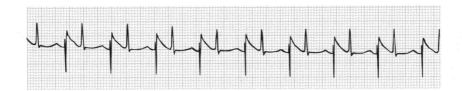

Figure 23.4 Atrial pacing. At the time of this recording, atrioventricular conduction was satisfactory so each pacing stimulus was followed by a narrow QRS complex after a PR interval of 0.22s.

Myocardial perforation

In general, temporary pacing leads are rather stiff and occasionally the electrode tip may perforate the thin right ventricular myocardium. Failure to pace, diaphragmatic stimulation, pericardial friction rub and pericardial pain may result. Cardiac tamponade is rare.

Exit block

Sometimes pacing failure occurs without electrode tip displacement or other cause. In these cases failure is attributed to 'exit block', which is caused by excessive tissue reaction at the junction between electrode tip and endocardium.

Electrical fracture

A break in the electrical connection or in the electrode itself can be the cause of intermittent or complete pacing failure. In contrast to exit block, no pacing stimuli will appear on the ECG.

Inappropriate inhibition

External inhibition of a demand pacemaker from electromagnetic waves being emitted from electrical equipment can occasionally inhibit a pacemaker and will result in absent pacing stimuli. This problem can be quickly solved by changing the pacemaker to fixed rate mode.

Failure to sense

Pacemakers are most often used in the 'demand' mode, whereby the pacemaker senses spontaneous cardiac activity and only discharges a stimulus if a spontaneous beat has not occurred within a pre-set period. In some patients, those with myocardial infarction, the signal generated by spontaneous activity may be too small for the pacemaker to sense. As a result, the pacemaker will function in a 'fixed rate' mode and pacing stimuli will be discharged at inappropriate times, and may fall on the T wave of a spontaneous beat (Figure 23.5). This is undesirable in acute myocardial infarction because of the risk of precipitating ventricular fibrillation (Figure 23.6).

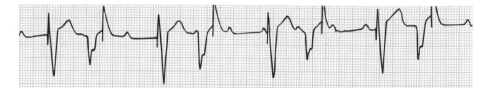

Figure 23.5 Failure to sense in a demand ventricular pacemaker. The first, third, fifth and seventh pacing stimuli capture the ventricles. The second, fourth, sixth and eighth stimuli fall on the T waves of spontaneous ventricular beats.

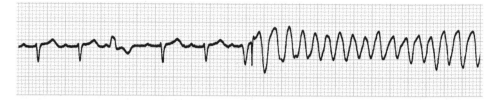

Figure 23.6 Failure to sense sixth ventricular complex, resulting in a pacemaker stimulus coinciding with the T wave and initiating ventricular fibrillation.

Infection

Infection can occur at the site of entry of a transvenous pacing electrode. Sometimes bacteraemia results, which is a serious complication if there is valve disease and thus the possibility of endocarditis. Infection will not clear without removal of the pacing electrode. If necessary, a new pacing electrode will have to be inserted at a different site.

ATRIOVENTRICULAR SEQUENTIAL PACING

Ventricular pacing results in dissociation between atrial and ventricular activity and a consequent reduction in cardiac output of up to one-third.

The atria and ventricles may be paced sequentially, enabling the normal sequence of cardiac chamber activation (Figure 23.7). In patients with a low cardiac output, AV sequential pacing can produce an important improvement in cardiac function. Usually, AV sequential pacing is achieved by passing two leads to the heart: one to

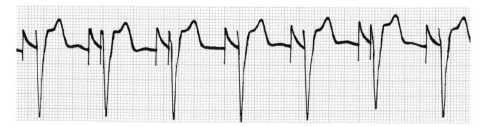

Figure 23.7 Atrioventricular sequential pacing. Pacing stimuli precede both atrial and ventricular complexes.

the atria and one to the ventricles. The best method of ensuring that an atrial lead is not displaced is to use one with a pre-formed J-shaped terminal portion. A lead of this type can easily be positioned in the right atrial appendage (see Chapter 24).

TEMPORARY TRANSCUTANEOUS AND OESOPHAGEAL PACING

Transcutaneous cardiac pacing was first attempted many years ago but was usually unsuccessful and caused severe discomfort due to skeletal muscle stimulation. Recently, considerable success with less discomfort has been achieved by using large surface area skin electrodes and stimuli of much longer duration than are used for endocardial stimulation (20–40 ms).

The latest generation of transcutaneous pacemakers function in the demand mode and have a maximum output in the region of 150 mA. One electrode is applied to the front of the chest and the other to the back over the right scapula. Pacing is likely to stimulate the atria at the same time as the ventricles. It is not always possible to ascertain from the ECG that the heart is being stimulated: monitoring of an arterial pulse may be necessary.

With oesophageal pacing, long impulse duration is necessary (10 ms). Atrial stimulation is more successful than ventricular stimulation.

As with transvenous pacing, transcutaneous and oesophageal pacing are unlikely to be successful after a prolonged period of cardiac arrest.

Main points

- Indications for temporary transvenous pacing include second- and third-degree AV block due to acute anterior infarction; 'complicated' second- and third-degree AV block due to acute inferior infarction; and recent syncope or near-syncope due to chronic disease of the sinus node or AV junction while awaiting implantation of a long-term pacemaker.

- Subclavian vein puncture is usually the best method of venous access for temporary pacing.

- The pacemaker stimulation threshold, battery function and electrical connections should be checked daily.

- AV sequential pacing improves cardiac output as compared with ventricular pacing.

Long-term cardiac pacing for bradycardias

This subject is discussed in detail to provide a concise account of the practical aspects of pacemaker implantation and the care of patients with pacemakers, which is often the remit of a cardiac department's more junior members.

An artificial cardiac pacemaker generates electrical stimuli which can initiate myocardial contraction. The stimuli are usually delivered to the heart by transvenous leads or much less commonly via epicardial electrodes.

The first pacemaker was implanted in 1958. Over the following years, rapid progress in technology and an increasing awareness of the benefits of pacing have led to pacemakers being widely used. People of all ages, from the newborn to patients over 100 years old, have been paced.

In the United Kingdom, which has a relatively low implant rate compared with other European countries and with North America, 26 000 pacemakers are implanted each year; the average age at first implantation is 76 years.

INDICATIONS FOR LONG-TERM CARDIAC PACING

The main reasons for implanting a pacemaker are to relieve symptoms or to improve prognosis. In some patients with asymptomatic impairment of the specialized cardiac conducting system, other factors may also be pertinent, such as the need for medication which may cause unwanted bradycardia, or concern in a motor vehicle driver that an accident might result should syncope occur.

There are published international guidelines relating to the indications for pacemaker implantation, some of which the author has found somewhat difficult to interpret! The indications below are largely in accordance with those guidelines.

COMPLETE ATRIOVENTRICULAR BLOCK

Syncope

The most common reason for pacemaker implantation is to prevent syncope or near-syncope due to complete AV block. A single episode is a sufficient indication and since the next blackout may cause injury or be fatal, delay should be minimal. Even in patients with a short life expectancy, pacing should be considered if by preventing syncope, independence may be preserved and serious injury avoided.

Dyspnoea and heart failure

Complete heart block can reduce cardiac output and thereby cause exertional dyspnoea and sometimes cardiac failure. Pacing usually improves these problems.

Prognosis

Without pacing, the prognosis in patients with complete heart block is poor. With an artificial pacemaker, life expectancy closely approaches that of the general population, though those with overt coronary heart disease or with heart failure have a less good outlook.

Pacemaker implantation should be considered in asymptomatic patients with complete AV block, particularly when the ventricular rate is 40 beats/min or less, on purely prognostic grounds. Furthermore, by preventing a first syncopal episode, pacing may well prevent major injury to the patient.

QRS breadth

Narrow ventricular complexes during complete AV block suggests that interruption in conduction is at AV nodal level and that, in contrast to infranodal block, a subsidiary pacemaker within the bundle of His will discharge reliably at a relatively rapid ventricular rate. However, in practice, patients with narrow ventricular complexes during complete heart block may experience syncope and impaired exercise tolerance. In the United Kingdom, one-third of patients who receive pacemakers for complete AV block have narrow QRS complexes.

Congenital heart block

Congenital heart block (i.e. complete AV block that is discovered as a neonate or child and is not caused by acquired disease) is widely regarded as benign. This is incorrect. Some patients do develop symptoms or die suddenly. If heart block has caused symptoms then pacing is indicated.

In young, asymptomatic patients the risks of not implanting a pacemaker have to be weighed against the possibility of complications associated with several decades of pacing. There are several documented risk factors: day-time ventricular rate less than 50 beats/min, broad QRS complexes, pauses more than 3.0 s, frequent ventricular ectopic beats and poor chronotropic response to exercise.

Unpaced patients should undergo ambulatory and exercise electrocardiography at regular intervals. In older patients who are found to have congenital heart block, the threshold for implanting a pacemaker should be low.

Cerebration

Mental impairment is sometimes attributed to heart block but is unlikely to improve with pacing. If there is doubt, it is best to undertake a trial of temporary pacing.

SECOND-DEGREE ATRIOVENTRICULAR BLOCK

Mobitz II AV block often progresses to complete AV block. The approach to Mobitz II is the same as that for complete AV block.

A study has refuted the previously held view that Mobitz I (Wenckebach) AV block is benign in that the incidence of symptoms, prognosis and influence of pacing were the same as for patients with Mobitz II block. However, Mobitz I block in young people with transient and often nocturnal Wenckebach block is due to high vagal tone. It is benign and pacing is not indicated.

Adult patients who are found to have AV Wenckebach block during daytime should be considered for pacing unless they undertake a lot of physical training, in which case their AV block may be attributable to high vagal tone.

FIRST-DEGREE ATRIOVENTRICULAR BLOCK

First-degree AV block is not usually an indication for cardiac pacing. If a patient presents with first-degree block and syncope or near-syncope it is quite possible that the symptoms are due to transient second- or third-degree AV block but a pacemaker should not be implanted without proof of this (e.g. by ambulatory electrocardiography).

Rarely, the PR interval is so long that the P wave immediately follows the preceding QRS complex. This may lead to the equivalent of the 'pacemaker syndrome' (see below) in which case dual chamber pacing is indicated.

BUNDLE BRANCH AND FASCICULAR BLOCKS

Bundle branch block

The risk of high-degree AV block developing in an asymptomatic patient with either left or right bundle branch block is small, and pacing is not indicated. In patients who present with syncope or near-syncope the approach should be the same as for first-degree AV block.

Bifascicular block

In bifascicular block the remaining functioning fascicle may fail to conduct, intermittently or persistently, and cause high-degree AV block. In patients with a typical history of Stokes–Adams attacks, pacemaker implantation is indicated to prevent syncope without further investigation. With atypical symptoms, high-degree AV block must be documented first. Some patients with bifascicular block have been shown to be prone to ventricular tachycardia.

In asymptomatic bifascicular block, the chances of progression to complete AV block is in the order of 2 per cent per year and the major determinants of prognosis are the presence of coronary artery or myocardial disease; prophylactic pacing is generally not indicated. Additional first-degree AV block or bundle of His electrographic evidence of prolonged infranodal conduction suggests that conduction in the functioning fascicle is also impaired. However, there is no evidence of a higher risk, though guidelines do recommend that patients with bifascicular block who are found to have a markedly prolonged HV interval are considered for pacing.

Alternating bundle branch block

'Alternating bundle branch block' (i.e. alternating patterns of left and right bundle branch block) or alternating left anterior and posterior fascicular block in patients with right bundle branch block is an indication for pacing.

Atrioventricular and bundle branch block after myocardial infarction

AV block due to inferior myocardial infarction usually resolves within a few days and almost always by three weeks. When anterior infarction is complicated by high-degree AV block, there is usually extensive myocardial damage and hence the prognosis is poor. Though block may persist, it is prudent to ensure that the patient is going to survive before implanting a pacemaker. Thus pacemaker implantation should not be considered unless second- or third-degree AV block is present three weeks after both inferior and anterior myocardial infarction.

Bifascicular block persisting after acute anterior infarction complicated by AV block raises the possibility that complete AV block might recur. However, there is little evidence that prophylactic pacing reduces mortality. Intermittent heart block has been demonstrated to occur in some patients with post-infarction bifascicular block and may necessitate pacing.

When a patient is admitted to hospital with heart block, there is often an unnecessary delay before referral for long-term pacing while myocardial infarction is excluded. Unless the patient has experienced typical cardiac pain or there are typical ECG changes of recent infarction, it is very unlikely that AV block has been caused by acute infarction.

SICK SINUS SYNDROME

Syncope

Sick sinus syndrome accounts for more than one-third of pacemaker implantations. Pacing is indicated when syncope or near-syncope are caused. It should be remembered that sinus bradycardia and pauses in sinus node activity for up to 3.0 s, particularly if nocturnal, can be physiological.

Bradycardia–tachycardia syndrome

In patients with the bradycardia–tachycardia syndrome, pacing may be required to avoid severe bradycardia caused by antiarrhythmic drugs. Atrial tachyarrhythmias which start during bradycardia may be prevented by atrial pacing.

Prognosis

Pacing for sick sinus syndrome is not usually indicated in asymptomatic patients. However, pauses in cardiac activity for several seconds might be considered an indication for pacing in those who operate machinery, including a motor car, to avoid an accident should syncope occur.

HYPERSENSITIVE CAROTID SINUS AND MALIGNANT VASOVAGAL SYNDROMES

Pacing will improve symptoms in these syndromes provided there is a significant cardioinhibitory component (see Chapter 17).

HYPERTROPHIC OBSTRUCTIVE CARDIOMYOPATHY

Dual chambered pacing with a short AV delay has been shown to reduce symptoms and left ventricular outflow tract gradient in some patients with hypertrophic obstructive cardiomyopathy who have a pressure gradient across the left ventricular outflow tract.

RESYNCHRONIZATION THERAPY

Biventricular pacing, a relatively new procedure, can markedly improve symptoms and also prognosis in many patients with poor left ventricular function who have marked prolongation of QRS duration and/or evidence of impaired left ventricular synchronization. The left ventricle is activated simultaneously by stimuli conducted via right and left ventricular leads, usually resulting in significant shortening of QRS duration.

Left ventricular pacing is achieved by passing a lead into a lateral branch of the coronary sinus. It can be technically challenging to introduce the lead into a suitable branch of the coronary sinus, achieve a satisfactory stimulation threshold and avoid diaphragmatic stimulation.

PACING MODES

The first generation of pacemakers functioned in a fixed rate mode. The pacemaker stimulated the ventricles regularly, usually at 70 beats/min, irrespective of any spontaneous cardiac activity (Figure 24.1). Competition with a spontaneous rhythm could cause irregular palpitation (Figure 24.2), and stimulation during ventricular repolarization could possibly initiate ventricular fibrillation (see Figure 23.6).

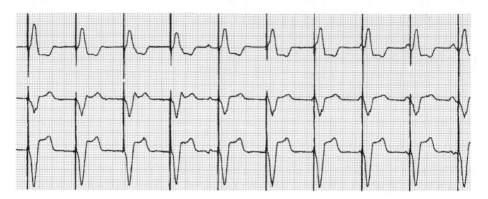

Figure 24.1 Fixed rate ventricular pacing (leads I, II, III). A large pacing stimulus precedes each ventricular complex. P waves dissociated from ventricular complexes can be seen.

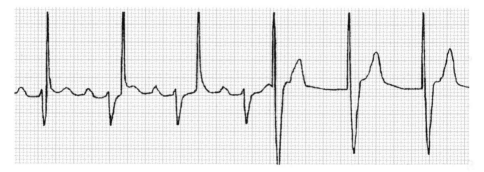

Figure 24.2 Fixed rate ventricular pacing in a patient with first-degree atrioventricular block. The first three stimuli fall during the refractory period and are ineffective. The fourth causes a premature contraction.

Subsequent developments enabled sensing of spontaneous activity via the stimulating lead to facilitate demand pacing. A sensed event resets the timing of delivery of the next pacemaker stimulus to avoid competition with spontaneous activity (Figure 24.3).

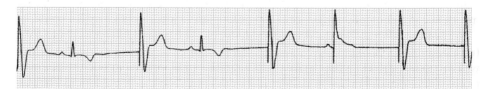

Figure 24.3 Demand ventricular pacemaker. The pacemaker is inhibited by the sinus beats (second and fourth complexes). The sixth complex is a fusion beat. A P wave can be seen to precede the pacing stimulus. By chance, a sinus impulse has arisen at the instant when the pacemaker was set to discharge and the ventricles have been activated by both stimulus impulse and pacemaker. Fusion beats should not be confused with failure to pace.

With the advent of reliable atrial transvenous pacing leads it became straightforward to pace and sense in the atrium as well as the ventricle, thus allowing atrial 'single chamber' pacing and also 'dual chamber' pacing, whereby stimulation and / or sensing can take place at both atrial and ventricular levels. These developments have facilitated a physiological approach to cardiac stimulation.

PACING SYSTEM CODE

A five-letter code is widely used to describe the various pacing modes:

- The first character identifies the chamber or chambers that are paced: 'A' for atrium, 'V' for ventricle and 'D' (for dual) if both atrium and ventricle can be stimulated.
- The second character indicates the chamber or chambers whose activity is sensed. In addition to the use of 'A', 'V' and 'D', 'O' indicates that the pacemaker is insensitive.
- The third character denotes the response to the sensed information. 'I' indicates that pacemaker output is inhibited by a sensed event, 'T' that stimulation is triggered by a sensed event and 'D' that ventricular sensed events inhibit pacemaker output while atrial sensed events trigger ventricular stimulation. 'O' indicates that there is no response to sensed events.
- A fourth character, 'R', is used if there is a rate responsive facility whereby the pacing rate is adjusted by a sensor that detects a physiological variable such as physical activity or respiration.
- The fifth character only relates to multisite pacing: 'O', none; A, V and D indicate a second atrial, ventricular or additional atrial and ventricular leads, respectively.

SINGLE CHAMBER PACING

Ventricular demand pacing (VVI)

In the absence of spontaneous ventricular activity, a ventricular demand pacemaker, like a fixed rate unit, delivers stimuli to the ventricles at a regular rate. However, if spontaneous activity is sensed via the ventricular lead, the timing of delivery of the next pacemaker output is reset to avoid competition.

In ventricular inhibited pacemakers (VVI) a sensed event terminates the current stimulation cycle, thus inhibiting pacemaker output, and starts a new cycle (Figure 24.3).

In contrast, a sensed event during the less commonly used mode of ventricular triggered (VVT) pacing immediately triggers delivery of a pacing stimulus which will consequently fall during the myocardial refractory period and will thus be ineffective. The subsequent cycle will then start from delivery of the triggered impulsive (Figure 24.4).

The pacemaker is rendered insensitive immediately after a paced or sensed event for an interval which approximates the duration of myocardial activation and recovery to prevent sensing the ventricular ECG which is produced by the event. This interval (250–300 ms) is referred to as the refractory period.

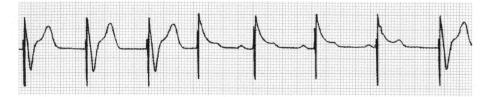

Figure 24.4 Ventricular triggered pacemaker. After the first three paced beats there is sinus rhythm. A pacing stimulus is discharged immediately after the onset of the QRS complex in these spontaneous beats.

Ventricular demand pacing is a commonly employed mode but its use is diminishing now its disadvantages – the inabilities to facilitate the normal sequence of cardiac chamber activation and to provide a chronotropic response to exercise – are widely appreciated (see below).

Indications for ventricular demand pacing include bradycardia associated with persistent atrial fibrillation, second- and third-degree AV block in patients who are limited by impaired cerebral or locomotor function and patients with infrequent bradycardia in whom the pacemaker is mainly on 'stand-by'.

Atrial demand pacing (AAI)

The timing cycles of atrial inhibited (AAI) and the less commonly used atrial triggered (AAT) modes are the same as for ventricular demand pacing, as described above (Figure 24.5). With atrial pacing, the refractory period is usually longer to avoid inappropriate inhibition of the pacemaker by sensing the 'far field' ventricular ECG via the atrial lead.

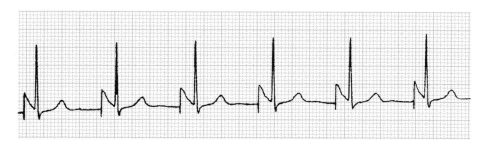

Figure 24.5 Atrial pacing. A pacing stimulus precedes each P wave. Atrioventricular conduction is normal and hence each paced P wave is followed by a normal QRS complex after a normal PR interval.

Atrial pacing is indicated for treatment of the sick sinus syndrome unless AV conduction is impaired. By stimulating the atria rather than the ventricles, the normal sequence of cardiac chamber activation is maintained, loss of which can reduce cardiac output by up to one-third.

In patients with the sick sinus syndrome, atrial pacing has been shown to reduce the incidence of heart failure, atrial fibrillation and stroke as compared with those patients in whom the ventricles are paced.

Sick sinus syndrome can sometimes be associated with impaired AV conduction. However, if there is no evidence of it at the time of pacemaker implantation the subsequent development of impaired AV conduction is uncommon. A dual chamber should, however, be implanted if there is also bifascicular or bundle branch block, or if during pacemaker implantation, atrial pacing at a rate of 120 beats/min causes second-degree AV block.

DUAL CHAMBER PACING

AV sequential pacing (DVI and DDI)

In AV sequential (DVI) pacing the atria are stimulated first and then, after a delay which approximates the normal PR interval, the ventricles are stimulated (Figure 24.6). The pacemaker is inhibited by spontaneous ventricular activity but no sensing occurs in the atrium. As with other dual chamber modes, both atrial and ventricular electrodes are required.

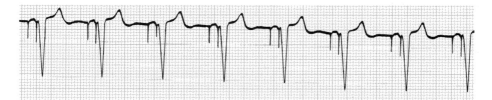

Figure 24.6 Atrioventricular sequential (DVI) pacing. Pacing stimuli precede both atrial and ventricular complexes.

Fusion beats (Figure 24.7) are commonly seen during DVI pacing and are sometimes misinterpreted as pacemaker malfunction. Whereas the pacemaker is inhibited by an event sensed in the ventricles, the first chamber to be stimulated is the atrium. Pacemaker output may therefore occur at the same time as spontaneous atrial activation because its resultant ventricular depolarization has not yet occurred.

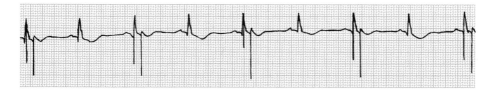

Figure 24.7 DVI pacing: fusion beats.

More recently, the mode of DDI pacing has been introduced. Sensing occurs at atrial as well as ventricular levels, thus avoiding competitive atrial pacing.

Unlike DDD pacing, sensed atrial events do not trigger ventricular stimulation and thus DVI and DDI pacing will not facilitate endless loop tachycardia (see below).

The main indications for DVI and DDI pacing are sick sinus syndrome associated with impaired AV conduction, and carotid sinus and malignant vasovagal syndromes.

Atrial synchronized ventricular pacing (VDD)

In this mode, ventricular stimulation is triggered by a sensed atrial event after an interval similar to the normal PR interval (Figure 24.8). It thereby maintains the normal sequence of cardiac chamber activation. In addition, provided sinus node function is normal, the sinus node rate will increase during exercise and thus lead to an increase in ventricular stimulation rate during exercise (i.e. a chronotropic response to exercise is facilitated).

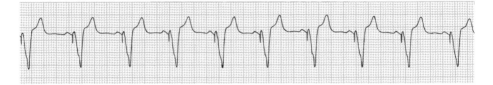

Figure 24.8 Atrial synchronized pacing. Each P wave triggers a paced ventricular beat.

If an atrial event is not sensed, ventricular stimulation continues at a fixed cycle length – otherwise atrial standstill might lead to ventricular asystole. To avoid atrial tachycardia or fibrillation triggering inappropriately fast ventricular pacing rates, there is an atrial refractory interval: the atrial channel is rendered insensitive during the AV delay and for a period after ventricular stimulation. Sensed atrial activity at a cycle length shorter than this period will not trigger ventricular stimulation.

The upper rate at which atrial activity will trigger ventricular output is determined by the 'total atrial refractory period', which consists of the AV delay plus the post-ventricular stimulus refractory period. For example, if the AV delay is 125 ms and the atrial refractory period is 250 ms, the upper rate limit will be 60 000/375 = 160 beats/min.

In earlier years, sensing only took place in the atrium and pacing only occurred in the ventricle (VAT). Thus ventricular ectopic beats or ventricular rhythms faster than the sinus node rate would not inhibit ventricular output. Subsequently, VDD pacing was introduced whereby sensing takes place in the ventricles as well so that spontaneous ventricular activity will inhibit the pacemaker (Figure 24.9).

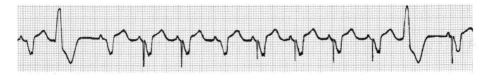

Figure 24.9 VDD pacing, showing chronotropic response to exercise and inhibition of ventricular pacing by ventricular ectopic beats.

Atrial synchronized ventricular pacing is indicated in second- and third-degree AV block when sinus node function is normal. It is contraindicated in the sick sinus syndrome or when there are atrial tachyarrhythmias.

Endless loop tachycardia

If a ventricular stimulus is conducted retrogradely to the atria via either the AV junction or, if present, an accessory AV pathway, and the timing of the resultant atrial activation is outside the pacemaker's atrial refractory period, it will trigger ventricular stimulation and hence initiate an 'endless loop tachycardia' (Figure 24.10), also referred to as 'pacemaker mediated tachycardia'.

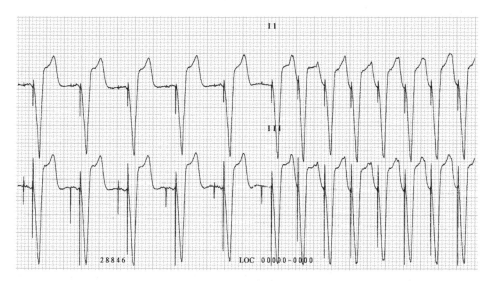

Figure 24.10 Pacemaker-mediated tachycardia after six cycles of dual chamber VDD pacing.

Ventriculoatrial conduction is present in approximately two-thirds of patients with the sick sinus syndrome and one-fifth of those with complete AV block. Endless loop tachycardia can usually be prevented by prolongation of the atrial refractory period but at the expense of reduction of the upper rate limit for ventricular stimulation. Endless loop tachycardia can be avoided in 90 per cent of patients by setting the AV delay to 125 ms and the post-ventricular atrial refractory period to 300 ms.

Most pacemakers can detect endless loop tachycardia and interrupt it, for example, by prolonging the atrial refractory period for one cycle.

Atrioventricular universal pacing (DDD)

In this mode (DDD), which all modern dual chamber pacemakers can facilitate, both sensing and pacing can take place at atrial and ventricular levels. Universal pacing allows the pacemaker to function in atrial demand (AAI), AV sequential

(DVI, DDI) or atrial synchronized (VDD) modes, depending on the spontaneous heart rhythm (Figure 24.11).

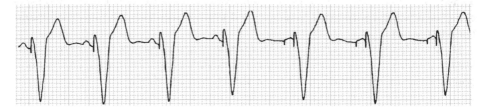

Figure 24.11 Universal (DDD) pacing. In the first four beats, spontaneous P waves trigger ventricular stimulation. There is then sinus node slowing to which the pacemaker responds by pacing the atria as well as the ventricles.

If there is sinus bradycardia it functions as an atrial demand pacemaker. If there is impaired AV conduction, ventricular pacing is triggered by either spontaneous atrial activity or by delivery of an atrial stimulus. When sinus node function is normal, it functions in the atrial synchronized mode, thus providing a chronotropic response to exercise. The pacemaker is inhibited by both atrial and ventricular ectopic beats. Endless loop tachycardia may occur if there is retrograde AV conduction.

DDD pacing is indicated in second- and third-degree AV block. Atrial tachyarrhythmias are a contraindication unless the pacemaker has a mode-switching facility (see below) because the rapid atrial rate would trigger an inappropriately fast ventricular pacing.

'PHYSIOLOGICAL PACING'

Physiological pacing systems facilitate a chronotropic response to exercise by maintaining AV synchronization as the sinus node rate varies and/or by a rate adaptive mechanism.

Atrial synchronized ventricular pacing

VDD and DDD modes both maintain AV synchronization and facilitate a chronotropic response to exercise. Cardiac output has been shown to increase at rest and during exercise as compared with ventricular pacing.

Exercise capacity has been measured on a double-blind basis during ventricular pacing at 70 beats/min and during atrial synchronized ventricular pacing. The latter mode has been demonstrated to increase maximal exercise capacity by approximately 30 per cent. However, individual patients varied in the degree by which they benefited: in a few there was little improvement, whereas in many there was a dramatic increase. Neither age nor cause of heart block predicted the amount of benefit. It used to be thought that 'physiological' pacing was of greatest value to patients with poor ventricular function. This is not the case; indeed, patients with high venous pressures may not benefit.

Atrial synchronized pacing improves parameters in addition to maximal exercise tolerance. Shortness of breath, dizziness and palpitation are less frequent whereas fixed rate pacing tends to impair the normal blood pressure response to exercise and leads to a higher respiratory rate and perceived exertion during submaximal exercise. The advantages of atrial synchronized pacing have been shown to be maintained long term.

There are limitations to atrial synchronized ventricular pacing. First, normal or at least near-normal sinus node activity is required. Second, the ventricular stimulation rate may increase in response to an atrial tachyarrhythmia.

Rate response systems

Several pacing systems are available that can facilitate a chronotropic response independent of atrial activity: a change in stimulation rate is achieved in response to a parameter that alters with exercise. In contrast to atrial synchronized pacing, normal sinus node activity is not required.

In terms of exercise capacity, the ability to increase heart rate is far more important than maintaining AV synchronization. This has been demonstrated by measuring exercise tolerance during three pacing modes: fixed rate, atrial synchronized and ventricular pacing at a rate equal to but not synchronized with atrial activity. Both the latter forms of chronotropic pacing increased exercise performance to a similar degree as compared with fixed rate pacing. Thus rate response ventricular pacemakers can enable an enhanced exercise tolerance without the need for an atrial lead.

Some patients with the sick sinus syndrome have chronotropic incompetence: there is little increase in sinus node rate in response to exercise. A rate responsive system will facilitate an appropriate rate response.

According to the pacemaker code, ventricular demand and dual chambered pacemakers with rate response facilities are termed VVIR and DDDR, respectively.

Activity sensor

Vibration resulting from physical activity is sensed by a piezoelectric crystal attached to the inside of the pacemaker can or an accelerometer bonded to the circuitry within the pacemaker. The stimulation rate increases in parallel with the level of sensed activity. An accelerometer is regarded as more physiological since it will respond to motion primarily in the antero-posterior direction.

The systems have been criticized because they are not truly physiological. For example, the same levels of vibration and hence the same heart rate will be generated by ascending and descending a flight of stairs though less work is required for the latter. There will be no response to non-exertional stresses such as emotion or illness. In addition, in the case of a piezoelectric crystal, the pacemaker rate may increase in response to pressure on the pacemaker can itself. However, in contrast to systems using other sensors, a very prompt and reliable chronotropic response to exercise is achieved and this is the most widely used sensor.

It is possible to modify how the sensor determines the pacing rate by externally programming a number of parameters. These include the reaction time, which is the time during which the initial increase in sensor driven pacing rate occurs; the recovery time, which is the time taken to return to standby rate after activity; and the slope, which determines the relation between sensor activity counts and pacemaker rate.

Evoked QT response

Though it has been known for many years that the QT interval decreases with increasing heart rate, it has only relatively recently been appreciated that sympathetic nervous system activity is a major independent determinant of QT interval duration: QT interval shortens during exercise even during fixed rate pacing.

The pacemaker senses, via a conventional ventricular pacing electrode, the interval between pacing stimulus and apex of the elicited T wave; a decrease in the interval leads to an increase in stimulation rate.

Since this system responds to sympathetic nervous system activity, it will increase the heart rate in response to emotion as well as exertion.

Respiration

There is a close relation between minute volume and heart rate. The system's discharge rate is governed by changes in intravascular impedance, a measure of respiratory minute volume, which is monitored by means of a conventional bipolar pacing lead.

Blood temperature

Skeletal muscle activity generates heat, which is transferred to the blood. There is a relation between level of exercise and right ventricular blood temperature. One problem, however, is that there is a latency in the system due to the delay of 1 or 2 min before blood temperature rises after the start of exercise.

Other sensors

Other parameters such as oxygen saturation and right ventricular pressure have been investigated for use in rate response pacing. Information on long-term reliability of sensors is not yet available. Rate response systems that can use a conventional lead have practical advantages over systems that require a lead incorporating a specialized sensor.

Multisensor pacing

Dual chamber pacemakers are available which, in addition to sensing atrial activity, will respond to parameters related to exercise such as activity or QT interval (DDDR). Thus, normal AV synchrony can be maintained and a chronotropic response to exercise can be provided even if sinus node function is impaired or if an intermittent atrial arrhythmia occurs.

Some newer pacing systems incorporate not one but two types of physiological sensor so that the limitations of each system can be minimized, for example, an activity sensor to provide a prompt response and a QT sensor to ensure the rate response is proportional to the workload.

Automatic mode switching

This relatively new, important facility allows implantation of DDD pacemakers in patients prone to paroxysmal atrial fibrillation and other atrial tachyarrhythmias. When rapid, abnormal atrial activity is sensed, the pacing mode automatically switches from DDD or DDDR to VVI or VVIR, respectively. Dual chamber pacing resumes on termination of the atrial arrhythmia (Figure 24.12).

'Pacemaker syndrome'

It is at rest or during standing that the disadvantage of loss of AV synchrony caused by single chamber ventricular pacing may be most apparent. Atrial contraction may occur against closed mitral and tricuspid valves. Atrial pressure will rise and impede venous return so that during the next diastolic period the ventricles will be underfilled with resultant reduction in stroke volume. Loss of properly timed atrial systole reduces cardiac output by up to one-third and may cause hypotension; near-syncope and syncope can result (Figure 24.13). Other symptoms include weakness, dizziness and dyspnoea.

Hypotension is likely to be more marked whilst standing. It is most severe during the first few seconds of ventricular pacing (Figure 24.14), before vasoconstrictor compensatory mechanisms can come into play, so ventricular pacing is particularly unsuitable for patients who are mainly in sinus rhythm but who often develop bradycardia at a rate less than the cycle length of the ventricular pacemaker (i.e. those with the sick sinus or carotid sinus syndromes). This has been demonstrated by recording ambulatory blood pressure in patients with ventricular demand pacemakers. The onset of ventricular pacing was followed by hypotension, which was greater in those who had complained of syncope and near-syncope.

Ventriculoatrial conduction (Figure 24.15) causes even greater haemodynamic upset; the resultant atrial distension may initiate a reflex vasodepressor effect. AV sequential pacing or, when AV conduction is not impaired, atrial pacing will avoid these problems.

Single chamber versus dual chamber pacing

In recent years, a number of clinical trials have been conducted comparing ventricular demand pacing with dual chamber pacing. Patients both with sinus node disease and with AV block were included. Perhaps not surprisingly, there was no significant difference in mortality or stroke between the two groups. This has led some to conclude that single lead ventricular pacing, which has the advantage of requiring somewhat cheaper hardware and which avoids the not very challenging task of positioning an atrial lead, is adequate. However, these studies showed that dual chamber pacing conferred better exercise tolerance, increased quality of life, reduced the incidence of new atrial fibrillation, and was cost-effective in that it avoided the necessity to upgrade a single chamber system when there were severe symptoms due to the pacemaker syndrome.

In general, single chamber ventricular pacing is *only* indicated in patients with persistent atrial fibrillation or other atrial arrhythmia, or in the very elderly and infirm patient with heart block whose mobility is very limited.

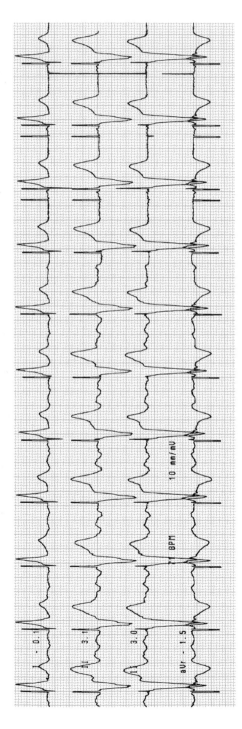

Figure 24.12 Automatic mode switching. During atrial fibrillation, there is VVIR pacing. DDDR pacing returns on termination of atrial fibrillation.

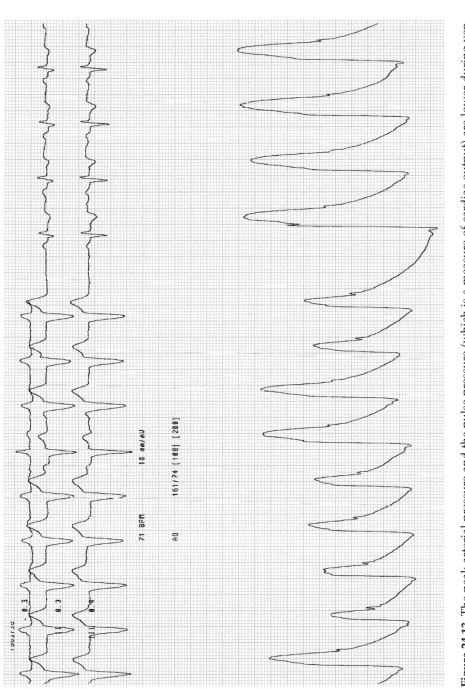

Figure 24.13 The peak arterial pressure and the pulse pressure (which is a measure of cardiac output) are lower during ventricular pacing (left side of panel) than during sinus rhythm (right side of panel). During ventricular pacing, the pressure varies depending on the relation between paced beats and dissociated P waves.

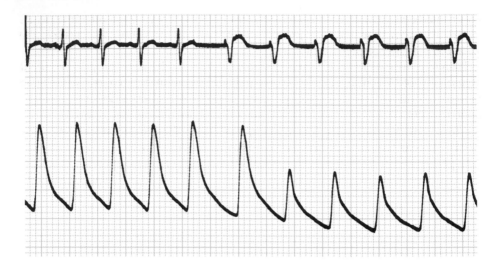

Figure 24.14 Pacemaker syndrome. There was symptomatic hypotension (lower trace) during ventricular pacing which occurs after the first four sinus beats.

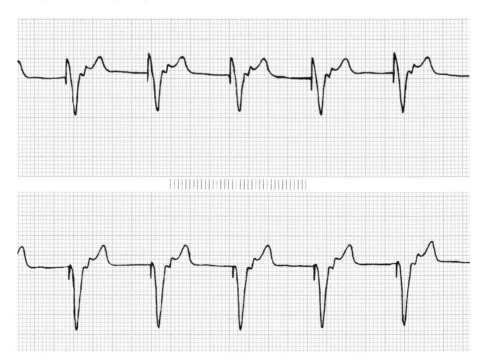

Figure 24.15 Ventricular pacing with retrograde activation (leads II and III). Each ventricular complex is followed by an inverted P wave.

Right ventricular apical pacing may cause heart failure

Several recent studies have clearly shown that long-term right ventricular apical pacing can impair ventricular function and cause heart failure. The incidence of failure has been shown to be related to the amount of pacing compared with normal ventricular activation (i.e. the greater the percentage of ventricular pacing the greater the incidence of heart failure).

Therefore, in patients with dual chamber systems with no or only intermittent abnormality of AV conduction, the AV delay should if possible be increased to facilitate normal ventricular activation (e.g. program the AV interval up to 250 ms). Another option is right ventricular outflow tract rather than apical pacing (see below).

Nuclear myocardial perfusion imaging has shown that apical pacing can cause perfusion defects even in patients with normal coronary arteries.

In patients with right ventricular apical leads who have developed heart failure, marked improvement can be achieved by upgrading to a biventricular pacemaker.

PACEMAKER HARDWARE

PULSE GENERATOR

A pulse generator consists of a power source together with electronic circuits to control the timing and characteristics of the impulses that it generates.

In the past, several power sources have been used, including mercury zinc cells, rechargeable nickel cadmium cells and nuclear energy. Now, lithium iodide cells are used almost exclusively. Lithium pacemakers have a lifespan of 4–15 years and predictable, progressive discharge behaviour. They are contained in a hermetically sealed titanium can, 35–50 g in weight, and generally have a maximum diameter of no more than 50 mm and a thickness of as little as 6 mm.

PACEMAKER LEADS

Stimuli produced by the pulse generator are conducted to the heart via a lead that consists of an insulated wire with an electrode at its tip which is attached to the heart.

Transvenous leads are used in virtually all pacemaker implantations. A modern lead consists of a multifilar, helically coiled wire that is insulated by a material that does not cause tissue reaction or thrombosis: silicone rubber or polyurethane. At the lead tip is the cathode, which is composed of an inert material such as platinum-iridium, Elgiloy, steel or vitreous carbon. For effective stimulation, this must be securely and closely attached to the endocardium. If fibrous tissue, which is non-excitable, develops between cathode and endocardium the amount of energy required to stimulate the heart will increase and may exceed the output capability of the pacemaker.

To achieve secure endocardial attachment and a low threshold for stimulation, several 'fixation devices' have been employed. 'Passive' fixation devices include tines, flanges or fins positioned proximal to the lead tip, which can become entrapped in the myocardial trabeculae. 'Active' devices involve a metal screw, usually retractable, that can be screwed into the endo-myocardium (Figure 24.16). 'Porous' metal or carbon electrodes are now widely used; the surface of the cathode consists of many microscopic

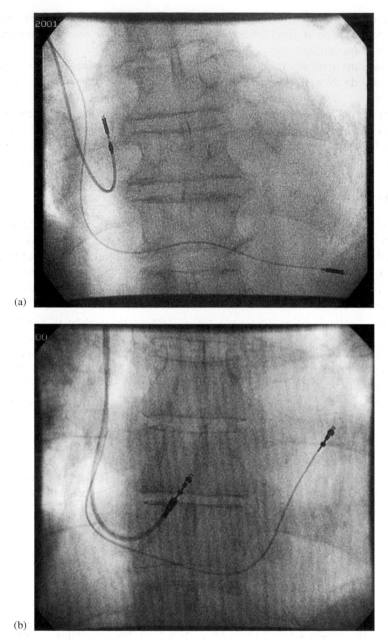

Figure 24.16 (a) X-ray showing 'screw-in leads' positioned in right ventricular apex and right atrial appendage. (b) X-ray showing 'screw-in leads' positioned in right ventricular outflow tract and on low atrial septum.

pores that promote rapid tissue ingrowth and hence very secure fixation. Movement between electrode and endocardium and thus generation of fibrous tissue is minimized. Many types of electrode elute dexamethasone to minimize local tissue reaction and hence stimulation threshold.

Attachment of atrial leads was impracticable until the advent of fixation devices. The distal portions of atrial leads are often 'J' shaped to facilitate positioning in the right atrial appendage.

The amount of energy required to stimulate the heart is related to the surface area of the cathode. Nowadays, low surface area electrodes are used, with a surface area of 6–12 mm^2.

Leads that are sewn on to the epicardium or screwed into the myocardium necessitate thoracotomy and are now, with the advent of reliable transvenous leads, rarely used unless pacemaker implantation is undertaken at the time of open heart surgery, or venous thrombosis or a tricuspid valve prosthesis preclude a transvenous approach.

Unipolar versus bipolar pacing

In unipolar pacing the anode is remote from the heart; it is usually the metal can that contains the pulse generator. In bipolar pacing, both anode and cathode are within the cardiac chamber to be paced, the anode positioned along the lead near to its cathodal tip. A commonly held view is that an electrogram sensed by a unipolar lead is larger than that from a bipolar lead. There is in fact usually no difference between bipolar and unipolar electrograms or stimulation thresholds.

Bipolar pacing has the advantage that inappropriate sensing of electromagnetic interference and skeletal muscle electromyograms is much less likely, as is extracardiac stimulation. Reasons for favouring unipolar pacing are that there is greater experience with unipolar leads, in the past bipolar electrodes have been less reliable and larger in calibre, and surface ECG unipolar pacemaker stimuli are larger, making ECG interpretation easier. Nowadays, bipolar pacing leads are reliable and are to be preferred.

COSTS

In the United Kingdom, the current approximate costs of a pulse generator plus leads for single chamber and dual chambered rate responsive pacing systems are £900 and £1700, respectively.

PACEMAKER IMPLANTATION

For pacemaker implantation, facilities for fluoroscopy, ECG monitoring and cardiopulmonary resuscitation are required. The procedure is usually carried out under local anaesthesia and takes 15–45 min. Conscious sedation, as discussed in Chapter 20, is often used. Strict aseptic technique is essential. Thorough handwashing is necessary: surgical gloves have been shown to be imperfect barriers.

SUBCLAVIAN APPROACH

The subclavian approach is now widely used and is especially useful if more than one lead is to be inserted. The pacemaker lead(s) are introduced via infraclavicular subclavian vein puncture and are connected to the pulse generator which is implanted in a subcutaneous pocket fashioned over pectoralis major.

Usually, the left subclavian vein is used. Occasionally, however, a persistent left-sided superior vena cava which will drain into the coronary sinus will be encountered, dictating that the atrial and/or ventricular leads will have to be positioned via the coronary sinus. This is almost always possible but is technically challenging. A left-sided superior vena cava is most commonly encountered in a patient with congenital heart disease, particularly atrial septal defect. If a patient is known to have congenital heart disease, the right subclavian vein is to be preferred.

An incision is made 2 cm below the junction of the middle and inner thirds of the clavicle and is extended in a lateral and inferior direction for approximately 6 cm. A subcutaneous pocket large enough to accommodate the pulse generator is created by blunt dissection.

Puncture of the subclavian vein is easier if the vein is distended: a slight head-down position will help or, alternatively, the legs should be raised. Dehydration, which can markedly reduce venous pressure and thereby make puncture more difficult, should be avoided or corrected.

A needle is introduced just below the inferior border of the clavicle at the junction of its middle and inner thirds and directed towards the sternoclavicular joint so that it passes behind the posterior surface of the clavicle. As the needle punctures the vein, venous blood will be aspirated easily; only a trickle suggests that the needle is not in the vein. Aspiration of air or bright pulsatile blood indicate puncture of the pleura or subclavian artery, respectively. If the patient has a 'deep' chest, and particularly if the clavicle bows anteriorly, it may be necessary to introduce the needle a little more laterally and to point it slightly posteriorly.

Cannulation of the vein is then achieved by introducing a flexible guidewire, preferably with a J-shaped tip, through the needle. Resistance to its passage indicates that the wire is not in the vein. The wire is passed into the superior vena cava and its position checked by fluoroscopy. (If screening demonstrates that the wire is in the centre of the chest it is likely that the subclavian artery has been entered and the tip of the wire is in the aorta.) The needle is then withdrawn and a sheath, within which is a vessel dilator, is passed over the wire into the vein. The guidewire and dilator are then removed and the pacing lead inserted into the sheath. If it is planned to introduce a second pacing lead, then the guidewire can be left in place to permit introduction of a second introducer and sheath. 'Peel-away' sheaths are used so that their removal is not prevented by the connector at the proximal end of the lead.

Cephalic vein approach

An alternative to subclavian vein puncture is to cut down onto the cephalic vein in the deltopectoral groove. This approach avoids the risks of subclavian vein puncture but sometimes the vein is not big enough to accommodate two leads and occasionally is even too small for one lead. It can sometimes be difficult to advance a lead from the cephalic into the subclavian vein. However, use of a hydrophilically coated guidewire, over which introducer and sheath are advanced, makes negotiation of the bends between the cephalic and subclavian veins very much easier.

POSITIONING OF A VENTRICULAR LEAD

To facilitate manipulation of a long-term pacing lead, which is very flexible, a wire stylet is passed down the centre of the lead. Bending the distal part of the stylet or slight withdrawal will often aid positioning.

The lead is passed into the right atrium (see Figure 23.1). Sometimes the lead can then be directly advanced through the tricuspid valve to the right ventricular apex. More often, it is necessary to form a loop in the atrium by impinging the lead tip on the atrial wall and then advancing the lead a little further. By rotating the lead its tip can then be positioned near the tricuspid valve. Slight withdrawal of the lead will allow it to 'flick' through the valve into the ventricle. Ventricular ectopic beats are almost always provoked as the valve is crossed. *If these do not occur then it is probable that the coronary sinus has been entered* (see Figure 23.1).

Entry into the ventricle can be confirmed by advancing the lead into the pulmonary artery. Once in the right ventricle, the lead tip is positioned in or near the ventricular apex by a process of lead rotation, advancement and withdrawal. A stable position should be ensured by checking for continuous pacing and for absence of excessive lead tip movement during deep inspiration and coughing. Additional measures to ensure lead stability include brief partial withdrawal of the lead so that there is only a little slack and then temporarily advancing the lead so that there is excessive slack in the body of the lead.

Once a satisfactory position has been achieved both in terms of stability and measurements (see below), it is essential that the lead is secured by placing a short sleeve around it near its point of entry into the vein and fixing it to the underlying muscle with a non-absorbable suture. It is important to check that the lead is securely fixed – otherwise lead displacement may occur.

Recently, there has been increasing interest in pacing the right ventricular outflow tract rather than apex. The author uses this approach routinely. There is evidence of haemodynamic advantage in some patients and no evidence of harm. An active fixation lead is required.

POSITIONING OF AN ATRIAL LEAD

The right atrial appendage is the usual site for atrial pacing. If necessary, atrial pacing may be performed by using a 'screw-in' lead to pace from the septal or free right atrial walls.

For pacing the right atrial appendage, a lead with a J-shaped terminal portion is usually used. First, using a straight stylet, the lead tip is straightened and advanced to the mid-right atrium. The lead is then rotated so that its tip is near the tricuspid valve. Partial withdrawal of the stylet causes the lead to assume its J shape and slight withdrawal of the lead itself allows the lead tip to enter the appendage. A straight lead may be positioned in the appendage by use of a stylet whose terminal 5 cm has been shaped into a tight J-shaped curve.

Correct positioning will be demonstrated by the lead tip moving from side to side with atrial systole. Lateral screening will demonstrate that the lead is pointing anteriorly. Lead stability should be confirmed by twisting the lead 45 degrees in either direction; the lead tip should not turn. It is important that there is the correct amount of slack in the lead. During inspiration the angle between the two limbs of the J should not exceed 80 degrees.

MEASUREMENT OF STIMULATION AND SENSING THRESHOLDS

Low stimulation and sensing thresholds are essential for satisfactory long-term pacing. High thresholds suggest that the cathode is not in close apposition to excitable tissue. Thresholds rise after pacemaker implantation, usually peaking three weeks to three months after surgery. If they become high they may exceed the stimulation and sensing capabilities of the pulse generator. Thresholds are usually measured with a commercially produced pacing systems analyser (PSA). It is preferable to match the analyser with the generator to be implanted so that they have similar impulse generating and sensing circuits. The unipolar or bipolar electrode configuration should be the same as that planned to be used in the implanted system.

Stimulation threshold

The stimulation threshold is the smallest electrical stimulus (delivered by the cathode outside the ventricular effective and relative refractory periods) that will consistently activate the myocardium.

To measure the stimulation threshold, the analyser is usually set to deliver impulses at 70 beats/min (or if there is no bradycardia at the time, 10 beats/min in excess of the spontaneous rate) with an impulse duration similar to that which the implanted pulse generator will deliver (often 0.5 ms) and a voltage output of 5 V. The threshold is then established by progressively reducing the output until failure of capture occurs. If the patient has no spontaneous rhythm, pacemaker output will have to be promptly increased to avoid asystole. It is very important to know that the stimulation threshold is substantially greater when increasing from a sub-threshold level. This phenomenon is known as the Wedensky phenomenon (Figure 24.17). Therefore, as soon as there is a failure to capture, output should be immediately increased by at least 2 V.

At a pulse duration of 0.5 ms, a voltage threshold of less than 1 V is satisfactory; often the threshold will be less than 0.5 V. It should be noted that with screw-in leads the threshold can initially be quite high but will fall within 3–4 min after fixation.

It is important that the distal and proximal poles of the electrode are connected to the pacemaker cathode (−) and anode (+), respectively. If the poles are reversed, the stimulation threshold will be significantly higher. The longer the duration of the pacing stimulus the more energy is delivered and hence the lower the stimulation threshold. However, the relationship is not linear: the range of efficient impulse duration, in terms of energy consumption, is 0.25–1.0 ms (Figure 24.18). (The output at which a further increase in pulse duration does not reduce the stimulation threshold is called the rheobase. Twice this value is termed the chronaxie.)

When measuring the stimulation threshold of a unipolar lead the distal pole of the electrode is connected to the pacemaker cathode (−) and the proximal electrode (+) is connected to a metal object such as a self-retaining retractor which is placed

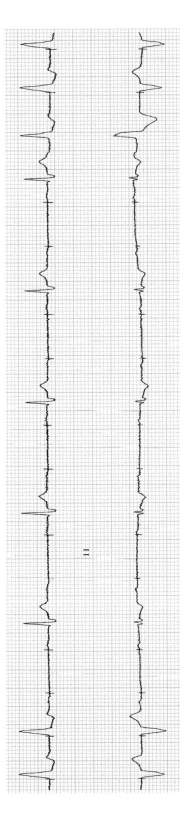

Figure 24.17 Wedensky phenomenon. The stimulation threshold is measured by progressively reducing the ventricular output by 0.1 V decrements until after the second paced beat there is failure to capture. The output is then increased by 0.1 V increments. Only after 10 increments is ventricular capture achieved. Had there not been a spontaneous rhythm while there was failure to capture there would have been an embarrassing and probably symptomatic period of asystole! The output should have been immediately increased by at least 2 V as soon as the stimulation threshold had been established.

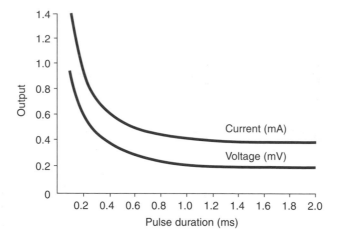

Figure 24.18 Typical strength-duration curve. The stimulation threshold is measured at different pulse widths. There is no significant reduction in stimulation threshold when the pulse duration is increased above 1.0 ms.

in the wound. It is important that the surface area of the anode approximates that of the pacemaker can, otherwise a falsely high threshold will be obtained.

Sensing threshold

To ensure satisfactory sensing it is important that the intracardiac electrogram resulting from spontaneous activity of the cardiac chamber to be paced is of sufficient amplitude. It is usually measured with a pacing systems analyser. Ventricular and atrial electrograms should be greater than 4 mV and 2 mV, respectively. In 'borderline' cases the slew rate (i.e. the rate of change of signal voltage) is also important: low rates may result in failure to sense.

Lead impedance

The pacing systems analyser can also be used to measure lead impedance, which is a measure of resistance to flow of current in the lead. It varies with lead type but is usually in the order of 400–1000 ohms.

A low impedance suggests a break in insulation and hence leakage of current, whereas a high impedance points to lead fracture.

Paced ventricular electrogram

Pacing the right ventricular apex will lead to a ventricular complex with left axis deviation and left bundle branch block configuration (Figure 24.19). Right ventricular outflow tract pacing results in right axis deviation and left bundle branch block configuration (Figure 24.20) as would occur with right ventricular outflow tract tachycardia (see Chapter 12). Inadvertent pacing of the left ventricle via a patent foramen ovale leads to a paced complex with right bundle branch block configuration.

Biventricular pacing for resynchronization therapy typically results in a relatively narrow ventricular complex (Figure 24.21, see pages 265 and 266).

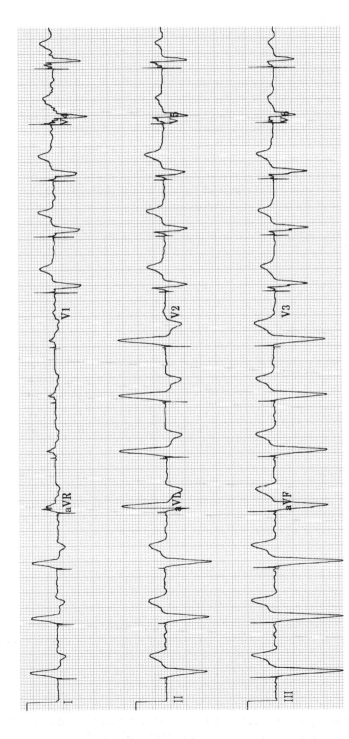

Figure 24.19 Right ventricular apical pacing: left axis deviation and left bundle branch block configuration.

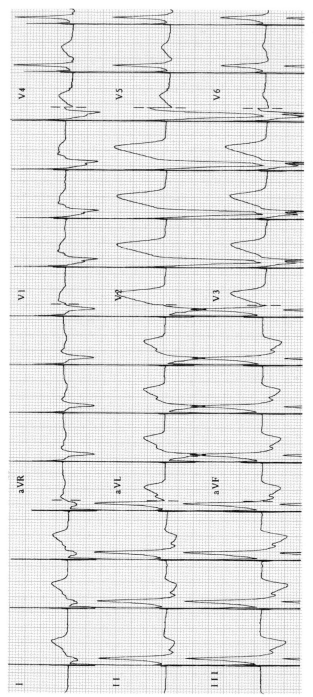

Figure 24.20 Right ventricular outflow tract pacing: right axis deviation and left bundle branch block configuration.

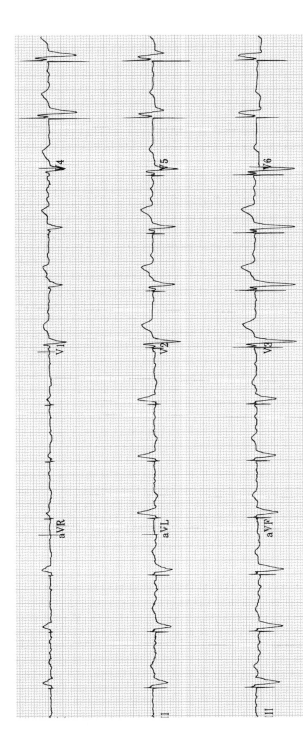

Figure 24.21 (a) Biventricular pacing resulting in shorter QRS duration than occurs with single lead stimulation.

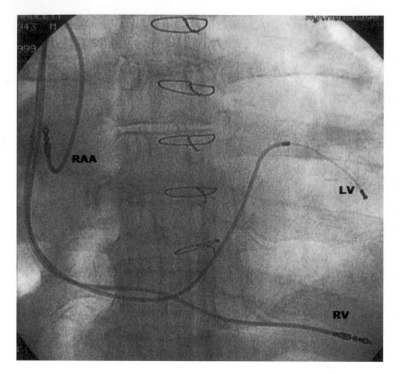

Figure 24.21 (b) Biventricular pacing leads. Radiograph showing leads in right atrial appendage (RAA), apex of right ventricle (RV), and lateral branch of coronary sinus (LV).

FASHIONING A PACEMAKER POCKET

It might appear that creating a pocket for the pacemaker is the least challenging part of the implantation procedure. However, unless done well wound complications are likely; often, they develop some months after implantation.

A subcutaneous space to accommodate the pacemaker is usually fashioned by blunt dissection. Extensive infiltration with local anaesthesia is required and even then some patients experience discomfort during the minute or so that the pocket is created. It is important that the wound is sufficiently deep so that the pacemaker is placed on the surface of the pectoral muscle. A common mistake is to site the pocket close to the clavicle where there is little subcutaneous tissue – inviting pacemaker erosion. The pocket should be positioned more inferiorly, enabling it to be covered by a thicker layer of 'flesh'.

Fashioning of a generator pocket that is too large may allow spontaneous or intentional repeated rotation of the pulse generator, which can cause dislodgement or fracture of the pacing lead – the 'twiddler's syndrome'. Too small a pocket and the skin over the pacemaker will be tense and erosion is likely.

In very thin patients or in those who are anxious for the generator to be as inconspicuous as possible, the device should be positioned beneath the pectoral muscle.

COMPLICATIONS OF PACEMAKER IMPLANTATION

Bleeding

Mild bruising is not uncommon but occasionally, poor haemostasis will result in a haematoma which, if tense, must be evacuated without delay.

Not infrequently, patients requiring pacemaker implantation are receiving warfarin. This drug will need to be stopped to allow the INR to fall to a value not more than 1.7. A small dose of *oral* vitamin K can be very effective at reducing the INR.

Lead displacement

Lead displacement was once a common problem but with modern leads it occurs in less than 1 per cent of implantations; it necessitates re-operation.

Subclavian vein puncture

Complications of attempted subclavian vein puncture are infrequent. They include pneumothorax, haemothorax, air embolism, brachial plexus damage and puncture of the subclavian artery. Surprisingly, inadvertent subclavian artery puncture only rarely leads to problems.

Infection

Infection should occur in less than 1 per cent of implantations and is virtually always staphylococcal. Unless it is only superficial, explantation will usually be required even if antibiotics appear to help initially. Ideally, the pacing lead(s) should be removed and this is very desirable if there has been systemic infection. It is usually easy to remove leads within the first few months of implantation by moderate, sustained traction. Clearly, with screw-in leads the metal tip needs to be retracted before removal. However, removal late after implantation can be difficult, particularly if the leads have a passive fixation device such as fins. Use of special lead extraction devices such as 'locking stylettes' are often effective and reduce the risk of cardiac tamponade. Rarely, it is necessary to resort to thoracotomy. Alternatively, the lead can be shortened so that it no longer lies in or close to the infected area. The proximal end should be capped and fixed with a suture. However, there is a risk of persistent infection and bacteraemia.

Several studies have shown that antibiotic cover, usually with flucloxacillin, reduces the risk of infection.

Erosion

Erosion of the skin overlying the pacemaker is a late complication but is often a consequence of implantation technique. Factors that predispose to erosion include creation of a pacemaker pocket that is too tight or too superficial, a very thin patient, and use of a generator with sharp corners. The skin will be found to be thinned around the site of erosion. Infection is often present but it is secondary to erosion. If the skin is broken, explantation will be necessary.

Thinned, reddened skin over the generator is a sign of 'threatened' erosion: *the generator should be re-sited without delay.*

COMPLICATIONS RELATED TO PULSE GENERATOR

Electromyographic interference

This common problem is virtually confined to unipolar pacing systems. Myopotentials generated from the underlying muscle are sensed by the pacemaker as spontaneous cardiac activity (Figure 24.22). In systems where sensed events inhibit output, inappropriate cessation of pacing will occur. Short periods of electromyographic inhibition are common and usually asymptomatic. Longer periods may cause syncope and necessitate adjustment to sensitivity, pacing mode or polarity.

Susceptibility to electromyographic inhibition can be demonstrated by asking the patient to extend his or her arms and then to press the hands firmly together. Inhibition is only significant if it lasts for several seconds, particularly if the patient's symptoms are reproduced.

Muscle stimulation

This complication is also related to unipolar pacing and is a consequence of the pacemaker can being the anode. Stimulation of the underlying pectoral muscle occurs.

Generator failure

Premature generator failure does occur occasionally. Very rarely, a device can malfunction such that it delivers pacing stimuli at an extremely fast rate with the risk of initiating ventricular fibrillation – a 'runaway pacemaker' (Figure 24.23).

COMPLICATIONS RELATED TO PACING LEAD

Exit block

The development of excessive fibrous tissue, which is non-excitable, around the cathode may increase the stimulation threshold to a level higher than the pacemaker's output. The result will be intermittent or persistent failure to pace without evidence of lead displacement (Figure 24.24). Exit block is most likely to occur in the first three weeks to three months after implantation, when stimulation threshold is at its highest. Sometimes exit block is transient, otherwise lead repositioning will be required unless generator output can be increased by reprogramming (see below). Modern leads with low surface area, porous surfaced electrodes and positive fixation devices rarely cause this complication.

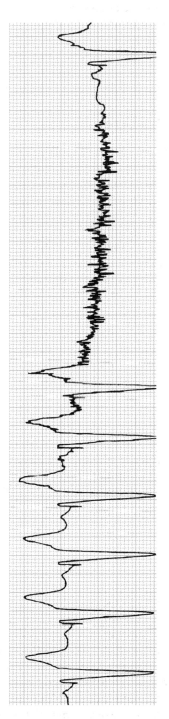

Figure 24.22 Electromyographic inhibition of a DDD pacemaker. Activities such as washing hands caused near-syncope. Corrected by decreasing pacemaker sensitivity.

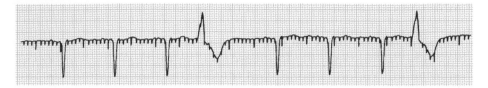

Figure 24.23 A runaway pacemaker. Fortunately, in this case the stimuli were sub-threshold.

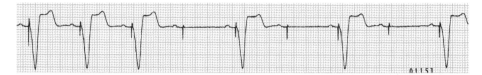

Figure 24.24 DDD pacing. After three paced ventricular complexes, there is intermittent exit block: pacing stimuli are not followed by ventricular complexes.

Lead fracture and insulation breakdown

With modern leads, fracture is rare. If it does occur it is usually at the point where the lead enters the venous system, at the site of a fixation suture or wherever there is excessive angulation of the lead. Lead fracture will cause intermittent or persistent failure to pace and sense. Lead impedance will be very high.

Lead fracture can often be detected radiographically but should not be confused with 'pseudofracture', in which the pressure of a tight ligature directly applied to the lead compresses the insulation and spreads the coils of wire inside without interfering with lead function.

Insulation breakdown will allow leakage of current, which may cause stimulation of adjacent muscles, and hence premature battery depletion. Lead impedance will be markedly reduced. A tight ligature anchoring the lead without use of a rubber sleeve is a common cause. Some types of polyurethane insulation are prone to this problem.

Lead fracture and insulation breakdown are less common with a cephalic vein approach.

Phrenic nerve and diaphragmatic stimulation

The phrenic nerve or diaphragm can sometimes be stimulated through the intervening thin myocardial walls by atrial and ventricular leads, respectively. Lead repositioning will be required unless, in programmable pacemakers, cessation of extracardiac stimulation can be achieved by output reduction.

Venous thrombosis

Clinically apparent subclavian vein thrombosis is rare and pulmonary embolism even rarer. Anticoagulant therapy is indicated. Angiographic studies have reported that asymptomatic venous thrombosis is not infrequent.

PACEMAKER PROGRAMMABILITY

A programmable pacemaker can be non-invasively adjusted in one or more of its functions by radiofrequency signals emitted from an external programming device. Programmability enables achievement of optimal pacemaker function for the individual patient and can also be used in the diagnosis and treatment of certain pacemaker complications; it reduces the need for pacemaker re-operation.

Simple programmable pacemakers permit alteration to rate and output. In multiprogrammable pacemakers a wide variety of parameters can be adjusted. These are listed below together with typical options:

1. Lower rate limit (30–150 beats/min)
2. Output (2.5–7.5 V)
3. Pulse duration (0.1–1.0 ms)
4. Sensitivity (0.25–8 mV)
5. Pacing mode (e.g. AAI, VVI, DDD, rate responsive)
6. Refractory period (200–500 ms)
7. Pacing polarity (uni- or bipolar)
8. Upper rate limits (100–180 beats/min) (for dual chamber and rate response pacemakers)
9. AV delay (0–300 ms) (for dual chamber pacemakers)

Some pacemakers are software based. Many functions are controlled by a microcomputer within the pacemaker which can be externally programmed; functions can be modified and new developments incorporated that had not even been anticipated at the time of implantation.

Some examples of the advantages of programmability are discussed below.

In patients who are mainly in sinus rhythm, reduction of the stand-by rate will allow sinus rhythm to be maintained for longer periods and will therefore help to avoid the haemodynamic disadvantages of ventricular pacing. Reduction of stimulation rate may occasionally help in the management of angina. Sometimes an increase in rate is helpful in the treatment of cardiac failure or arrhythmias.

Usually, the stimulation threshold is a lot lower than the maximum output of a pacemaker; a reduction in output will prolong battery life. At regular intervals, the threshold can be measured by progressive reduction in output and then the output programmed to the threshold value plus a safety margin. Extracardiac stimulation can often be stopped by reduction in output without approaching the threshold level. Some pacemakers have a high output facility (e.g. ability to increase output from 5 to 10 V): use of this may avoid the need for re-operation should exit block, which may be a temporary problem, occur.

Increase in sensitivity of the amplifier circuits may help with undersensing whereas inappropriate sensing of T waves or after-potentials may be dealt with by reduction in sensitivity or prolongation of refractory period.

Reduction in sensitivity may prevent electromyographic inhibition. Alternatively, reprogramming from inhibited to triggered mode will at least prevent bradycardia even if the electromyographic potentials reset the stimulation cycle. Another solution is to change from unipolar to bipolar pacing in systems that have this facility.

Atrial pacemakers require a higher sensitivity, because the atrial electrogram is usually of lower amplitude than its ventricular counterpart, and a longer refractory period to avoid sensing the far-field ventricular electrogram. A multiprogrammable generator can be adjusted for use as either an atrial or a ventricular pacemaker.

In dual chamber pacing systems, prolongation of the atrial refractory period may prevent endless loop tachycardia. Sometimes endless loop tachycardia can be prevented by reducing sensitivity of the atrial channel so that the atrial electrogram during sinus rhythm is sensed but the atrial electrogram resulting from retrograde conduction, which is usually of lower amplitude, is not detected. In patients with the sick sinus syndrome, reprogramming from DDD to DDI or DVI modes will prevent endless loop tachycardia. Alteration from DDD to VVI may be required should atrial fibrillation develop.

Many pacemakers have the facility of rate hysteresis. The interval after a sensed event which would trigger delivery of a pacemaker stimulus can be greater than the interval between paced beats. For example, a pacemaker can be programmed to stimulate the heart at 70 beats/min only if the spontaneous rate falls below 40 beats/min, thus helping to avoid problems that might occur with loss of AV synchrony.

TELEMETRY DATA

With most modern pacemakers, real-time and stored intracardiac electrograms can be obtained by telemetry (Figures 24.25 and 24.26).

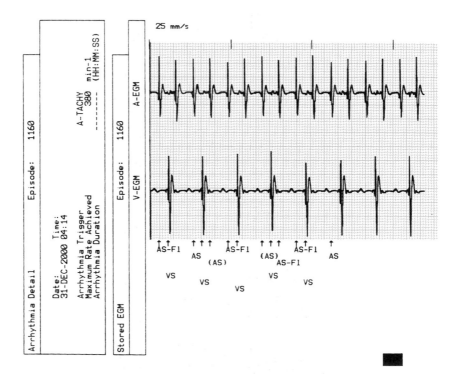

Figure 24.25 Real-time intra-atrial and intraventricular electrograms obtained by telemetry showing atrial fibrillation in a patient with a mode-switching pacemaker.

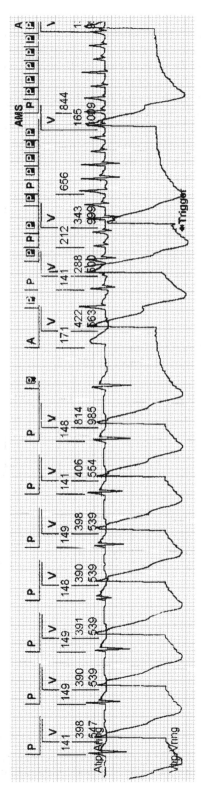

Figure 24.26 Stored electrogram showing intracardiac atrial ($A_{tip}A_{ring}$) and ventricular ($V_{tip}V_{ring}$) electrograms at the onset of an episode of atrial fibrillation resulting in almost immediate mode switching (AMS).

Other telemetered information includes how the pacemaker has been programmed; lead impedance; battery impedance and status; the percentages of time during which there has been pacing or inhibition; and range of paced and sensed heart rates that have occurred. These latter data can be helpful in programming rate responsive systems to ensure that the sensor facilitates an appropriate chronotropic response.

PACEMAKER CLINIC

FOLLOW-UP

Patients with implanted pacemakers should regularly attend a follow-up clinic. The purposes are to check that the pacemaker is working satisfactorily; to ensure that there are no pacing complications; to detect impending battery depletion so that generator replacement can be carried out before the patient is at risk; to adjust pacemaker output to at least twice stimulation threshold; and to maintain a record of patients' locations should a recall of a particular generator or lead be necessary.

Occasionally, a manufacturer reports that a fault has occurred in some of its pacemakers. Usually, the failure rate is very low but regulations dictate that a report is made and those suspect pacemakers monitored more closely. Sometimes a recommendation is made that generator replacement should be considered. One has to balance the risk of pacemaker failure against the not insignificant morbidity (especially infection) associated with generator change. Clearly the case is more compelling in a pacemaker-dependent patient.

BATTERY DEPLETION

There are several indicators of impending battery depletion. First, a reduction in the stimulation rate, which has to be measured precisely during fixed rate pacing, usually initiated by placing a magnet over the pacemaker. Each type of pacemaker has its own characteristic 'end of life' rate; it is usually in the order of 5–10 per cent less than the 'beginning of life' rate.

In addition, most pulse generators have the facility to transmit data to the programmer (i.e. telemetry). Marked reduction in battery voltage and increase in battery internal resistance are indicators of imminent battery depletion (Figure 24.27). There are two stages towards the end of battery life: 'recommended replacement time' (RRT) and 'end of life' (EOL). Some pacemakers will automatically revert to the VVI mode when EOL is reached, in order to minimize battery consumption.

Because of the likelihood of a delay before a patient can be admitted to hospital for generator change, it is desirable to make a decision based on careful analysis of battery data as to the timing of generator replacement before RRT is reached and certainly before EOL is reached.

Some pacemakers provide conflicting and confusing data so that it may be difficult to predict when generator change should be undertaken. It is important that pacemaker clinics are thoroughly familiar with the types of pacemaker implanted in

Basic Parameters

	Initial	Present	
Mode	DDI	DDI	
Base Rate	70	70	min^{-1}
A-V Delay	150	150	ms
Vent Pulse Configuration	Unipolar	Unipolar	
V. Pulse Width	0.4	0.4	ms
V. Pulse Amplitude	3.0	3.0	V
V. Sense Configuration	Unipolar Tip	Unipolar Tip	
V. Sensitivity	2.0	2.0	mV
V. Refractory	250	250	mV
Atrial Pulse Configuration	Unipolar	Unipolar	
A. Pulse Width	0.4	0.4	ms
A. Pulse Amplitude	2.5	2.5	V
A. Sense Configuration	Unipolar Tip	Unipolar Tip	
A. Sensivity	0.50	0.50	mV
A. Refractory	275	275	ms
Blanking	38	38	ms
Vent. Safety Option	Enabled	Enabled	
Rate Resp. A-V Delay	Disabled	Disabled	
Magnet Response	Off	Off	

Sensor Parameters

	Initial	Present	
Sensor	Off	Off	
Max Sensor Rate	140	140	min^{-1}
Threshold	2.0	2.0	
Meas Average Sensor	2.4	2.4	
Slope	8 Normal	8 Normal	
Reaction Time	Fast	Fast	
Recovery Time	Medium	Medium	

Measured Data

Measured Rate	62.9	min^{-1}
Ventricular		
Pulse Amplitude	2.9	V
Pulse Current	5.3	mA
Pulse Energy	5	μJ
Pulse Charge	2	μC
Lead Impedance	552	Ω
Atrial		
Pulse Amplitude	2.1	V
Pulse Current	3.9	mA
Pulse Energy	3	μJ
Pulse Charge	1	μC
Lead Impedance	538	Ω
Battery Data ......(W.G. 8077 - nom. 1.8 Ah)		
Voltage	2.26	V
Cuttent	11	μA
Impedance	21	$k\Omega$

Warning: The Elective Replacement Indicator has been reached.

Figure 24.27 Telemetered pacemaker data indicating how the pacemaker has been programmed and satisfactory lead impedances. The battery voltage is very low and the battery impedance exceptionally high, indicating that generator change should have been performed several months previously!

their centre and that they are able to receive prompt advice from the manufacturer if there is any doubt as to data obtained.

In general, the latest pacemakers last less long than past generations because the pacemakers and therefore batteries are smaller, and because the many sophisticated functions that pacemakers now provide increase current drain.

ELECTROMAGNETIC INTERFERENCE

External electromagnetic interference may affect pacemakers and cause either inhibition or reversion to the fixed rate mode, reprogramming or damage to the pacemaker circuitry. The many sources include electric motors in household devices, internal combustion engines, microwave ovens, radio transmitters, theft and weapon detection systems, arc welding apparatus and radar. In practice, because pacemakers are well shielded and because of the use of appropriate filters, very few problems are encountered and patients should be reassured that the risks are minimal. Clearly, if a patient feels dizzy near electrical equipment they should quickly walk away from it.

If a patient's work brings him or her into close proximity with strong sources of electromagnetic interference, a bipolar pacemaker should be implanted. If necessary, pacemaker function can be assessed by a site visit to ensure the device will not be influenced by electromagnetic interference. Arc welders should wear non-conductive gloves, should not work in a wet area, should avoid high current settings and never exceed 400 A, and connect the ground clamp to the metal as close as possible to the welding point.

ELECTRONIC ARTICLE SURVEILLANCE SYSTEMS (EAS) AND METAL DETECTORS

These could transiently inhibit or possibly reprogram a pacemaker. However, there are only a few reports of adverse incidents and no patient has been harmed. Current advice to patients is:

1. Do not stay near an EAS system or metal detector longer than is necessary and do not lean against the system. It is sufficient to pass the system at an ordinary pace.
2. Be aware that EAS systems may be hidden or camouflaged in entrances and exist in many commercial establishments.
3. If scanning with a hand-held metal detector is necessary, warn the security personnel that you have an electronic medical device and ask them not to hold the metal detector near the device any longer than is absolutely necessary; or you may wish to ask for an alternative form of personal search.

MAGNETS

A magnet held directly over a pacemaker can activate its reed-switch and thereby make it function in a fixed rate mode. The effect should only last as long as the magnet is applied. Patients should be advised to avoid clothing and accessories that contain magnets.

DIATHERMY

Diathermy may damage a pacemaker, cause inappropriate inhibition or possibly precipitate ventricular fibrillation. If possible, a bipolar system should be used. If a unipolar system has to be used, output should be kept as low as possible. The active electrode should be kept at least 15 cm from the generator and the indifferent electrode sited as far away as possible so that its dipole is perpendicular to the pacing system. The pulse should be monitored so that diathermy can be interrupted if prolonged inhibition occurs. Ideally, the pacemaker should be checked prior to surgery. Some pacemakers are more prone to external interference when the batteries are approaching end of life. A pacemaker check should be performed soon after surgery.

RADIATION

Radiation for diagnostic purposes will not affect a pacemaker but therapeutic levels may cause damage. The pacemaker should be shielded, and if this is not possible re-siting of the generator should be considered.

MAGNETIC RESONANCE IMAGING

Limited experience with magnetic resonance imaging (MRI) indicates that pacemakers will revert to fixed rate mode and some may pace at a dangerously fast rate. In general, pacemaker patients should not undergo MRI. However, there are a now a number of reports that patients with pacemakers have undergone MRI scanning without ill-effect. If there is a compelling case for an MRI scan advice from the pacemaker manufacturer should be sought. If a scan is performed the pacemaker's sensor and magnet responses should both be programmed off.

OTHER PRECAUTIONS

CARDIOVERSION AND DEFIBRILLATION

Pacemaker damage can be prevented if the paddles are at least 15 cm from the generator and preferably are positioned so they are at right angles to the pacing system. Pacemaker function should be checked after the procedure.

LITHOTRIPSY

Shocks should not be focused directly over the pacemaker. The pacemaker should be programmed to non rate-responsive VVI mode.

ELECTROCONVULSIVE THERAPY

Electroconvulsive therapy is safe.

TRANSCUTANEOUS ELECTRICAL NERVE STIMULATION (TENS)

Unipolar pacemakers can be inhibited and it is recommended that the heart rhythm is monitored during initial TENS application in patients with bipolar systems.

CELLULAR PHONES

Mobile telephones may possibly cause transient interference of pacemaker function. It is recommended that a mobile telephone is kept at least 15 cm from the pacemaker and when the phone is in use to put it to the ear opposite to the implant site. A number of manufacturers claim their devices are 'phone-proof'.

DRIVING

In the United Kingdom, driving must cease if a patient has sinoatrial disease or AV block and the arrhythmia has caused or is likely to cause incapacity. Patients may resume driving ordinary motor cars and motor cycles one week after implantation of a pacemaker or generator change provided there is no other disqualifying condition. Heavy goods and public service vehicle drivers are disqualified from driving for six weeks after pacemaker implantation. Licensing may be permitted thereafter provided there is no other disqualifying condition.

DIVING

The increased hydrostatic pressure underwater can compress pacemaker cans and cause device failure. Many pacemakers are affected at depths of 11 m. Manufacturers' advice should be sought.

CREMATION

A pacemaker must be explanted before cremation to avoid explosion, which may well lead to structural damage. Relevant staff need to be aware that occasionally the patient will have more than one pulse generator in situ and occasionally generators migrate to unusual locations!

Main points

- Long-term pacing is indicated in cases of symptomatic bradycardia and should also be considered in asymptomatic patients with second- or third-degree AV block or long pauses in sinus node activity.

- Ventricular demand pacing prevents normal AV synchrony and does not permit a chronotropic response to exercise.

- Loss of normal AV synchrony during ventricular demand pacing may cause symptomatic hypotension (pacemaker syndrome) and can be prevented by atrial or AV sequential pacing.

- Absence of a chronotropic response to exercise can markedly reduce exercise tolerance. Atrial synchronized ventricular pacing and rate response systems sensitive to physiological parameters can facilitate a chronotropic response to exercise.

- The modern pacemaker is small, reliable and has a long battery life. Pacemaker infection is the commonest reason for re-operation. Many other complications can be resolved without operation if the pacemaker is programmable.

- Electromagnetic interference from household devices and from electronic surveillance equipment is unlikely to affect the modern pacemaker.

CHAPTER 25

Automatic implantable cardiovertor defibrillator

The automatic implantable cardiovertor defibrillator is a device that can recognize and automatically terminate ventricular fibrillation or tachycardia by delivering an appropriate electrical therapy. It has been shown to improve prognosis in patients at high risk of sudden cardiac death due to ventricular arrhythmias.

The three therapies are:

1. Rapid ventricular pacing stimuli to terminate ventricular tachycardia (see Figure 12.14).

2. Low energy (0.5–10 J) DC shock to terminate ventricular tachycardia (i.e. cardioversion) (Figure 25.1).
3. Higher energy (10–34 J) DC shock to terminate ventricular tachycardia or fibrillation (i.e. defibrillation) (Figure 25.2).

In addition, the device can act as a pacemaker to prevent bradycardia and to provide a chronotropic response to exercise.

The first defibrillator was implanted in 1980. Since then there have been great strides in technology. Early devices were very large, necessitating implantation abdominally in the rectus sheath, and employed epicardial leads.

Current devices are somewhat bigger than a pacemaker and can be implanted subcutaneously over, or in the case of very thin patients beneath, pectoralis major. A single ventricular transvenous lead, introduced via the cephalic or subclavian vein, is required: the can of the device acts as the indifferent electrode. A DC shock is delivered between a coil positioned on the distal portion of the lead and the can. Some leads have a second coil positioned more proximally so that it lies in the superior vena cava, enabling a shock to be delivered between the distal coil (cathode) and the can together with the proximal coil (anodes).

In patients without persistent atrial fibrillation, dual chamber devices are usually employed necessitating the addition of an atrial lead. Dual chamber devices provide the same benefits as dual chamber pacemakers for the management of bradycardia. In addition, atrial sensing enables better discrimination between supraventricular and ventricular arrhythmias.

Devices last approximately five to eight years.

DEFIBRILLATOR IMPLANTATION

The procedure is similar to that for a pacemaker and is usually carried out under local anaesthesia.

In addition, it is necessary to ensure that the device can terminate ventricular fibrillation. Hefty short-acting intravenous sedation is given and then ventricular fibrillation is initiated by delivering via the implanted device a DC shock coincident with the preceding T wave (Figure 25.3), or by a burst of alternating current (50 or 60 Hz), or by a brief, very rapid train of ventricular stimuli.

It is desirable that the device is effective at an output at least 10 J less than its maximum output, which is in the region of 30 J. Many centres will program the device to an initial output of 18–20 J and ensure that it is effective at two consecutive inductions of ventricular fibrillation. Some centres will only induce on one occasion. A single successful 14 J shock has been shown to have the same predictive accuracy as two consecutive 18 J shocks. The device is programmed to deliver a second higher energy shock if the first one fails: if the second shock delivered by the device fails, immediate external defibrillation is carried out.

If a high defibrillation threshold is encountered then sometimes programming reversal of polarity such that the distal coil is the anode can reduce it.

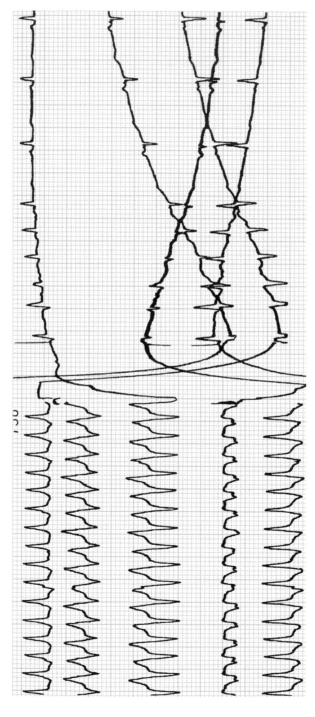

Figure 25.1 Transvenous cardioversion of ventricular tachycardia.

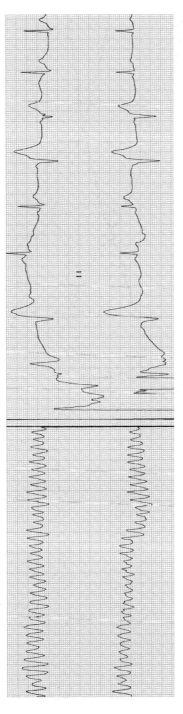

Figure 25.2 Termination of ventricular fibrillation by implanted defibrillator.

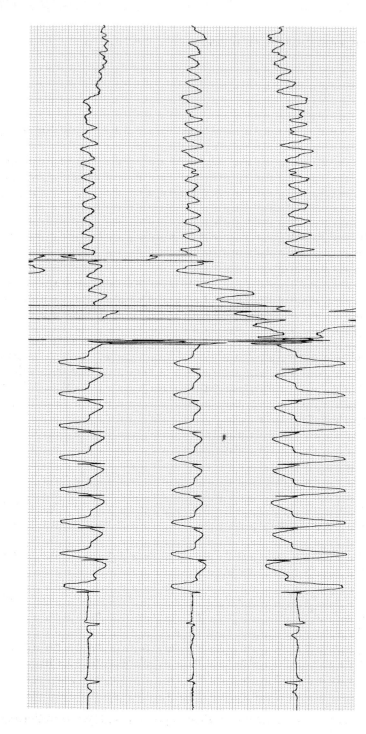

Figure 25.3 Initiation of ventricular fibrillation by delivering a low-energy DC shock on the T wave of the eighth paced beat.

INDICATIONS

Indications are considered in terms of primary and secondary prevention.

SECONDARY PREVENTION

Secondary prevention is therapy to deal with a recurrence of ventricular tachycardia or fibrillation.

In accordance with current United Kingdom guidelines, defibrillator implantation should be considered for patients who present with the following, provided the arrhythmia is not due to acute myocardial infarction and there is no correctable cause:

1. Survivors of sudden cardiac death caused by ventricular fibrillation or tachycardia.
2. Spontaneous sustained ventricular tachycardia causing syncope or significant haemodynamic compromise.
3. Sustained ventricular tachycardia without syncope or cardiac arrest in patients who have a left ventricular ejection fraction less than 35 per cent but are no worse than class III of the New York Heart Association functional classification of heart failure.

Several major clinical trials have demonstrated that in the above groups of patients, the automatic cardiovertor defibrillator reduces mortality as compared with antiarrhythmic drug therapy. Overall, these studies have shown a reduction in death due to cardiac causes of approximately 50 per cent and a reduction in 'all cause mortality' of approximately 25 per cent.

PRIMARY PREVENTION

Primary prevention is therapy for patients who are at high risk of death or collapse from ventricular tachycardia or fibrillation who have *not yet* sustained these arrhythmias.

In accordance with current United Kingdom guidelines, defibrillator implantation should be considered for patients with:

1. Previous myocardial infarction (more than four weeks) with symptoms no worse than class III of the New York Heart Association and
All of the following:
   (i) Non-sustained ventricular tachycardia on ambulatory electrocardiography
   (ii) Inducible ventricular tachycardia at electrophysiological testing
   (iii) Left ventricular ejection fraction less than 35 per cent.

Or:
   Left ventricular ejection fraction less than 30 per cent and QRS duration equal to or more than 120 ms.

These recommendations are based on studies that have shown that mortality in patients with the above characteristics is reduced by the automatic cardiovertor defibrillator as compared with antiarrhythmic drug therapy, mainly amiodarone.

2. A cardiac condition in which it is recognized that the patient is at high risk of sudden death including:
    (i)   long QT syndrome,
    (ii) hypertrophic cardiomyopathy,
    (iii) Brugada syndrome,
    (iv) arrhythmogenic right ventricular dysplasia,
    (v)   following repair of tetralogy of Fallot.

In terms of primary prevention, the main indicators of high risk in conditions i–iv are discussed in earlier chapters. Following repair of Fallot's tetralogy, prolonged QRS duration and ventricular dysfunction have been reported to be predictors of sudden death.

FURTHER INDICATIONS FOR PRIMARY PREVENTION

Three recent important studies have shown that in patients with poor left ventricular function (ejection fraction <35 per cent), whether due to coronary artery disease or to cardiomyopathy, and New York Heart Association class II or III heart failure, prognosis can be improved by defibrillator implantation even without there being non-sustained ventricular tachycardia or a positive ventricular stimulation study.

Analysis of these studies has shown that a policy of defibrillator implantation in patients with poor ventricular function will prolong life, on average, by two to six years and is 'cost-effective'. The studies had fairly short follow-up periods; an average of two to four years. It is likely that with a longer period of follow-up increased benefit will be seen.

These studies have also clearly shown that antiarrhythmic therapy, mainly amiodarone, though it may reduce the incidence of ventricular arrhythmia, does not improve prognosis.

Recent myocardial infarction

In the studies referred to above, patients who had recently sustained a myocardial infarction were excluded. A study of patients early after myocardial infarction with an ejection fraction <35 per cent and indicators of higher risk of ventricular arrhythmia failed to show that defibrillator implantation within six weeks of acute myocardial infarction improved prognosis.

Biventricular implantable defibrillator

Biventricular pacing in patients with heart failure and prolonged QRS duration has been shown to improve prognosis as well as symptoms. However, devices are now available which combine biventricular pacing with the functions of an automatic implantable defibrillator with further prognostic benefit.

RESERVATIONS CONCERNING DEFIBRILLATOR IMPLANTATION FOR PRIMARY PREVENTION

In contrast to clinical trials that study a large group of patients, clinical practice involves advice to the individual patient. One has to discuss with the patient the negative aspects of defibrillator implantation as well as the significant benefits.

Disadvantages include the complications of defibrillator implantation, the possibility of inappropriate shock delivery, possible psychological effects and also implications in connection with driving (see below).

The patient needs to understand that though clinical trials have shown a significant prognostic benefit with defibrillator implantation, only approximately one in 12 defibrillator recipients is going to receive life-saving therapy from their device within the first few years of implantation.

With increasing age, patients are progressively more susceptible to non-cardiac diseases that may shorten life such as stroke and cancer. Thus, the elderly patient with poor ventricular function may be less likely to benefit from a defibrillator than a younger patient.

A further difficulty is raising the question of possible sudden death in a patient who has not had a major arrhythmia. Depending on the result of a ventricular stimulation study and the patient's own feelings about whether he or she feels a defibrillator is worthwhile, the patient may not proceed to implantation and yet has had to come to terms with the possibility of sudden death.

DEFIBRILLATOR FUNCTION

DEVICE COUNTERS

The device can store data indicating the number of episodes of arrhythmia that have occurred, and the number of therapies that have been delivered and whether they were successful or unsuccessful.

ELECTROGRAM RECORDING

Implantable defibrillators can store intra-atrial and intraventricular ECGs prior to and immediately after the device has delivered therapy. Thus it is possible to ensure that appropriate therapy was initiated and that the device had not responded to a supraventricular tachycardia (Figures 25.4 and 25.5).

TIERED THERAPY

Some ventricular tachycardias can be terminated by 'antitachycardia pacing' (i.e. delivery of 6–12 ventricular stimuli in rapid succession). Ventricular fibrillation can

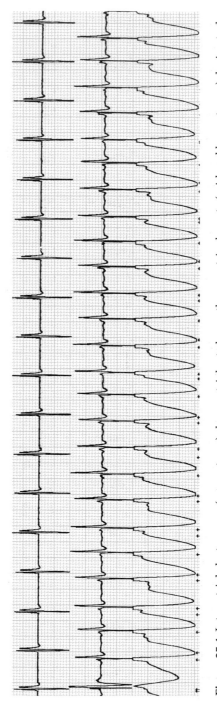

Figure 25.4 Intra-atrial electrogram (upper trace) shows atrial rate lower than ventricular rate (mid and lower traces) during tachycardia indicating ventricular origin.

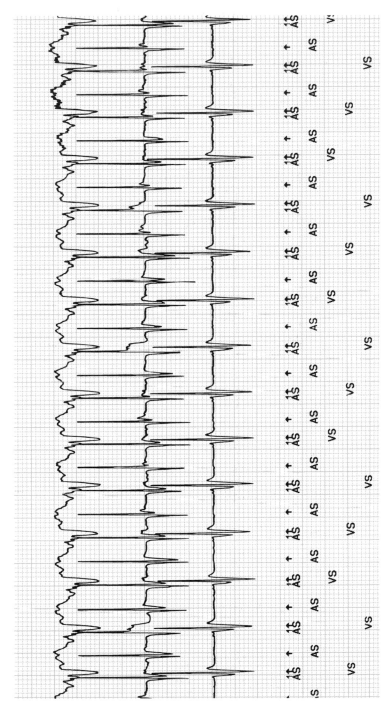

Figure 25.5 Intra-atrial (middle trace) and intraventricular electrograms (lower trace) recorded during tachycardia show that the atrial rate exceeded the ventricular rate indicating an atrial arrhythmia.

only be terminated by delivery of a high-energy shock. The advantages of terminating ventricular tachycardia by antitachycardia pacing are that it is painless and battery energy is conserved. However, antitachycardia pacing is not always effective and may sometimes accelerate the tachycardia.

Detection of ventricular tachycardia and fibrillation is based mainly on the rate of sensed ventricular electrograms. Usually, rate criteria are used to place the arrhythmia in one of three zones:

Slow ventricular tachycardia zone

Ventricular tachycardia at a rate of 130–170 beats/min is termed 'slow'. There is a good chance that antitachycardia pacing will be effective (Figure 25.6).

It is usual to program the device to attempt to terminate the tachycardia several times before proceeding to cardioversion (i.e. delivering a synchronized 5–10 J shock). Either 'burst' or 'ramp' pacing can be used. With the former, the interval between stimuli is constant, whereas with the latter, the interval between successive stimuli is decreased by approximately 8–10 ms. For most patients, burst and ramp pacing are in fact equally effective. Initial attempts at pacing typically employ a train of six impulses at 81–88 per cent of the tachycardia cycle length. If ineffective, the device will then deliver more aggressive therapies (e.g. up to 12 impulses with shorter cycle lengths, 78–81 per cent of tachycardia cycle length).

It is important to ensure that the lower limit of the range of tachycardia detection does not overlap with a heart rate that the patient is likely to achieve during sinus rhythm – otherwise the device will deliver therapy inappropriately.

Fast ventricular tachycardia zone

'Fast ventricular tachycardia' is usually defined as a rate between 170 and 200 beats/min. There is a moderate chance that it can be terminated by pacing but often little time can be allowed for pacing because it is likely that a tachycardia in this range will cause collapse. It is usual to program the device to attempt antitachycardia pacing up to four times. If unsuccessful the device will then proceed to deliver a 10 J shock and if necessary a further shock at maximum energy (Figure 25.7).

Ventricular fibrillation zone

A rate in excess of 200 beats/min is assumed to be ventricular fibrillation. Electrograms during ventricular fibrillation are of low amplitude. To avoid failure to detect ventricular fibrillation, only 80 per cent of sensed electrograms over a period of approximately 6 s are required to meet the rate criteria. Ventricular fibrillation is assumed and a high-energy shock (e.g. 30 J) will be discharged after a further 6 s (Figures 25.8 and 25.9). If fibrillation is redetected, further shocks will be delivered.

It has been shown that antitachycardia pacing may be effective, even with very fast ventricular tachycardias. If within the ventricular fibrillation zone, *each* cycle length is more than 240 ms (i.e. <250 beats/min) then ventricular tachycardia rather than fibrillation is assumed. A single burst of eight paced beats at 88 per cent of the

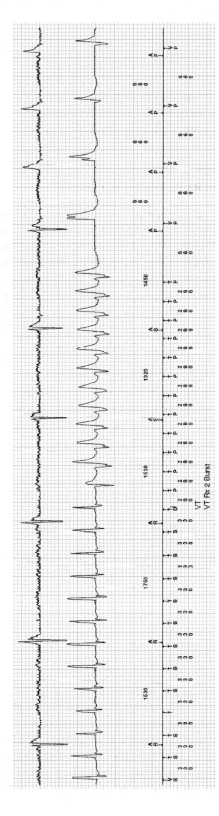

Figure 25.6 Lower electrogram shows ventricular tachycardia with a cycle length of 330 ms interrupted by a train of ventricular stimuli at a cycle length of 280 ms. Upper electrogram shows independent atrial activity during tachycardia.

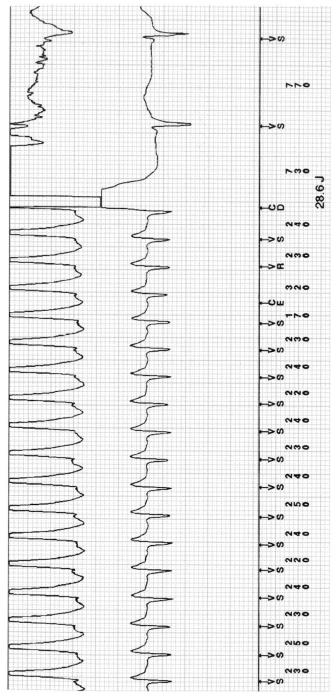

Figure 25.7 Ventricular electrograms recorded before and after termination of ventricular tachycardia (fast ventricular tachycardia zone) by delivery of a 28.6 J shock.

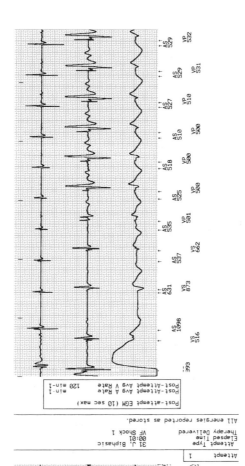

Figure 25.8 Detection of ventricular fibrillation while atrial channel (upper trace) records normal atrial rate. A 31 J shock terminates ventricular fibrillation, after which the device paces the ventricles to prevent bradycardia.

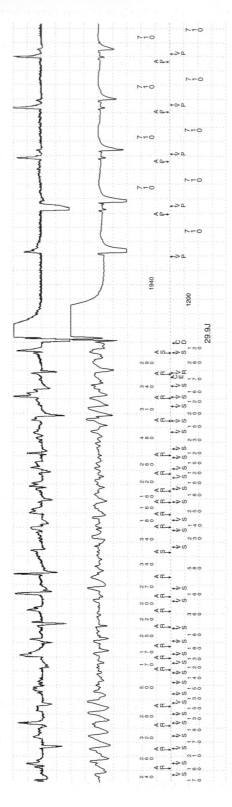

Figure 25.9 Delivery of 29 J shock terminates ventricular fibrillation (lower channel) and also fortuitously atrial fibrillation (upper channel).

measured cycle length has been reported to terminate the arrhythmia in 80 per cent of cases, thereby avoiding a painful DC shock.

PACING MODE

Choice of pacing mode (e.g. AAIR, VVIR, DDIR) is as for implanted pacemakers (see Chapter 24). As with pacemakers, unnecessary ventricular pacing should be avoided to prevent right ventricular apical pacing causing heart failure. Where possible, AAIR or DDIR pacing with a long AV delay should be employed.

AUDIBLE ALERT ALARMS

Most devices can be programmed to deliver an audible alarm if lead impedance becomes abnormal (suggesting lead fracture or insulation breakdown) or if there is abnormal battery function. On hearing such an alarm, the patient should contact his or her cardiology centre.

DEACTIVATION OF DEVICE

Occasionally it is necessary to deactivate a defibrillator either because it is delivering inappropriate shocks or because a patient has become terminally ill and resuscitation is no longer indicated.

The device can be deactivated using an external programmer. If not available, deactivation can be achieved with most devices by placing a magnet over the generator and taping it in place. It should be noted that with some devices, defibrillator and antitachycardia functions continue to be disabled after magnet removal and reprogramming is required.

DEFIBRILLATOR CLINIC

Patients are usually seen every three to six months. Device function is checked and battery status measured in terms of battery voltage and capacitor charge time.

LIMITATIONS

Discharge of a DC shock in a conscious patient usually results in sudden, marked chest discomfort and may cause considerable distress! Patients describe experiencing sensations such as 'a blow to the chest' or 'a spasm making the whole body jump'. The device therefore is not suitable for patients with frequently recurrent or incessant arrhythmias since it would be activated too often. A minority of patients report experiencing only minor discomfort on defibrillator discharge.

An implantable defibrillator is often regarded as an alternative to antiarrhythmic drugs. However, to almost lose consciousness from ventricular fibrillation and then be defibrillated is not a pleasant experience. Ideally, the implantable defibrillator should act as a 'backup' device. Often, antiarrhythmic drugs are required to minimize the frequency of ventricular arrhythmia (see below).

Inappropriate discharge may occur in response to a rapid ventricular rate during atrial fibrillation or other supraventricular tachycardia, or as a result of lead malfunction. A recent study showed that 15 per cent of patients received inappropriate therapy.

Many patients benefit psychologically from the peace of mind that the potentially life-saving facility of an implantable defibrillator offers. However, some patients, particularly those who have received inappropriate or frequent shocks, dread further shocks and are psychologically disturbed as a consequence.

Device or lead malfunctions occur in a minority of patients. The rate is somewhat higher than is encountered with implanted pacemakers.

DRUG THERAPY IN PATIENTS WITH DEFIBRILLATORS

PROGNOSIS

There are a number of drugs that have been shown to improve prognosis in patients with poor ventricular function which clearly should, unless contraindicated, be prescribed whether or not a defibrillator has been implanted: beta-blockers, angiotensin-converting enzyme inhibitors, eplerenone and statins. Smoking cessation is, of course, essential.

ARRHYTHMIA REDUCTION

Often, amiodarone, beta-blockers or sotalol are required to reduce the frequency of ventricular arrhythmias that might lead to shock delivery, or to prevent supraventricular arrhythmias.

These drugs, if not effective in preventing ventricular tachycardia, may prolong the cycle length and may therefore increase the chances of success with antitachycardia pacing. However, occasionally, antiarrhythmic drugs, especially amiodarone, may slow the rate during tachycardia such that it is below the device's detection rate and antitachycardia pacing is not delivered (Figure 25.10).

ATRIAL ARRHYTHMIAS

A very rapid ventricular response to atrial fibrillation and less commonly to atrial flutter and tachycardia can sometimes lead to inappropriate shock delivery (Figure 25.11).

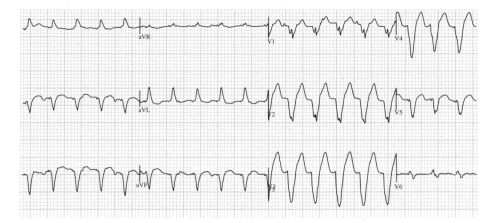

Figure 25.10 Symptomatic but relatively slow ventricular tachycardia (130 beats/min) which did not meet the defibrillator's detection criterion to initiate antitachycardia pacing.

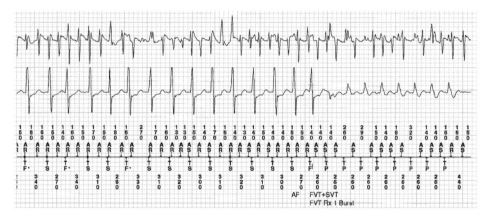

Figure 25.11 Intra-atrial (upper ECG) and intraventricular (lower ECG) demonstrating atrial fibrillation. The annotations at the bottom of the trace indicate that the rapid ventricular rate has led to an inappropriate diagnosis of ventricular tachycardia (TS) which initiated futile antitachycardia pacing (TP).

It is important to ensure that the ventricular rate is controlled by AV nodal blocking drugs. Occasionally, these are ineffective and catheter ablation is required.

DEFIBRILLATION THRESHOLD

It should be noted that amiodarone may raise the defibrillation threshold and possibly render the device ineffective if the threshold was already high. Sotalol has been reported to reduce the defibrillation threshold.

Other drugs that are reported to sometimes increase defibrillation threshold include lignocaine, mexiletine and flecainide.

ELECTRICAL STORMS

Some patients will experience a period when there are frequent episodes of ventricular arrhythmia necessitating defibrillation. Causes include hypokalaemia, worsening ventricular dysfunction, myocardial ischaemia and proarrhythmic drugs. Clearly, the cause should be dealt with if possible. Intravenous amiodarone, beta-blockers and occasionally mexiletine may be effective.

A similar situation, though not strictly an electrical storm, can be precipitated by supraventricular arrhythmias, by sinus tachycardia due to hyperthyroidism (a possible consequence of amiodarone therapy) and by lead malfunction (Figure 25.12, see page 298).

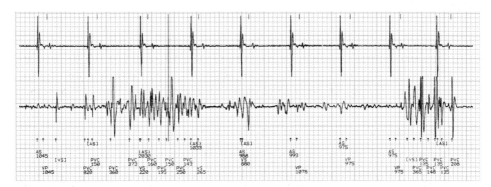

Figure 25.12   Electrical noise resulting from partial lead fracture registered on intraventricular electrogram (lower channel) that could lead to an incorrect diagnosis of ventricular tachycardia or fibrillation.

HARDWARE COSTS

In the United Kingdom, implantation costs are in the region of £16 000.

PRECAUTIONS

Implantable defibrillators are subject to electromagnetic interference in the same way as pacemakers are, as discussed above. Application of a magnet over a defibrillator will inactivate it. Clothing and accessories containing magnets should not be worn.

A defibrillator should be inactivated during implantation or removal otherwise the operator may possibly receive an electric shock.

DRIVING

Discharge of a defibrillator during motor vehicle driving will at very least cause distraction and will probably result in temporary incapacity. It may save the driver's life but could endanger others' lives. Furthermore, the device may be triggered by ventricular arrhythmias that would not have caused collapse, and inappropriate discharge might result from supraventricular tachycardia or technical failure such as lead fracture.

Approaches to licensing drivers vary from country to country. The somewhat complex United Kingdom regulations which have recently been revised can be found at www.dvla.gov.uk/at_a_glance/ch2_cardiovascular.htm.

Main points

- The automatic cardiovertor defibrillator is an implantable device that can recognize and automatically terminate ventricular tachycardia or fibrillation by delivering a train of ventricular pacing stimuli or a DC shock. The device can also act as a pacemaker to prevent bradycardia and to provide a chronotropic response.

- Implantation procedures for defibrillators and pacemakers are similar.

- Patients at high risk from a recurrence of ventricular tachycardia or fibrillation (i.e. secondary prevention) or at high risk from a condition which might cause death from ventricular tachycardia or fibrillation (i.e. primary prevention) are candidates for implantation of an automatic cardiovertor defibrillator.

Catheter ablation

Catheter ablation has transformed the treatment of many rhythm disturbances, particularly those of supraventricular origin. For several common arrhythmias it is not just another therapeutic option but first-line treatment, offering a cure and obviating the need for antiarrhythmic drugs with their associated unwanted effects. Success rates well over 90 per cent are being widely achieved. The risks are low. The purpose of this chapter is to illustrate briefly some of the main applications of catheter ablation.

PROCEDURE

The procedure is usually carried out under local anaesthesia, with intravenous sedation, in a cardiac catheterization laboratory. The sequence of cardiac activation during normal and abnormal rhythms is studied by recording electrograms from various intracardiac sites using multipolar catheter electrodes introduced via percutaneous puncture of the femoral vein and, if necessary, the femoral artery. The electrodes also facilitate introduction of pacing stimuli that can initiate and terminate tachycardias.

Mapping during normal and paced rhythms, and/or during tachycardia, enables location of the re-entrant circuit or focus causing the arrhythmia. Radiofrequency energy, which is high frequency alternating current, is delivered via a special catheter electrode. This has a deflectable end, enabling the tip to be precisely positioned at the target site. Radiofrequency energy is delivered for 30–120 s. The endocardium in contact with the tip and the myocardium beneath is heated to 50–70°C and is thereby coagulated. Surrounding myocardium is not damaged.

Cryothermy is being evaluated as an alternative energy source.

NORMAL SINUS RHYTHM

Figure 26.1 shows typical findings during normal sinus rhythm. Recordings are usually made at a paper speed of at least 100 mm/s. Below the six surface ECG leads are recordings from three intracardiac sites: high right atrium, tricuspid valve and the coronary sinus.

HIGH RIGHT ATRIAL ELECTROGRAM

An electrode positioned in the high right atrium is close to the sinus node. It records the earliest atrial activity during each cardiac cycle. It coincides with the onset of the P wave seen on the surface ECG.

HIS BUNDLE ELECTROGRAM

The His bundle electrogram is recorded by positioning an electrode across the tricuspid valve. Three waves can be seen:

1. The A wave due to activation of the adjacent low right atrium.
2. The H wave: the electrogram resulting from activation of the His bundle. The interval between A and H waves indicates the speed of conduction through the AV node.
3. The V wave, which is the ventricular electrogram. It coincides with the QRS complex on the surface ECG. The HV interval indicates the time of transmission by the His bundle and bundle branches from the AV node to the ventricular myocardium. It is normally 35–55 ms in duration. Often, as in this example, electrograms are recorded from two pairs of electrodes on the multipolar catheter across the tricuspid valve so proximal and distal His bundle electrograms can be obtained.

Figure 26.2 shows a markedly prolonged HV interval in a patient with bifascicular block.

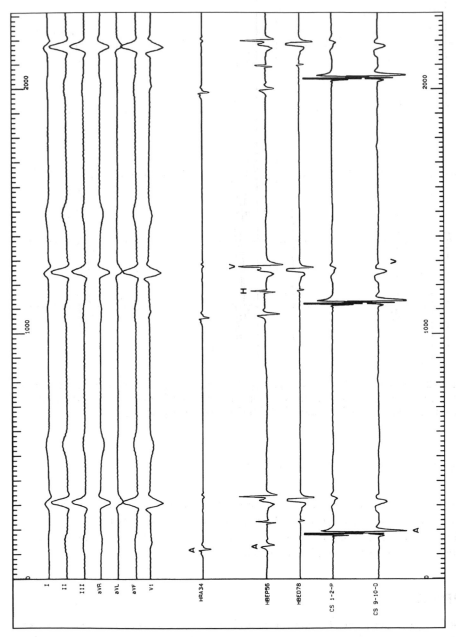

Figure 26.1 Six surface ECGs, and intracardiac ECGs from the high right atrium (HRA), from the His bundle (HBEP = proximal, HBED = distal) and coronary sinus (CS.P = proximal, CS.D = distal). A, H and V = atrial, His bundle and ventricular electrograms, respectively).

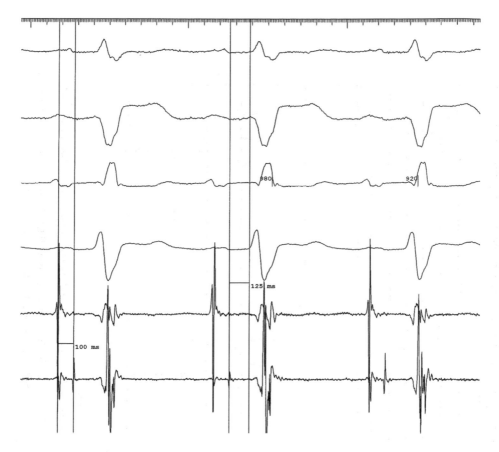

Figure 26.2 Surface leads I, II, V1 and V6 together with a bundle of His electrogram (bottom trace) in a patient with bifascicular block and a long PR interval. The AH interval (100 ms) is normal but the HV interval (125 ms) is markedly prolonged.

CORONARY SINUS ELECTROGRAMS

The coronary sinus runs in the groove between the left atrium and left ventricle. Activity from both the left atrium and left ventricle can be recorded.

In Figure 26.1, a large left atrial electrogram can be seen, which is followed by a smaller wave resulting from left ventricular activity.

Mapping

Figure 26.1 provides a simple example of how the path of an activating impulse can be 'mapped'. It shows how the atrial impulse originates in the high right atrium (i.e. close to the sinus node), passes to the low right atrium, near to the AV node, and then to the left atrium as recorded by the coronary sinus electrodes.

WOLFF–PARKINSON–WHITE SYNDROME

An accessory pathway is located by identifying the site of earliest ventricular activation during sinus rhythm (or atrial pacing) for that must be the site where the accessory pathway connects with ventricular myocardium. An electrogram at this site will precede the onset of the delta wave in the surface ECG (Figure 26.3). Sometimes, it is possible to actually demonstrate an accessory pathway potential (Figure 26.4).

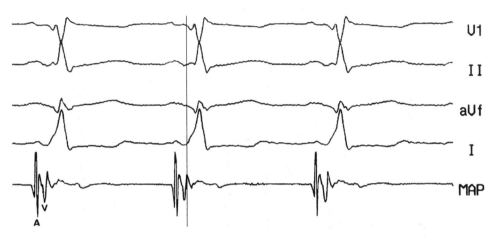

Figure 26.3 Wolff–Parkinson–White syndrome. The vertical line marks the onset of the delta wave on the surface ECG. The tip of the mapping electrode has been positioned at the site of successful ablation. Both A and V waves can be seen in the mapping electrogram. The V wave precedes the onset of the surface ECG delta wave by 25 ms.

Figure 26.5 shows how the surface ECG and electrogram at the site of radiofrequency delivery change as the accessory pathway is ablated by radiofrequency energy.

Left-sided pathways are ablated by introducing a catheter into the left ventricle via the femoral artery (Figure 26.6), or by transseptal puncture via the femoral vein, and positioning its tip across the mitral valve ring. Free right wall accessory pathways are ablated by introducing a catheter from the femoral vein and positioning across the tricuspid valve ring. Postero-septal and antero-septal pathways are also ablated by a catheter in the right ventricle. Postero-septal pathways are found near the mouth of the coronary sinus. Antero-septal pathways are located close to the bundle of His.

There is a small risk that antero-septal and, to a much lesser extent, postero-septal pathway ablation might cause complete heart block and the need for long-term pacing.

Sometimes, T wave memory following successful ablation causes unnecessary concern (Figure 26.7, see pages 308 and 309).

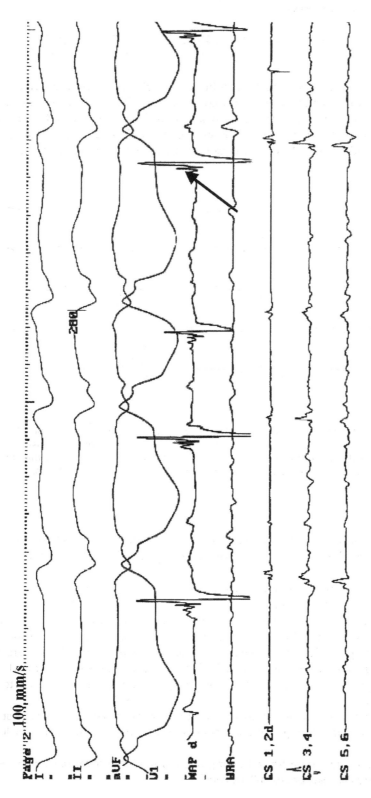

Figure 26.4 Wolff–Parkinson–White syndrome during atrial fibrillation. The arrow indicates a potential arising from an accessory pathway which precedes the onset of the delta wave on the surface ECG.

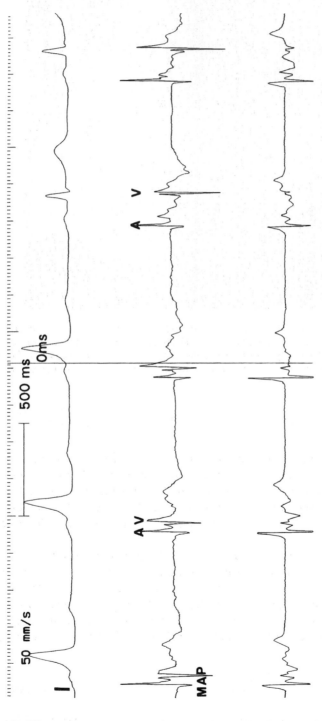

Figure 26.5 Wolff–Parkinson–White syndrome. Radiofrequency energy is delivered after the first three beats and interrupts accessory pathway conduction. The vertical line demonstrates that before ablation, ventricular activity in the mapping electrogram (MAP) precedes the onset of the surface ECG delta wave. After ablation, the delta wave disappears and ventricular activity in the mapping electrogram succeeds rather than precedes the surface ECG QRS complex.

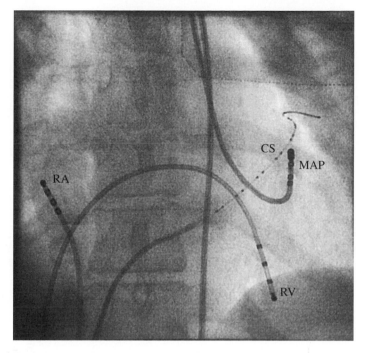

Figure 26.6 Ablation of left-sided accessory pathway. Electrodes are positioned in the right atrium (RA) and right ventricle (RV). There is a multipolar electrode in the coronary sinus (CS). The mapping electrode (MAP) has been introduced via the femoral artery, passed across the aortic valve and positioned across the mitral valve ring.

CONCEALED ACCESSORY PATHWAYS

A concealed accessory pathway can transmit impulses from ventricles to atria and therefore facilitate AV junctional re-entrant tachycardia, but cannot conduct from atria to ventricles and thus there will be no delta wave during sinus rhythm.

Concealed pathways have to be located during AV re-entrant tachycardia or ventricular pacing. The site of earliest atrial activation will indicate the location of the accessory pathway.

For example, in Figure 26.8 (see page 310) electrograms are recorded from a multipolar electrode in the coronary sinus during AV re-entrant tachycardia. Earliest atrial activity is found in the mid coronary sinus, thereby demonstrating a concealed left-sided free wall pathway. An electrode (MAP) positioned across the mitral valve close to coronary sinus electrode CS 9,10 showed even earlier atrial activity. Delivery of radiofrequency energy at that site blocked the accessory pathway.

ATRIOVENTRICULAR NODAL TACHYCARDIA

The hallmark of typical AV nodal re-entrant tachycardia (AVNRT) is the very short conduction time from ventricles to atria during tachycardia (<60 ms). Atrial activity

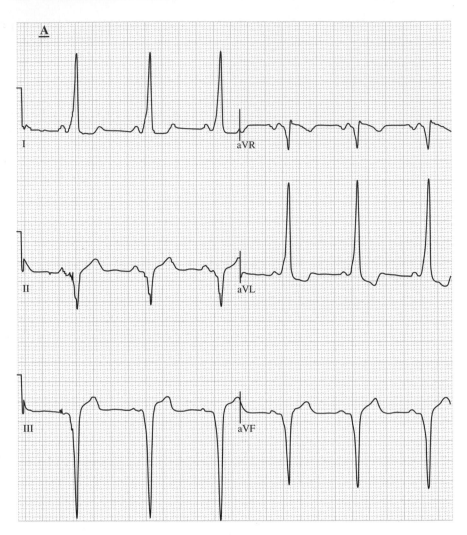

Figure 26.7 (A) ECG prior to successful ablation of postero-septal accessory pathway.

coincides with, or just precedes or just follows the ventricular complex. This is reflected by all intracardiac atrial electrograms (Figure 26.9, see page 311).

'Slow pathway ablation' is the most common approach to AVNRT. The slow pathway is one of the two limbs of the re-entrant. It is usually located just superior and anterior to the mouth of the coronary sinus. A typical slow pathway electrogram can be recorded (Figure 26.10, see page 312). If successful, radiofrequency energy delivered to the site at which this electrogram is recorded will lead to a period of junctional rhythm, after which the tachycardia can no longer be induced.

There is a 1–2 per cent risk of causing complete heart block when attempting slow pathway ablation. Patients should be informed of the small possibility that the procedure will lead to pacemaker implantation. This risk can be minimized by *immediately* interrupting delivery of radiofrequency energy if a junctional tachycardia rather

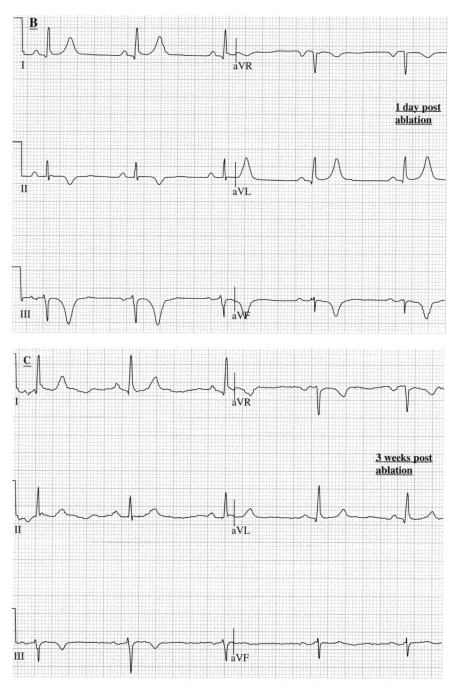

Figure 26.7 (B) ECG on next day showed absence of pre-excitation but deep T wave inversion in inferior leads caused concern about ischaemic damage. In fact it was due to 'T wave memory' (i.e. the T wave continues in the same direction as the QRS complex in that lead prior to ablation). (This phenomenon is not seen after ablation of concealed accessory pathways.) (C) The ECG had returned to normal within two weeks.

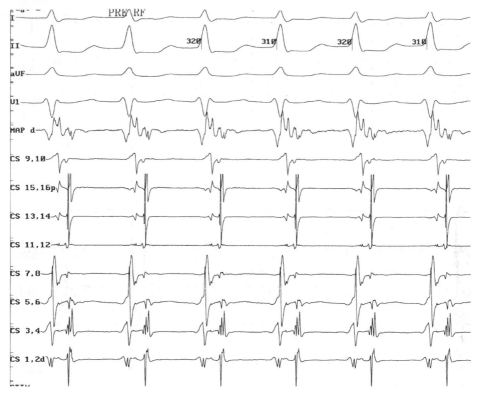

Figure 26.8 Concealed left-sided accessory atrioventricular pathway. The trace is recorded during atrioventricular re-entrant tachycardia. It shows four surface ECGs, electrograms from a mapping electrode (MAP) placed across the mitral valve, and a series of eight coronary sinus electrograms from proximal (CS 15, 16) to distal positions (CS 1, 2). The sequence of atrial electrograms in the coronary sinus indicates a left-sided free wall accessory pathway.

than junctional rhythm occurs or if there is loss of ventriculoatrial conduction during junctional rhythm (Figure 26.11, see page 312).

ATYPICAL ATRIOVENTRICULAR RE-ENTRANT TACHYCARDIA

In AV re-entrant tachycardia, the direction of the circuit is reversed so that conduction to the ventricles is via the fast AV nodal pathway and conduction from ventricles to the atria is via the slow pathway. This results in a long ventriculoatrial conduction time (Figure 26.12, see page 313).

As a result of the long ventriculoatrial conduction time, the surface ECG will show that the interval between the retrograde P wave and the following QRS complex is shorter than the subsequent interval between QRS complex and next retrograde P wave (Figure 26.13, see page 314). Hence the term 'long RP short PR tachycardia'. (For the record, there are three causes of a long RP short PR tachycardia: atypical AV

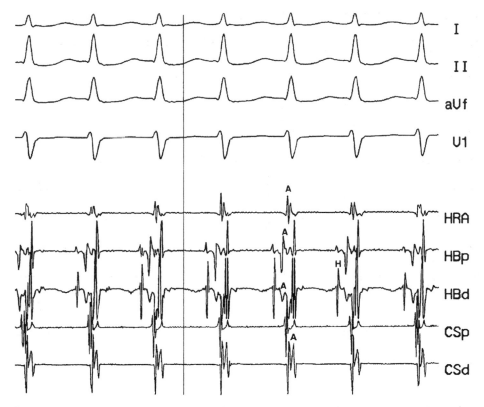

Figure 26.9 Typical atrioventricular nodal re-entrant tachycardia. The A waves in the high right atrial (HRA), His bundle (HB) and coronary sinus (CS) electrograms are almost coincident with ventricular activation. The His bundle electrogram (H) precedes the A and V waves.

NRT, atrial tachycardia with 1:1 AV conduction (see Figure 8.6) and AVRT with a slowly conducting accessory pathway (usually postero-septal).)

ATRIAL TACHYCARDIA

The site of origin of atrial tachycardia is located by mapping of the right and, if necessary, left atrium to identify the point of earliest activation during tachycardia. This will precede the onset of the P wave in the surface ECG. Sometimes, a complex electrogram will be recorded at this site – a sign of myocardial damage (Figure 26.14, see page 315).

ATRIAL FLUTTER

Typical atrial flutter is caused by a re-entrant circuit in the right atrium (see Chapter 7). It is possible to ablate myocardium in this circuit and thereby prevent atrial flutter.

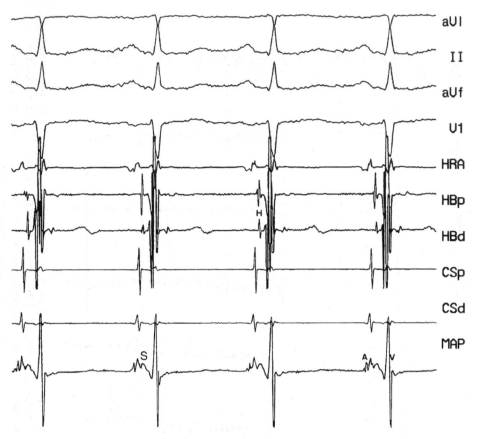

Figure 26.10 Recordings during sinus rhythm in a patient prone to atrioventricular nodal re-entrant tachycardia. The mapping electrode is positioned just superior and anterior to the mouth of the coronary sinus. A typical slow pathway electrogram (S) has been recorded: a small A wave followed by continuous electrical activity and then a large V wave.

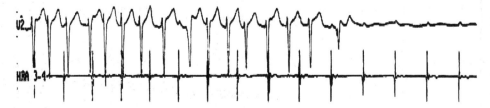

Figure 26.11 Slow pathway ablation. Trace shows surface lead V2 and high right atrial electrogram (HRA). Delivery of radiofrequency energy was not stopped in spite of junctional acceleration and loss of ventriculoatrial conduction. Complete heart block resulted. (Recording obtained from another cardiac unit!)

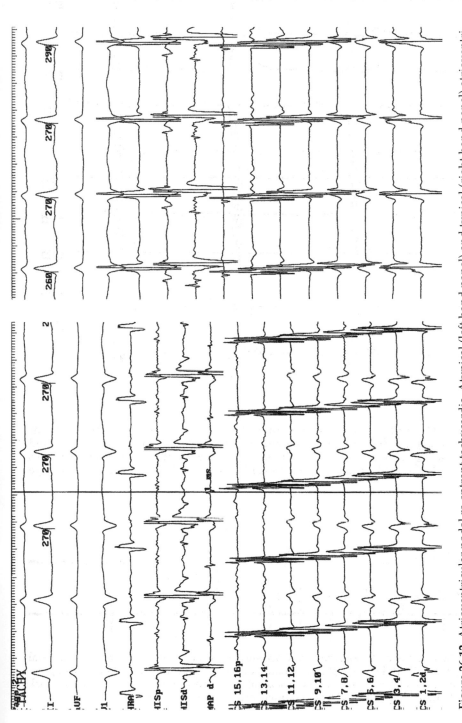

Figure 26.12 Atrioventricular nodal re-entrant tachycardia. Atypical (left hand panel) and typical (right hand panel) atrioventricular nodal re-entrant tachycardia recorded from the same patient. The traces show surface leads I, aVF and V1, high right atrial (HRA), His bundle and a series of coronary sinus (CS) electrograms. Ventriculoatrial conduction is very short during typical atrioventricular nodal re-entrant tachycardia but long during atypical atrioventricular nodal re-entrant tachycardia.

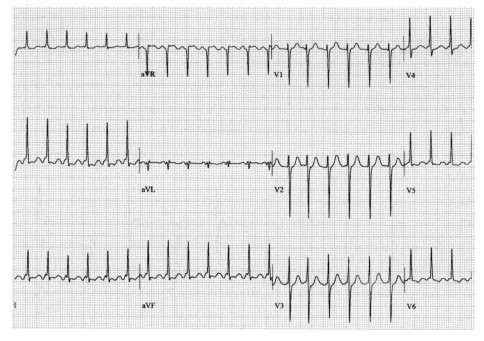

Figure 26.13 'Long RP short PR' tachycardia. Inverted P waves precede each QRS complex.

The narrowest part of the circuit, termed the isthmus, is between the posterior part of the tricuspid valve and the inferior vena cava. Radiofrequency energy is delivered to points along a line between these two sites (Figure 26.15, see page 316). Delivery of radiofrequency energy in the region of the inferior cava can be painful. Generous analgesia should be given. Cryothermy is not painful and its role in ablation for atrial flutter is being evaluated.

There is a significant recurrence rate necessitating a repeat procedure, and atrial fibrillation occasionally develops after successful ablation. Nevertheless, ablation compares very favourably with medical treatment of atrial flutter.

ATRIAL FIBRILLATION

In recent years, the application of catheter ablation to cure atrial fibrillation, the most common cardiac arrhythmia, has become the subject of intense interest. It has been shown that the abnormal electrical activity that initiates atrial fibrillation usually arises from the junction of one or more of the pulmonary veins with the left atrium. Success has been achieved in preventing atrial fibrillation by delivering radiofrequency energy to the circumferences of the ostia of the pulmonary veins in order to electrically isolate them from the left atrium. Currently, success rates are moderately high, antiarrhythmic drugs are still sometimes required, and asymptomatic atrial fibrillation has been shown to occur in some patients who have undergone apparently successful ablation.

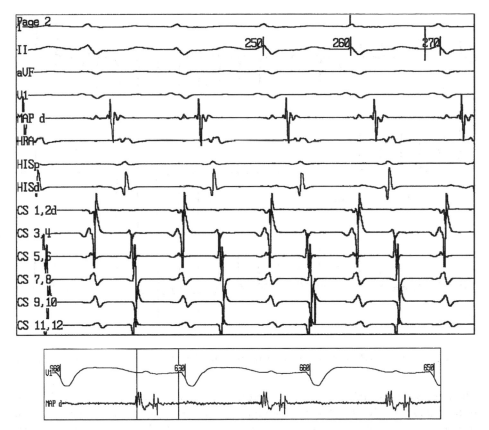

Figure 26.14 Atrial tachycardia. In the upper panel, atrial electrograms have been recorded from the high right atrium (HRA), region of the His bundle (HIS) and from sites within the coronary sinus (CS). Earliest atrial activation was recorded by the mapping electrode (MAP) positioned on the lateral wall of the right atrium. The lower panel shows a fractionated, complex atrial electrogram (MAP) recorded from the site of origin of an atrial tachycardia. Its onset precedes the beginning of the P wave in surface lead V1.

The procedure involves trans-septal catheterization to gain access to the left atrium. The hazards involved with this procedure are greater than for most types of ablation. There are small but significant risks of very serious complications: stroke, atrial wall perforation and pulmonary vein stenosis.

Compared with other widely performed forms of ablation, the success rates are lower and the risk of serious complication higher. At present, it would seem prudent to reserve this treatment for patients with severe symptoms from paroxysmal atrial fibrillation who have not responded to other forms of therapy. It may well be that further developments will improve the effectiveness and reduce the risks of the procedure, allowing its application to be more widespread.

A circumferential ablation procedure with delivery of radiofrequency energy lesions that encircle the left- and right-sided pulmonary veins has been reported to restore normal rhythm to a modest proportion of patients with persistent atrial fibrillation.

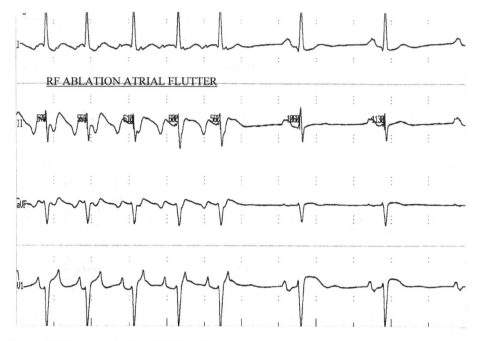

Figure 26.15 Leads I, II, aVF, V1 (100 mm/s) during atrial flutter as a line of radiofrequency lesions between tricuspid valve and inferior vena cava is completed: sinus rhythm returns.

ATRIOVENTRICULAR NODAL ABLATION

In some patients, atrial arrhythmias can not be controlled by medication and ablation is either not indicated or has failed. Radiofrequency energy can be used to ablate the AV node and to thus isolate the ventricles from the rapid atrial activity caused by these rhythm disturbances. AV node ablation will of course lead to complete heart block. In contrast to ablation for other arrhythmias, AV nodal ablation is palliative rather than curative since the procedure necessitates pacemaker implantation.

Ablation of the AV node is usually easy and failure is rare. The ablating electrode is positioned across the tricuspid valve to record a large His bundle electrogram. The tip of the electrode is then withdrawn slightly in order to record a large A wave with a smaller H wave (Figure 26.16). Delivery of radiofrequency energy usually first causes a junctional tachycardia and then complete AV block (Figure 26.17).

Occasionally, it is not possible to ablate the AV node via the right heart. In these cases, a left-sided approach is invariably successful. The ablating electrode can be passed across the aortic valve into the left ventricle. A large His bundle electrogram can be easily found below the aortic valve on the interventricular septum.

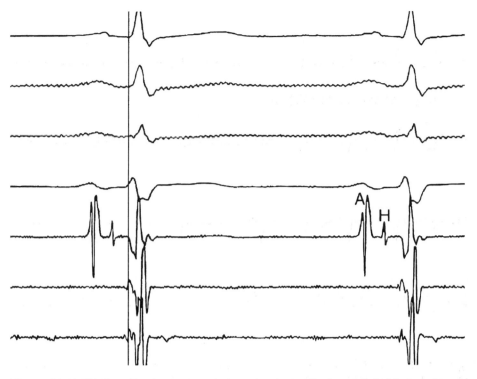

Figure 26.16 His bundle electrogram prior to atrioventricular nodal ablation showing large A wave and smaller H wave.

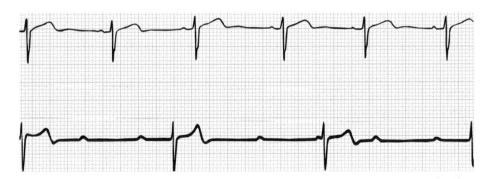

Figure 26.17 Patient with paroxysmal atrial fibrillation before (upper trace) and after (lower trace) atrioventricular node ablation.

CARDIAC PACING

Choice of appropriate pacing mode is important. The pacemaker must provide a chronotropic response. A VVIR pacemaker should be used in persistent atrial fibrillation or flutter. In patients with paroxysmal atrial arrhythmias, a DDDR pacemaker with mode switching facility is required (see Chapter 16).

Patients with poor ventricular function are at a small risk of ventricular fibrillation within the first few days after ablation (Figure 26.18). This risk can be minimized by programming the lowest pacing rate to at least 80 beats/min for the first few weeks after ablation.

Heart failure has been reported to occur in some patients as a result of right ventricular apical pacing following AV nodal ablation. This complication may well be avoided by pacing the right ventricular outflow tract (see Chapter 24).

There are advantages in implanting the pacemaker prior to AV node ablation. One can ensure that there are no pacemaker complications before committing the patient to the need of a pacemaker. Furthermore, in some patients with paroxysmal atrial fibrillation, it has been found that pacing (plus or minus an antiarrhythmic drug) will prevent or markedly reduce the frequency of atrial fibrillation and thereby obviate the need for AV node ablation. Pacing the atrial septum appears to be more effective than pacing the atrial appendage.

RIGHT VENTRICULAR OUTFLOW TRACT TACHYCARDIA

The origin of this tachycardia is just below the pulmonary valve. It can be located by seeking the earliest site of ventricular activation (Figure 26.19) and by pace-mapping (Figure 26.20, see page 321).

FASCICULAR VENTRICULAR TACHYCARDIA

Fascicular tachycardia arises from the posterior fascicle, or rarely, anterior fascicle of the left bundle branch. The appropriate site for delivery of radiofrequency energy can be found by seeking the earliest area of left ventricular activation and is confirmed by the demonstration of a fascicular potential (Figure 26.21).

VENTRICULAR TACHYCARDIA DUE TO STRUCTURAL HEART DISEASE

Ablation of ventricular tachycardias due to myocardial infarction or cardiomyopathy is challenging. Success rates are lower and procedure times much longer than for ablation of other arrhythmias. Identification of the optimal ablation site is usually performed during tachycardia. Therefore, ablation is usually only attempted in patients with slower, well-tolerated tachycardias.

BUNDLE BRANCH RE-ENTRY

This form of ventricular tachycardia typically occurs in patients with a dilated cardiomyopathy who have partial or complete bundle branch block during normal

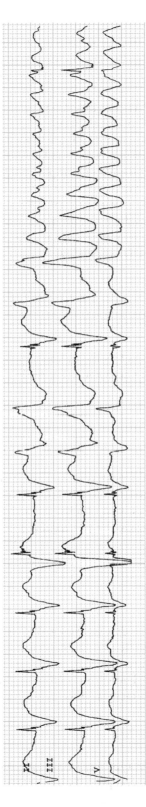

Figure 26.18 Patient with severe heart failure who had undergone atrioventricular nodal ablation a few hours earlier. After three ventricular ectopic beats, one of which was not sensed by the pacemaker, ventricular fibrillation was initiated.

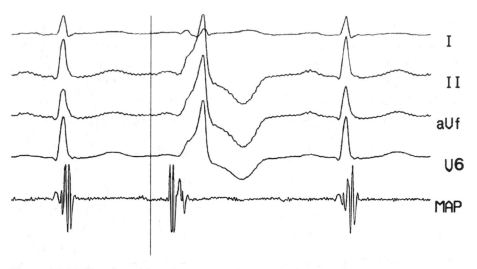

Figure 26.19 The second beat is a ventricular ectopic beat arising from the site of origin of right ventricular outflow tract tachycardia. In contrast to the normal sinus beats before and after, the mapping electrode records ventricular activity earlier than seen on the surface ECGs.

rhythm. During the arrhythmia, a circulating impulse is usually conducted from atria to ventricles via the right bundle and returns to the atria via the left bundle. Typically, the complexes during tachycardia are of left bundle branch block configuration. Each is preceded by a His potential but in contrast to supraventricular tachycardias with bundle branch block, atrial activity is dissociated from ventricular activity (Figure 26.22, see page 324).

Delivery of radiofrequency energy to the right bundle branch will prevent the arrhythmias, though sometimes heart block necessitating a pacemaker results.

CATHETER ABLATION: WHAT SHOULD THE PATIENT EXPECT?

The patient should be reassured that a local anaesthetic and intravenous sedation will be administered and that little or no discomfort will be experienced. It should be emphasized that it is not possible to feel the electrodes as they are advanced from the femoral vein to the heart.

It should be explained that tachycardia will usually be initiated on one or more occasions during the procedure; that onset of tachycardia does not mean that anything is going wrong and important diagnostic information is obtained; and that the tachycardia can be promptly terminated by an external pacemaker.

The patient should be given an estimate as to how long the procedure will last. For example, usually less than 1hour for ablation of AVNRT, atrial flutter or straightforward accessory pathway and approximately 2 hours for more complex arrhythmias.

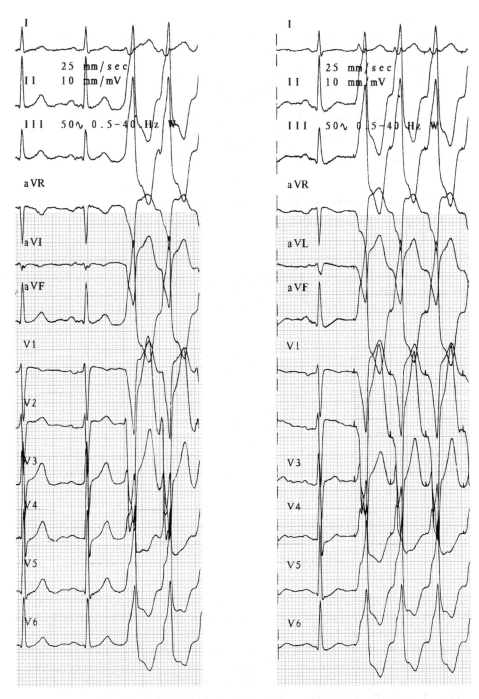

Figure 26.20 Pace-mapping. The left hand panel shows two spontaneous beats arising from the right ventricular outflow tract. In the right-hand panel, pacing at a site just inferior to the pulmonary valve resulted in an almost identical configuration. Radiofrequency energy to that site abolished right ventricular outflow tract tachycardia.

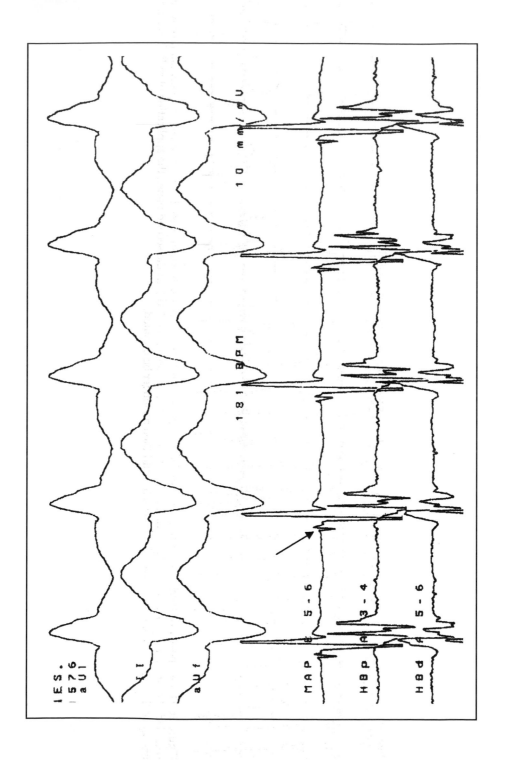

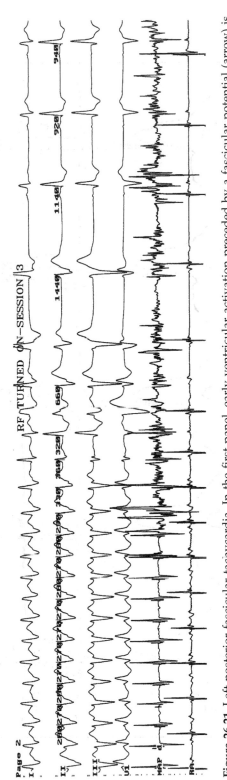

Figure 26.21 Left posterior fascicular tachycardia. In the first panel, early ventricular activation preceded by a fascicular potential (arrow) is recorded at a site in the postero-apical portion of the left interventricular septum (MAP). In the second panel, the application of radiofrequency energy to this site terminates the arrhythmia which could then no longer be initiated.

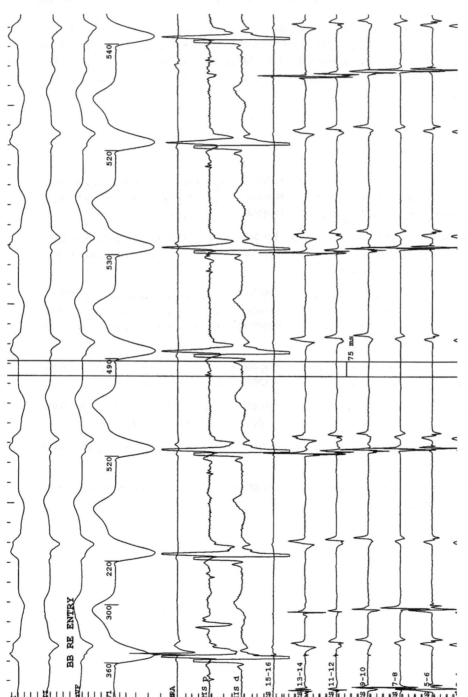

Figure 26.22 Ventricular tachycardia due to bundle branch re-entry. Each ventricular complex is of left bundle branch configuration and is preceded by a His potential (HIS p). Independent atrial activity is demonstrated in a series of coronary sinus (CS) electrograms.

Patients must be aware that ablation for some arrhythmias such as AVNRT and septal accessory pathways is associated with the small risk of heart block and the need for a pacemaker.

Patients often experience ectopic beats ('as though my tachycardia is about to start') and sinus tachycardia in the weeks following ablation. They should be informed that these do not indicate that the procedure has failed: only a recurrence of the identical symptoms experienced prior to ablation would point to the procedure having been unsuccessful.

Main points

- Catheter ablation can be used to treat many cardiac arrhythmias and has become a first-line treatment for supraventricular tachycardias and ventricular tachycardias not caused by structural heart disease.

- An accessory pathway is located by seeking the earliest site of ventricular activation during sinus rhythm or the earliest site of atrial activation during AV re-entrant tachycardia.

- AV nodal tachycardia is characterized by very short ventriculoatrial conduction times as measured at all atrial sites. Slow AV nodal pathway ablation is achieved by delivery of radiofrequency energy to a site close to the coronary sinus.

- Atrial flutter can be treated by ablating the isthmus in the right atrial re-entrant circuit. Success rates compare favourably with medical therapy.

- AV nodal ablation is very effective in atrial arrhythmias that cannot be controlled by medication. It necessitates pacemaker implantation.

- Fascicular and right ventricular outflow tract ventricular tachycardias can be cured by ablation.

- Pulmonary vein isolation techniques are effective at preventing paroxysmal atrial fibrillation.

Arrhythmias for interpretation

Interpretations 401

One hundred ECGs are presented. Their interpretations can be found at the end of the chapter. As is often the case in practice, there may be more than one observation to make about each example.

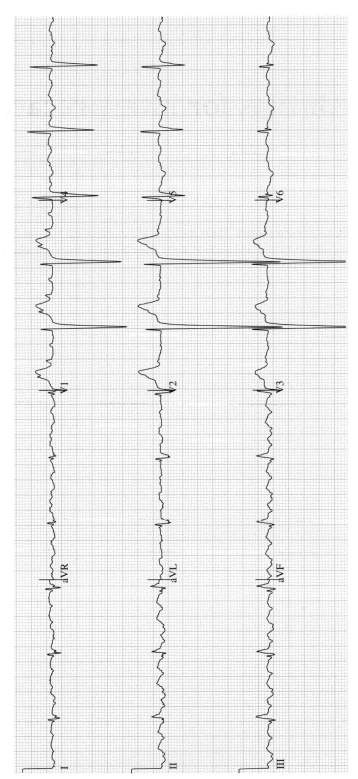

Figure 27.1

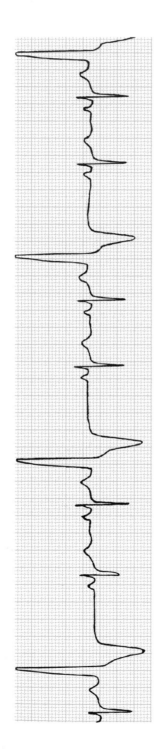

Figure 27.2

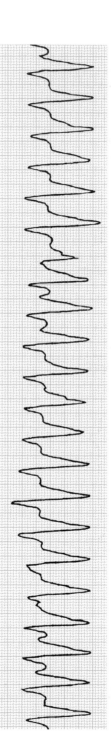

Figure 27.3

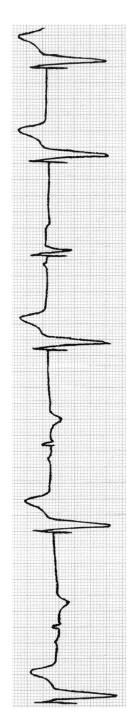

Figure 27.4

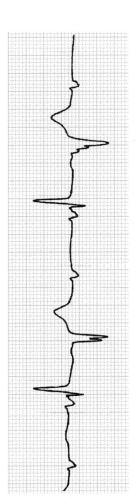

Figure 27.5

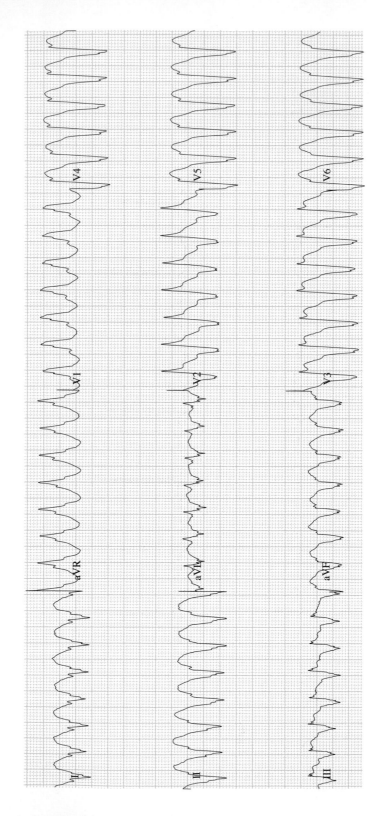

Figure 27.6

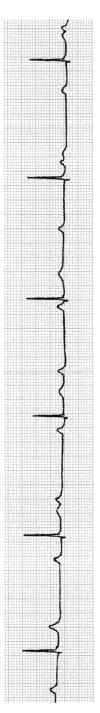

Figure 27.7

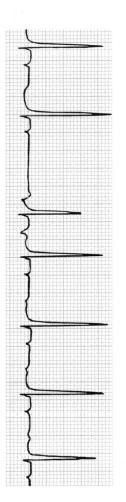

Figure 27.8

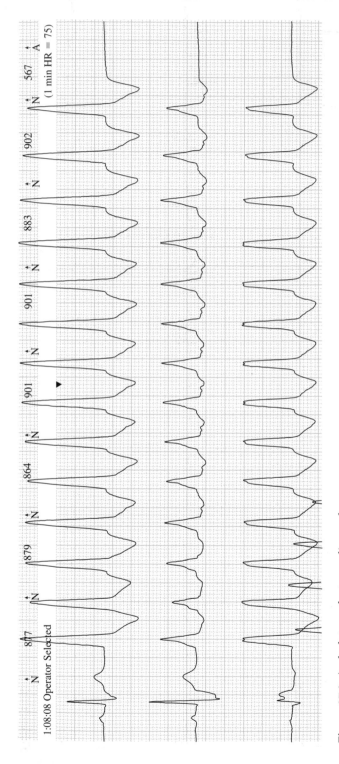

Figure 27.9 Ambulatory electrocardiography.

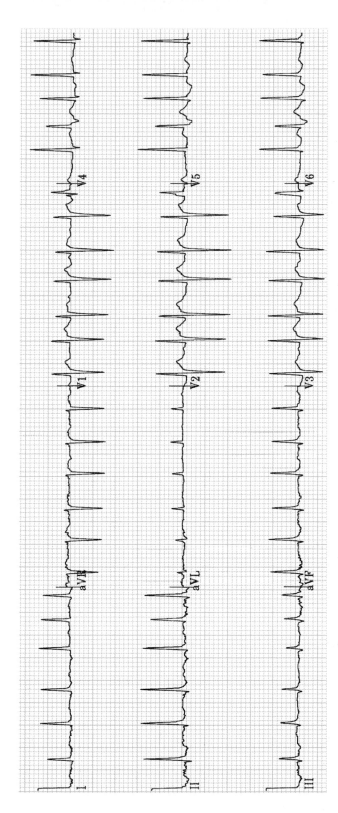

Figure 27.10

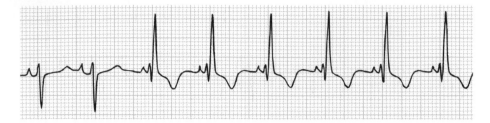

Figure 27.11

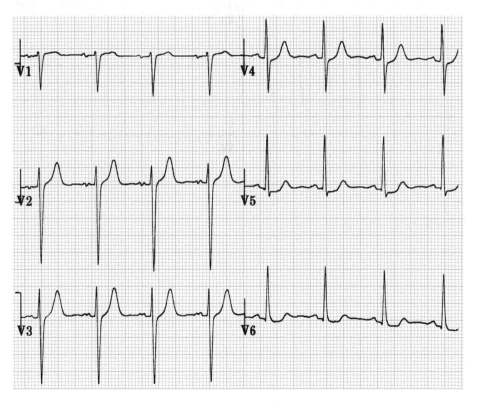

Figure 27.12 (Continued on page 335) Both ECGs from same patient.

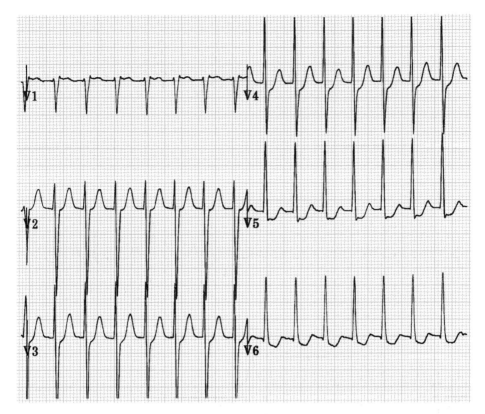

Figure 27.12 (Continued)

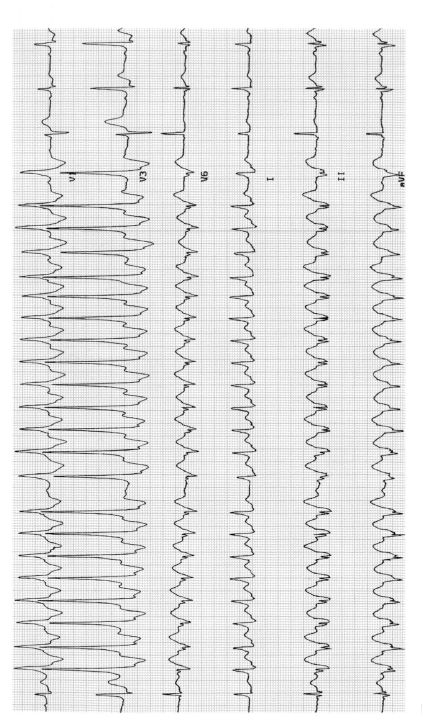

Figure 27.13

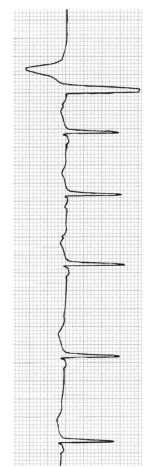

Figure 27.14

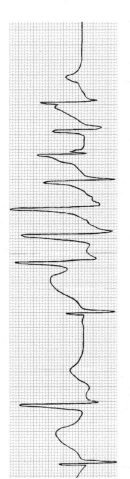

Figure 27.15

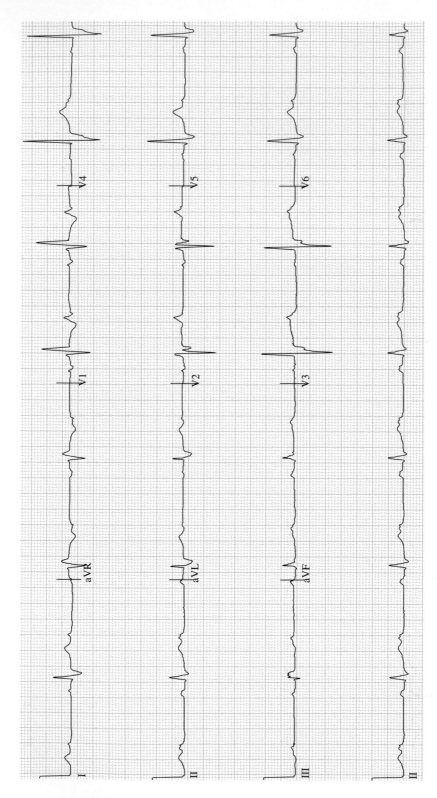

Figure 27.16

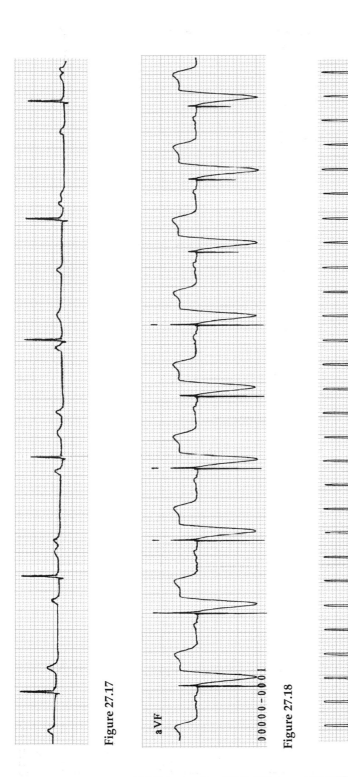

Figure 27.17

aVF

00000-0001

Figure 27.18

Figure 27.19

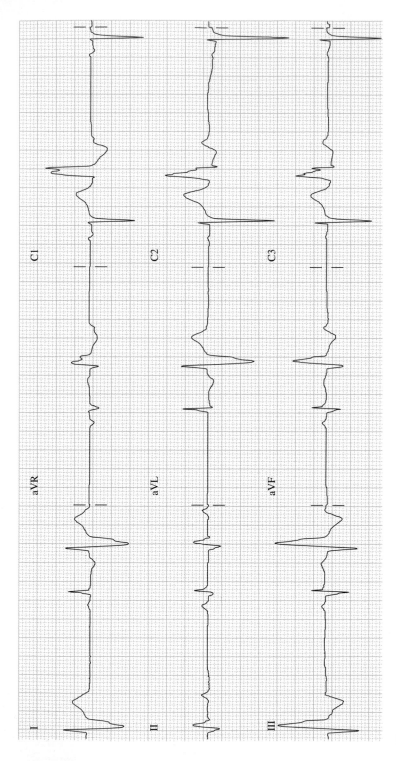

Figure 27.20

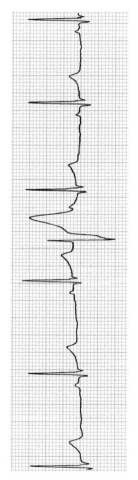

Figure 27.21

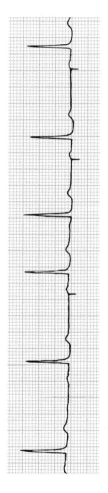

Figure 27.22

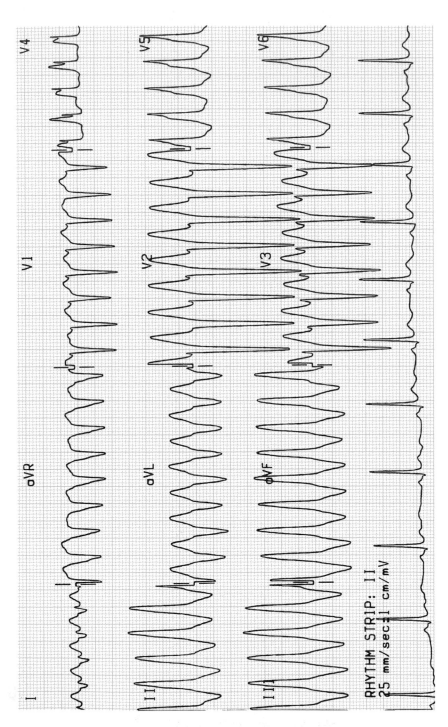

Figure 27.23

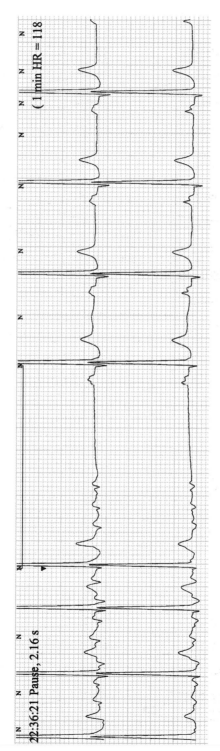

Figure 27.24

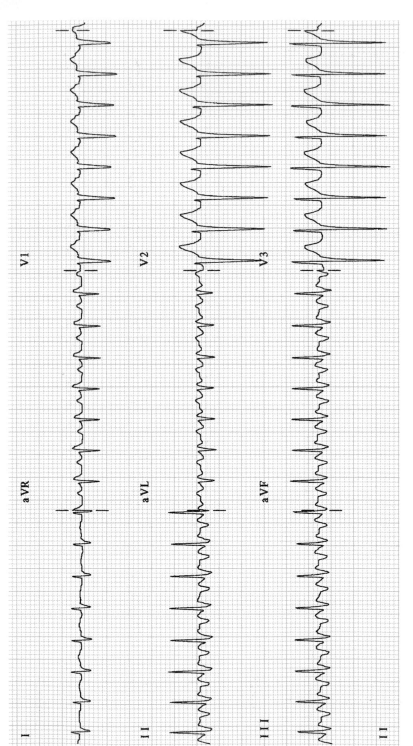

Figure 27.25

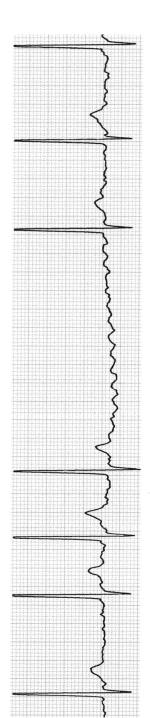

Figure 27.26

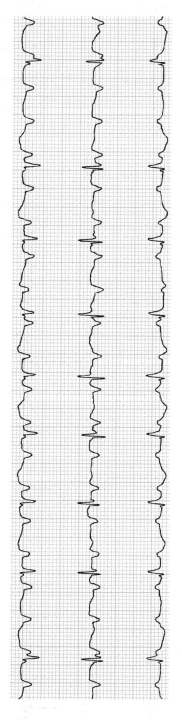

Figure 27.27

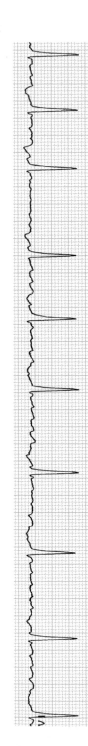

Figure 27.28

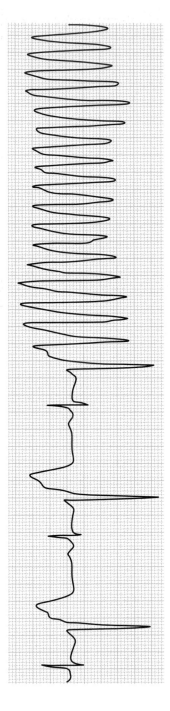

Figure 27.29

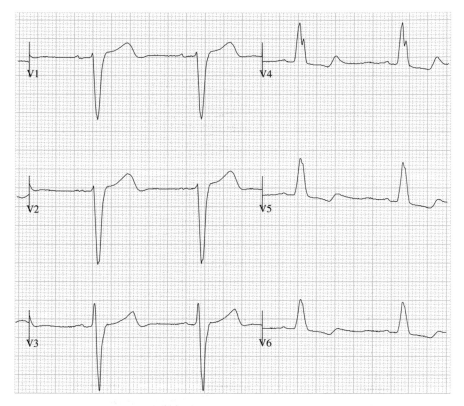

Figure 27.30

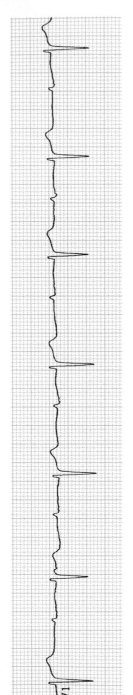

V1

Figure 27.31

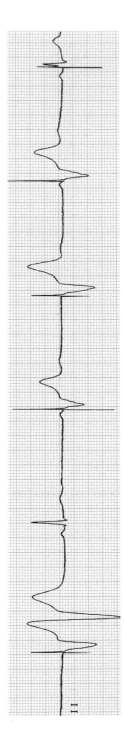

II

Figure 27.32

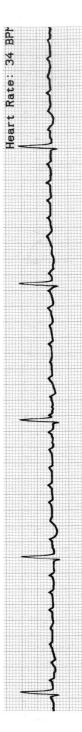

Heart Rate: 34 BP

Figure 27.33

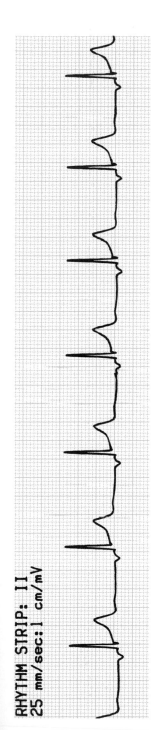

Figure 27.34

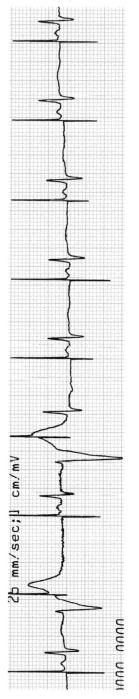

25 mm/sec;1 cm/mV

Figure 27.35

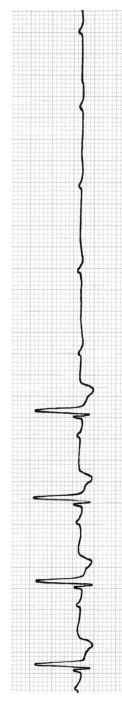

Figure 27.36

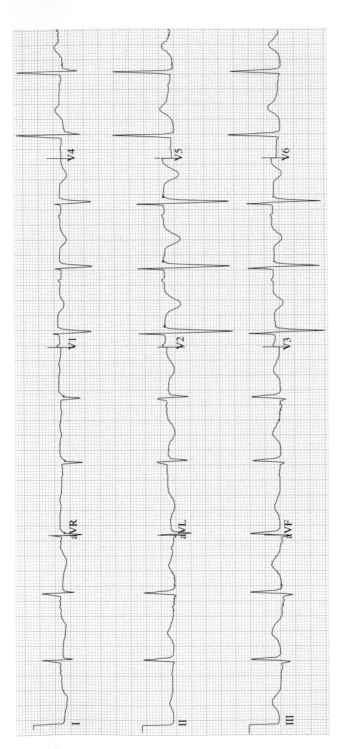

Figure 27.37 Patient was receiving an antibiotic.

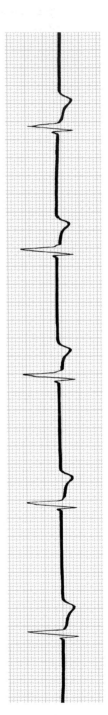

Figure 27.38

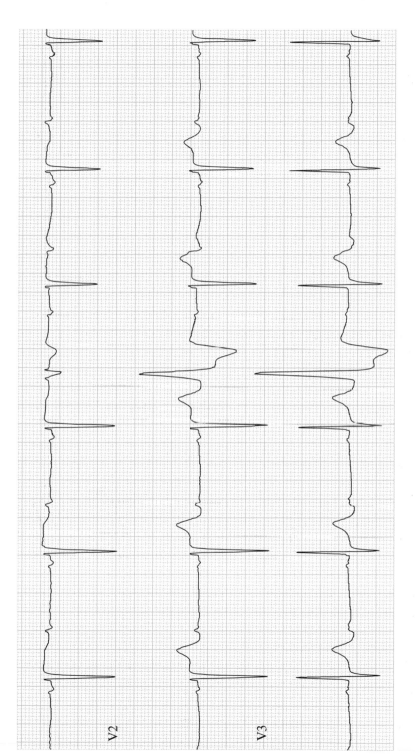

Figure 27.39

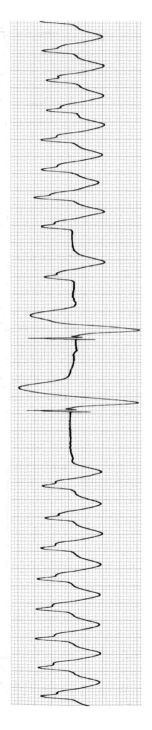

Figure 27.40

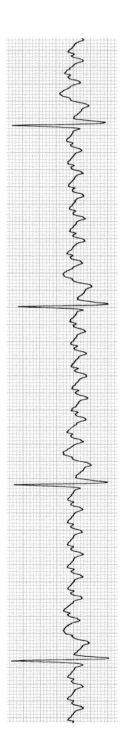

Figure 27.41

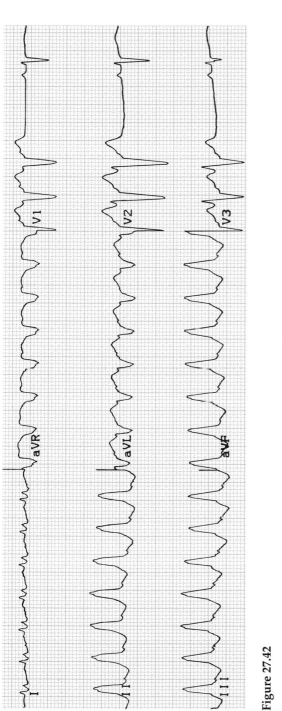

Figure 27.42

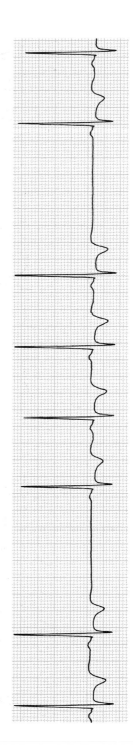

Figure 27.43

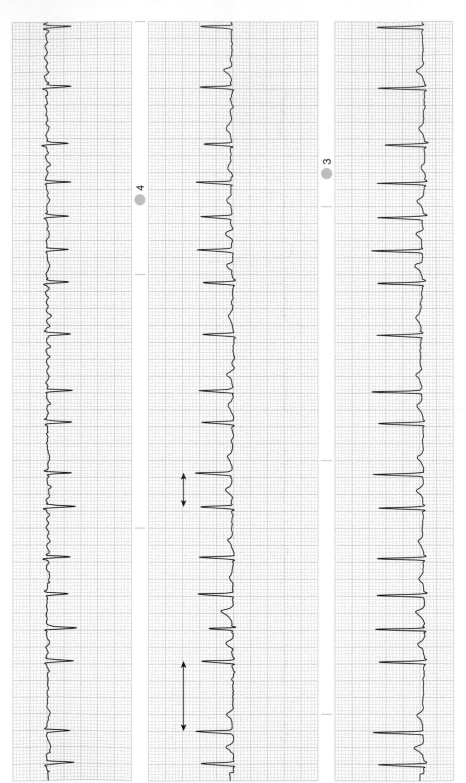

Figure 27.44

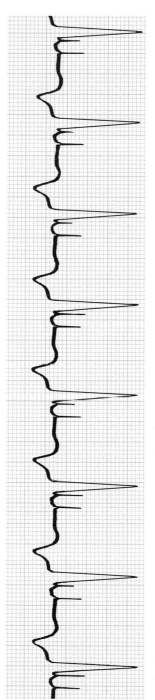

Figure 27.45

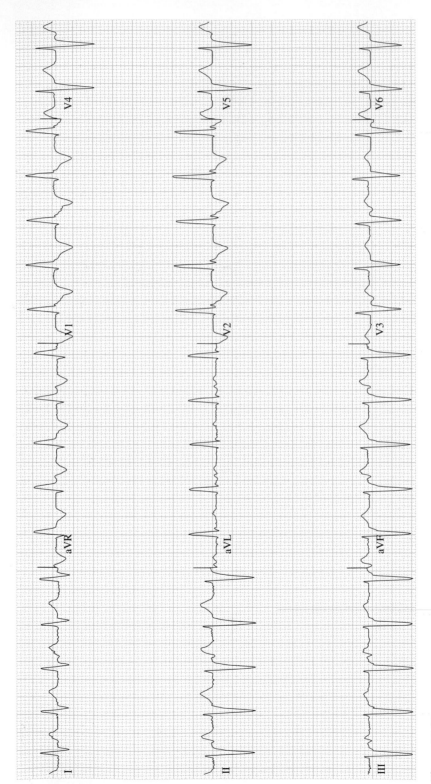

Figure 27.46

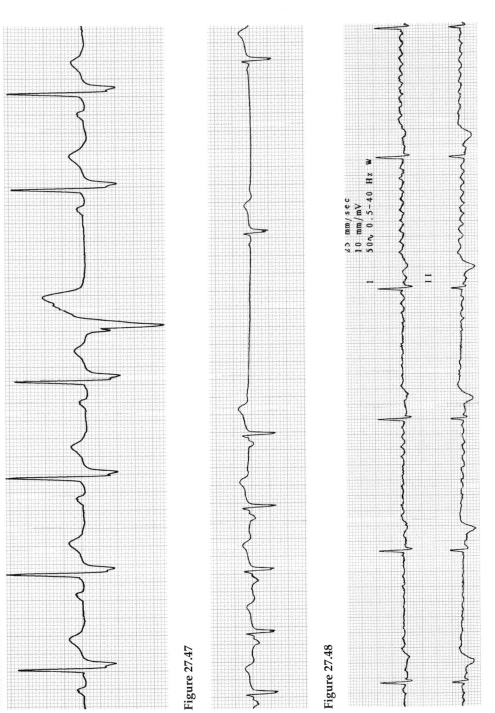

Figure 27.47

Figure 27.48

Figure 27.49

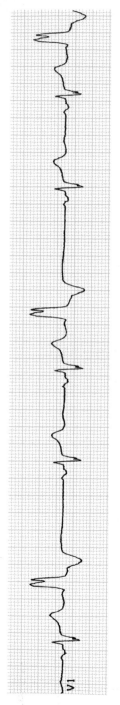

Figure 27.50

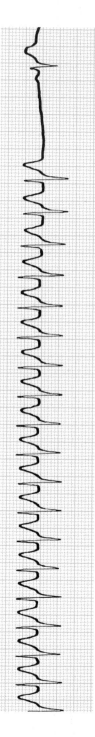

Figure 27.51

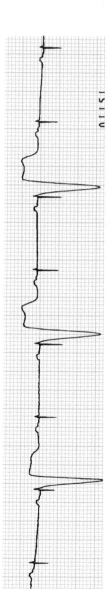

Figure 27.52

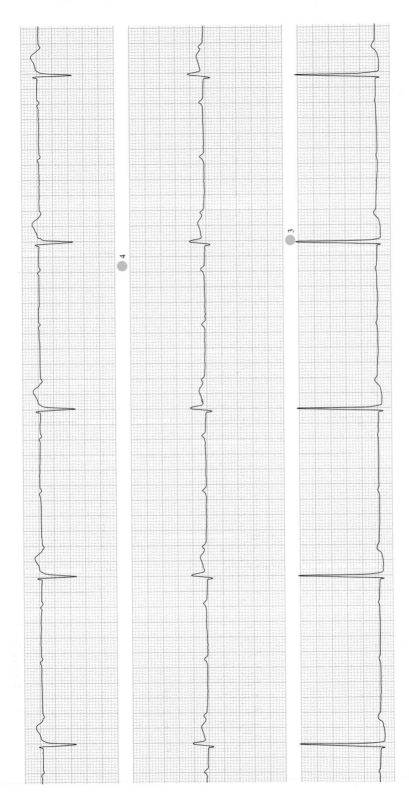

Figure 27.53

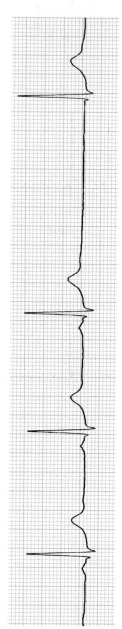

Figure 27.54

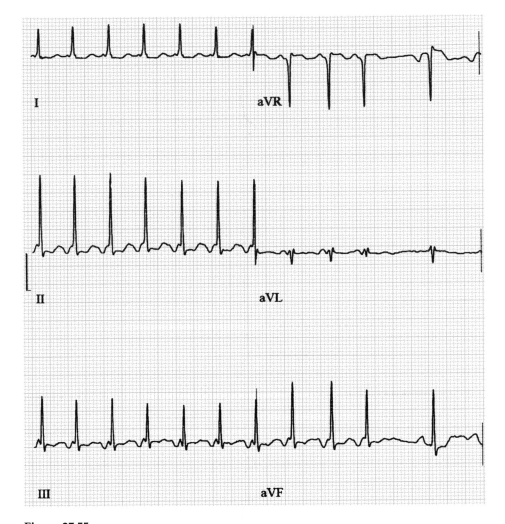

Figure 27.55

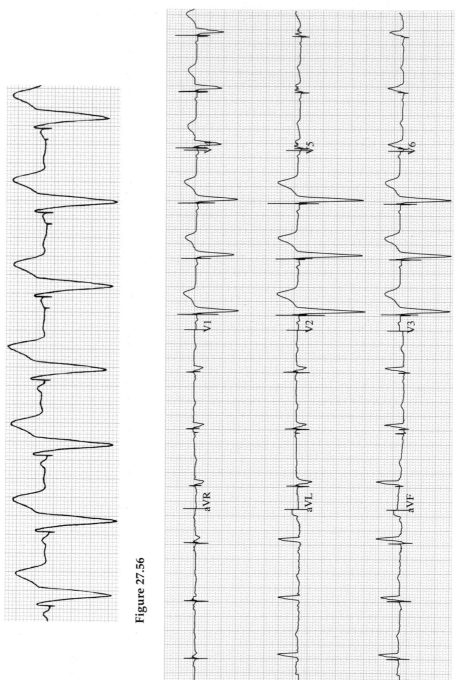

Figure 27.56

Figure 27.57

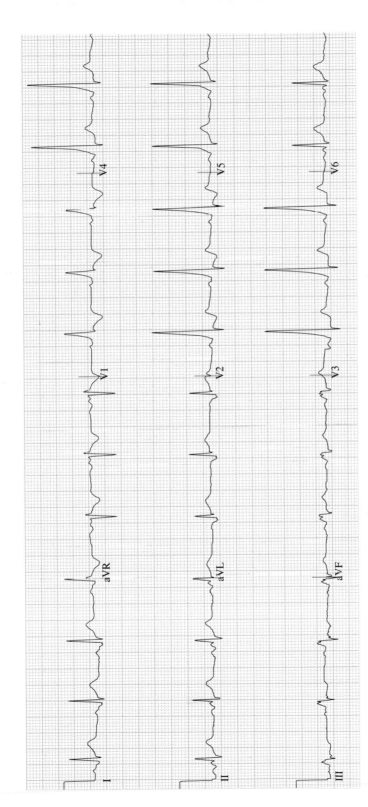

Figure 27.58

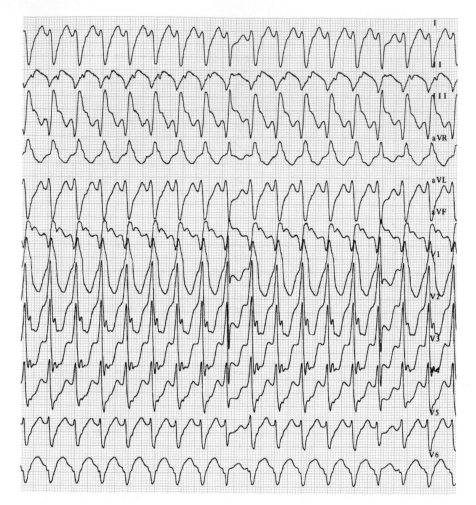

Figure 27.59

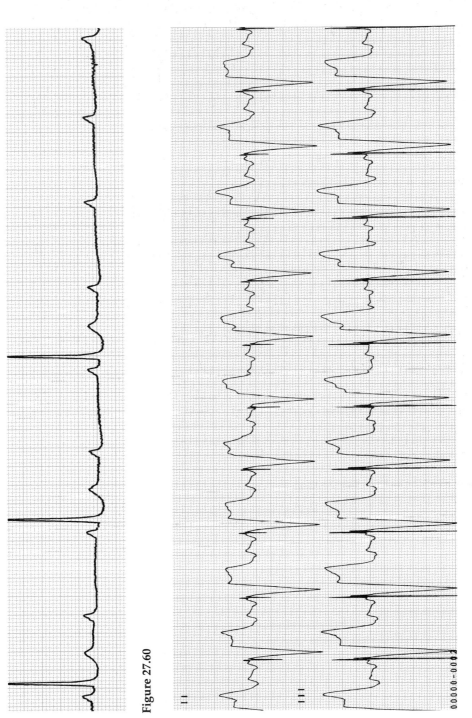

Figure 27.60

Figure 27.61

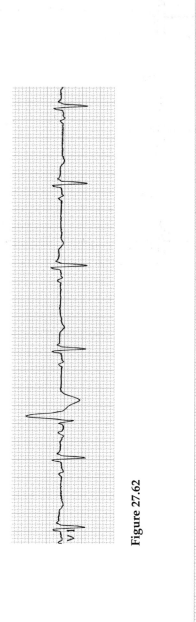

Figure 27.62

Figure 27.63

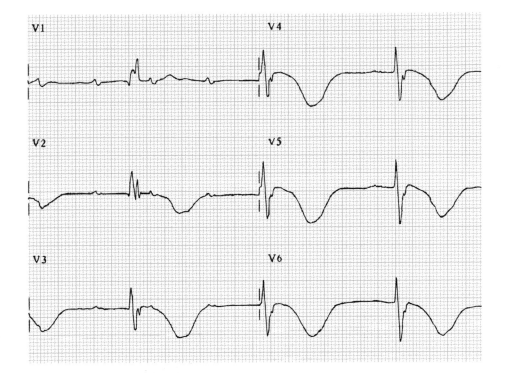

Figure 27.64

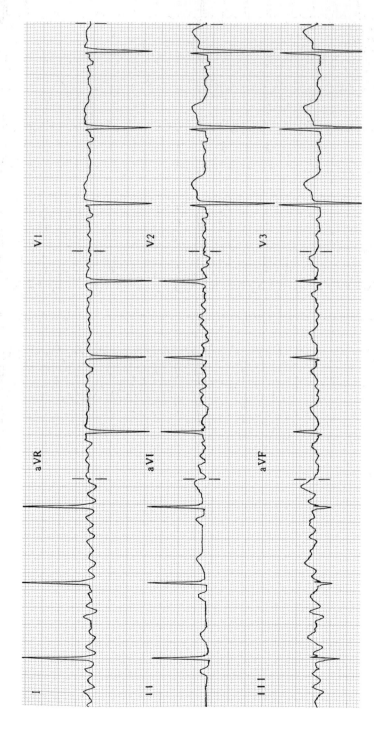

Figure 27.65

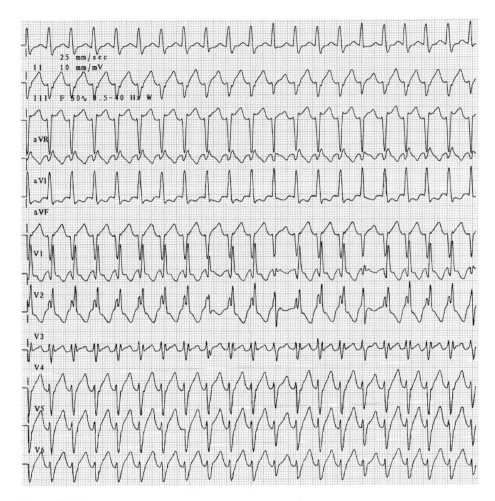

Figure 27.66

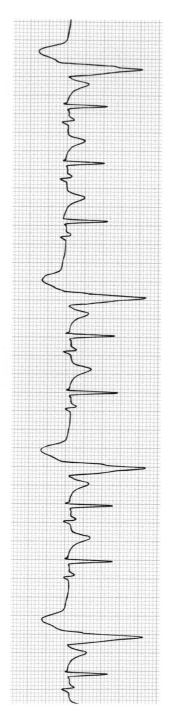

Figure 27.67

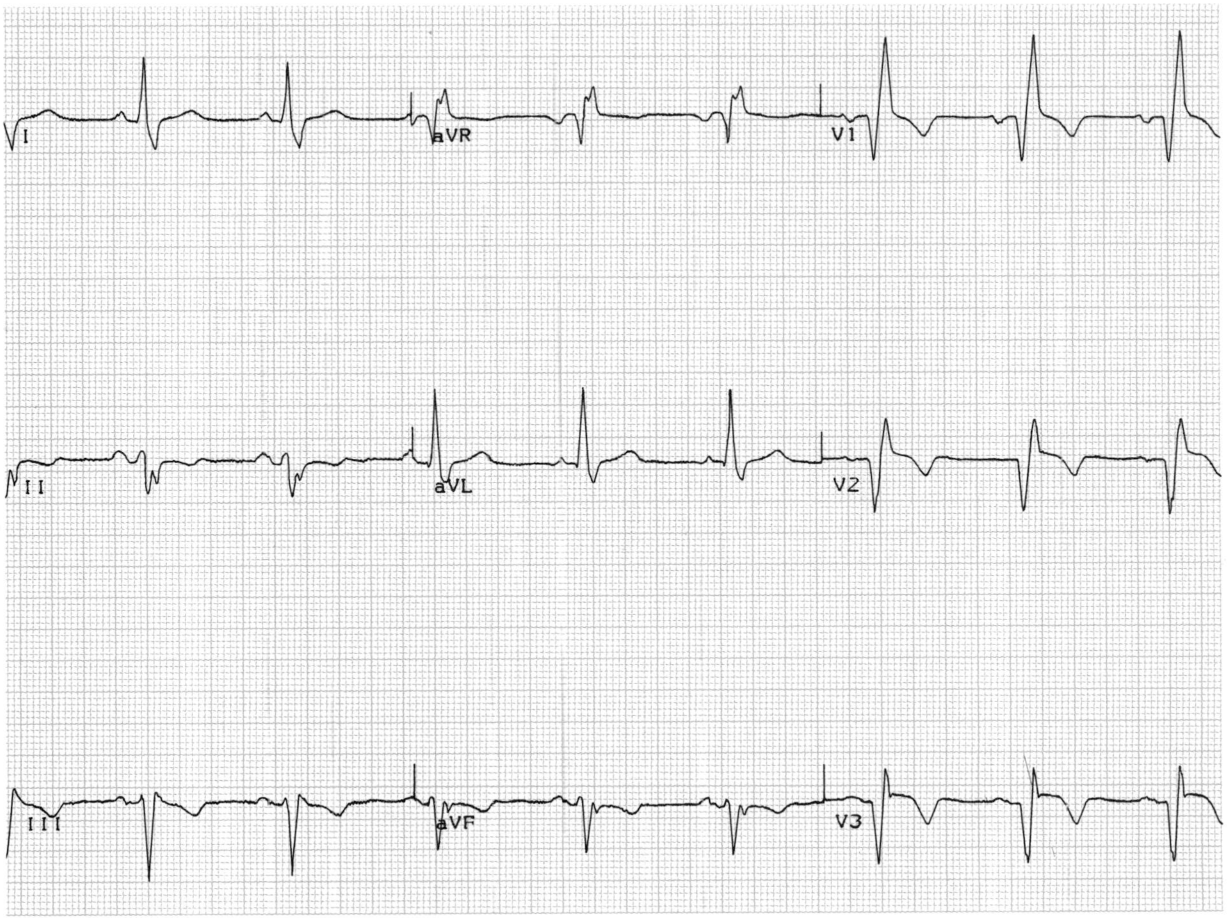

Figure 27.68

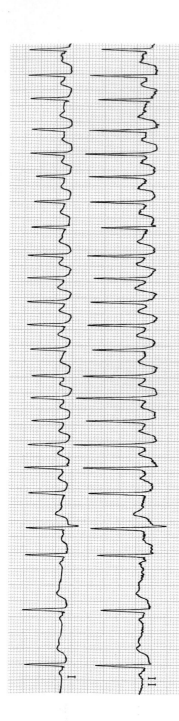

Figure 27.69

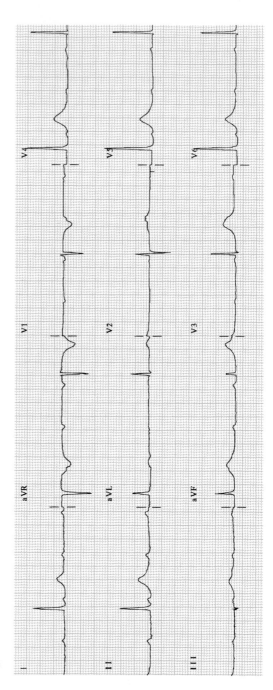

Figure 27.70

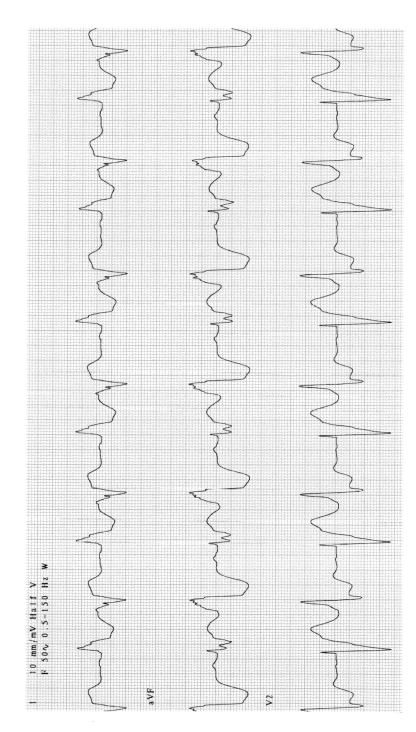

Figure 27.71

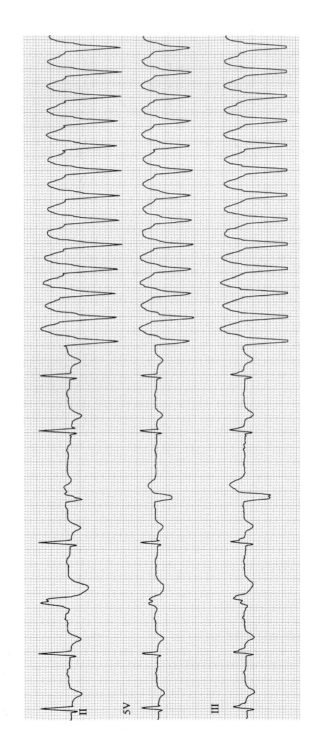

Figure 27.72

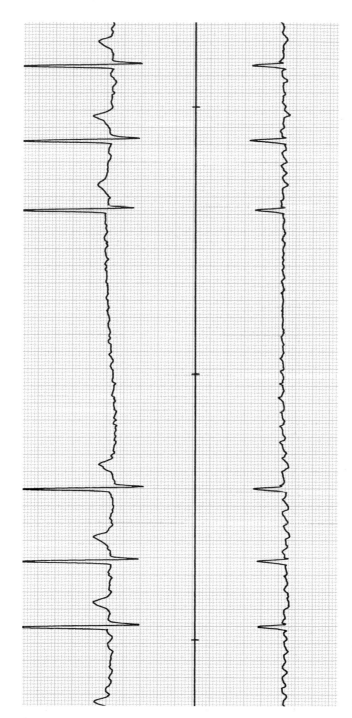

Figure 27.73

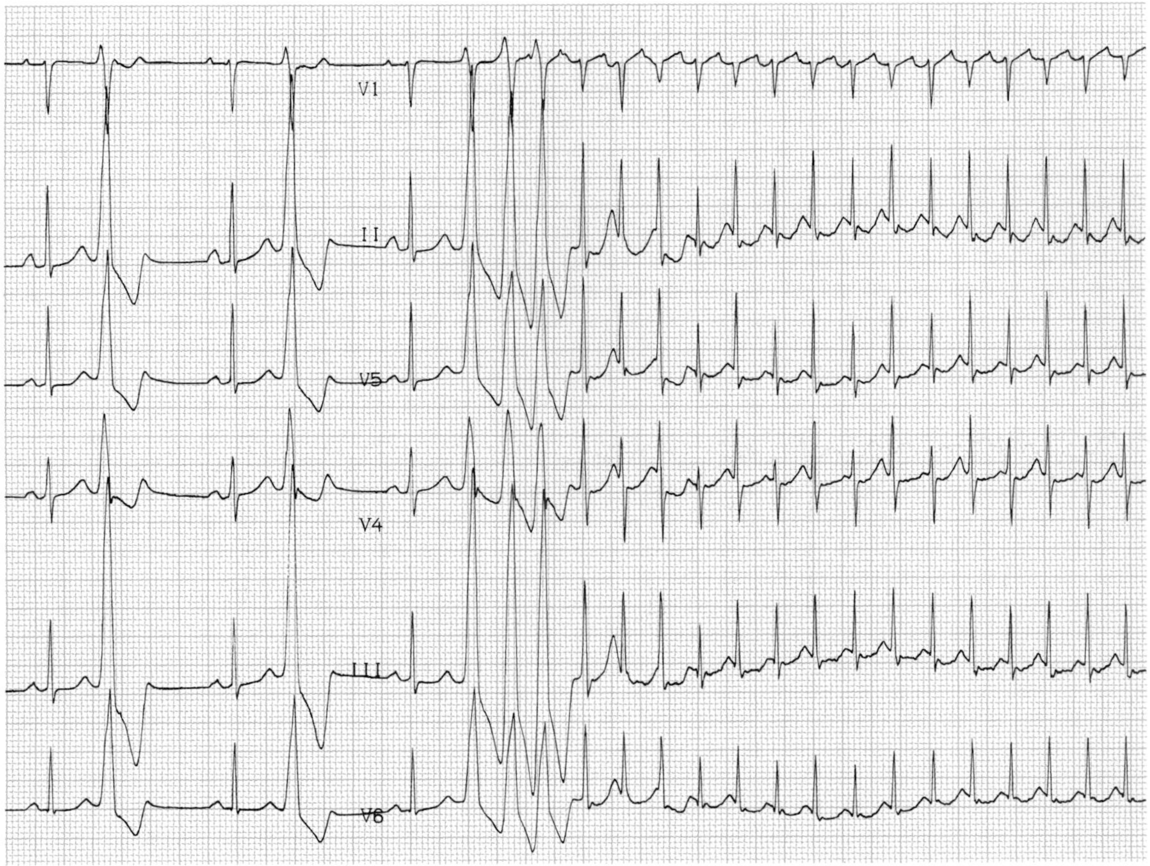

Figure 27.74

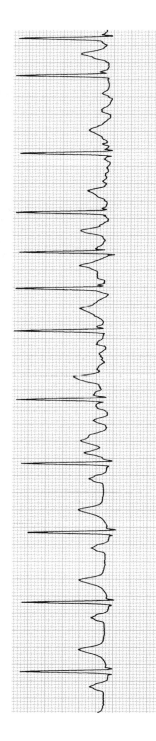

Figure 27.75

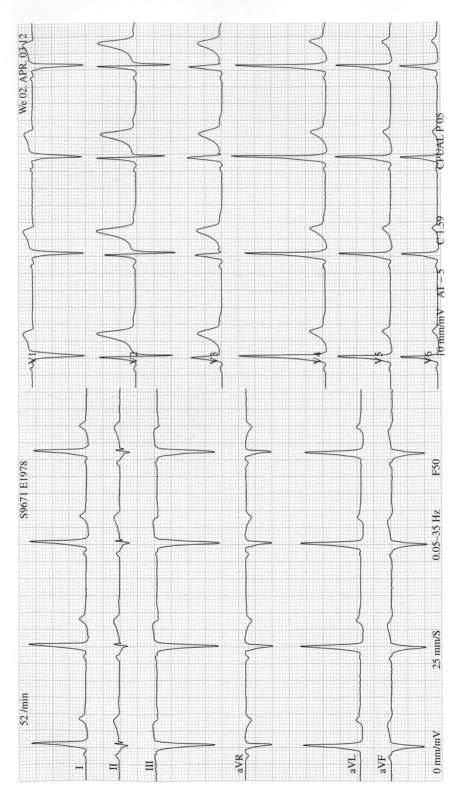

Figure 27.76

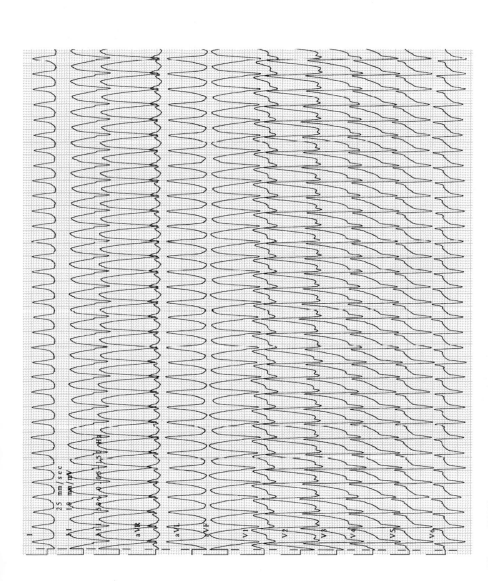

Figure 27.77

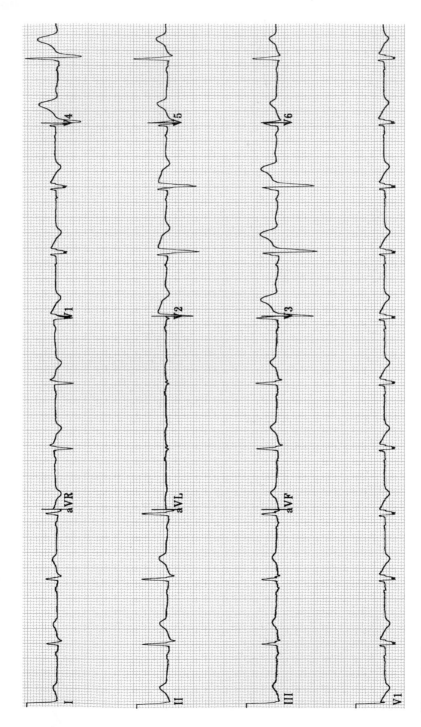

Figure 27.78

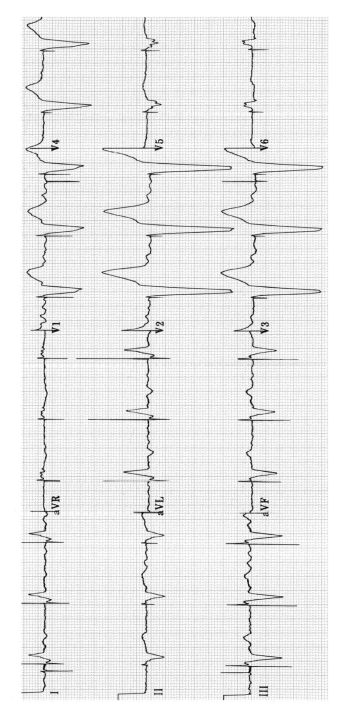

Figure 27.79

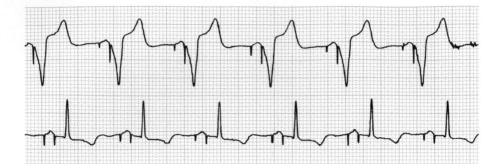

Figure 27.80

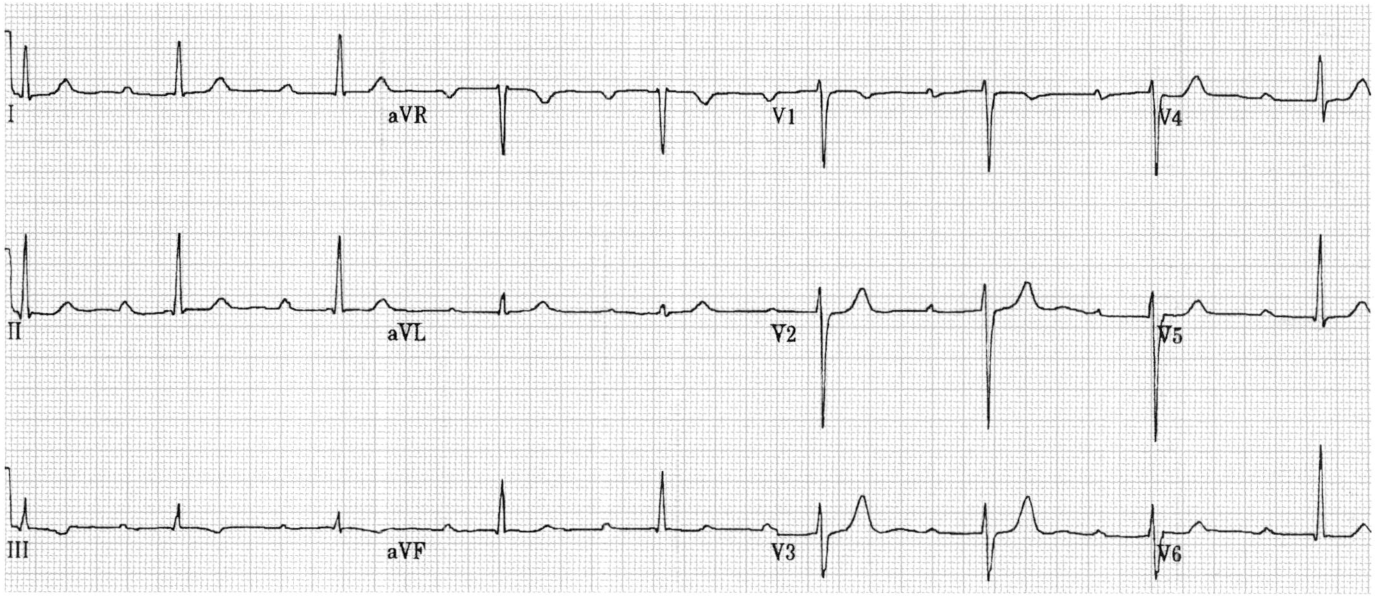

Figure 27.81

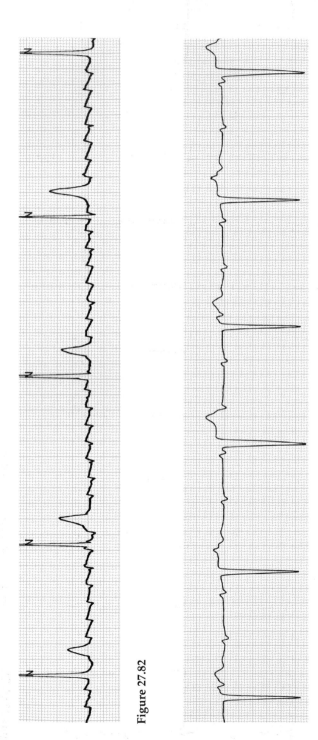

Figure 27.82

Figure 27.83

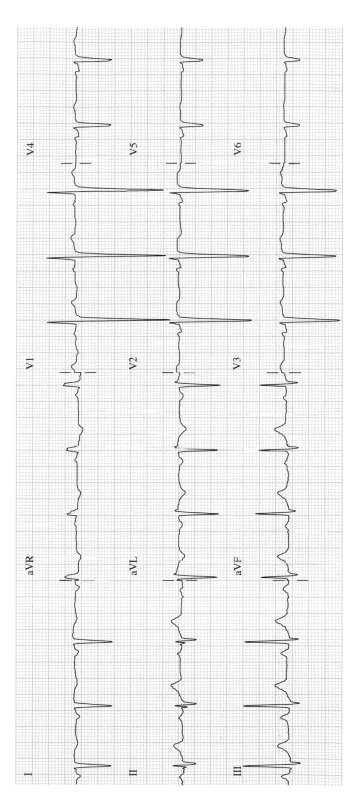

Figure 27.84 There is no arrhythmia or conduction defect.

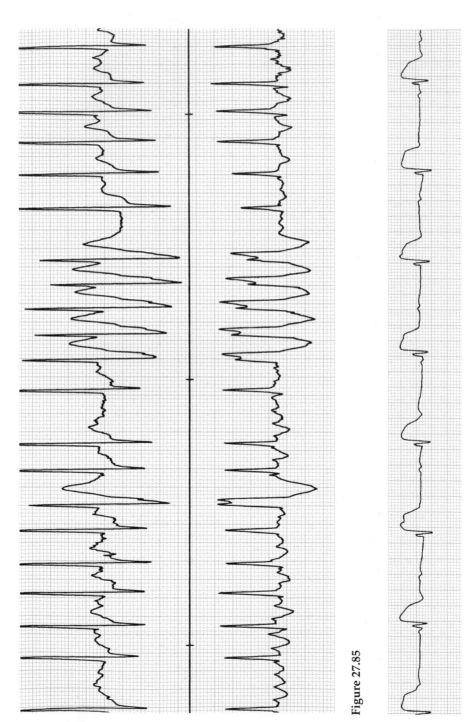

Figure 27.85

Figure 27.86

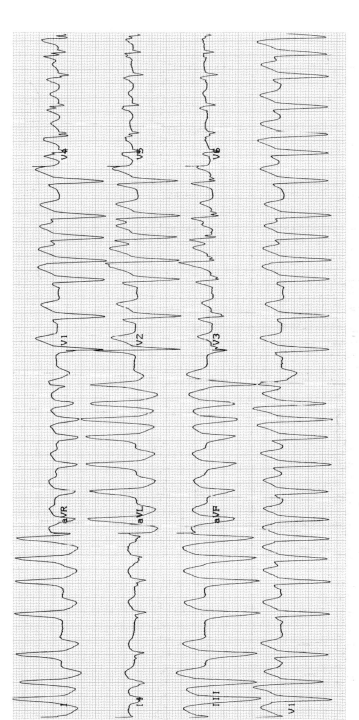

Figure 27.87

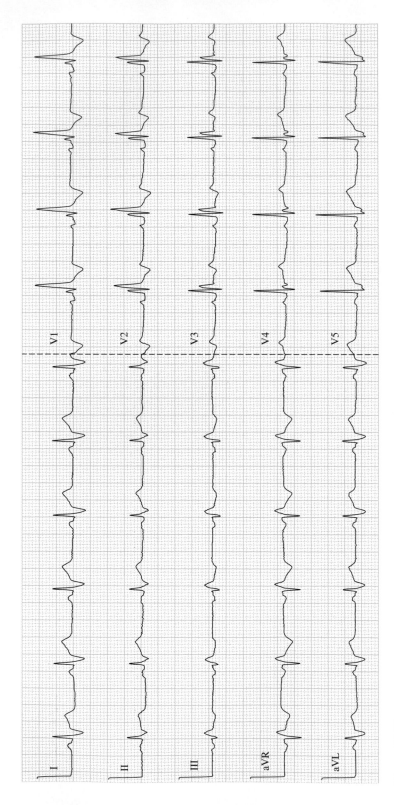

Figure 27.88

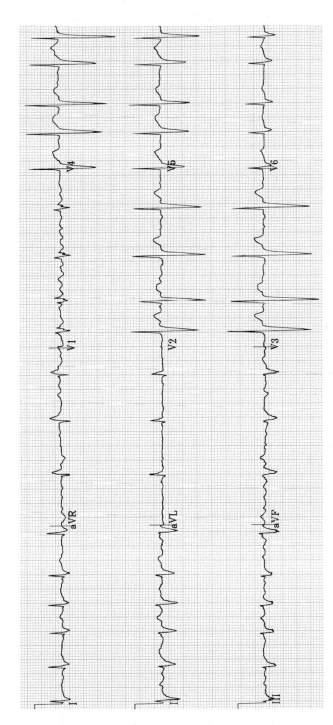

Figure 27.89

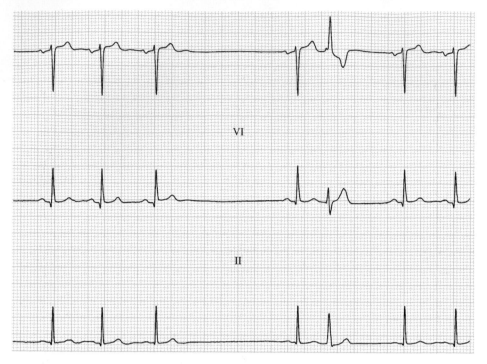

Figure 27.90

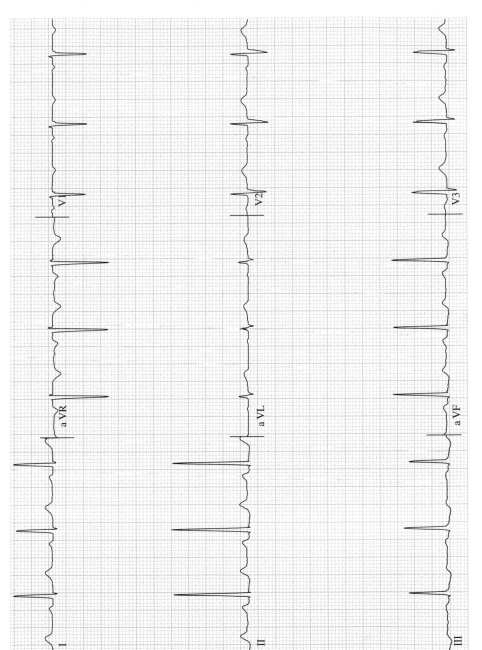

Figure 27.91

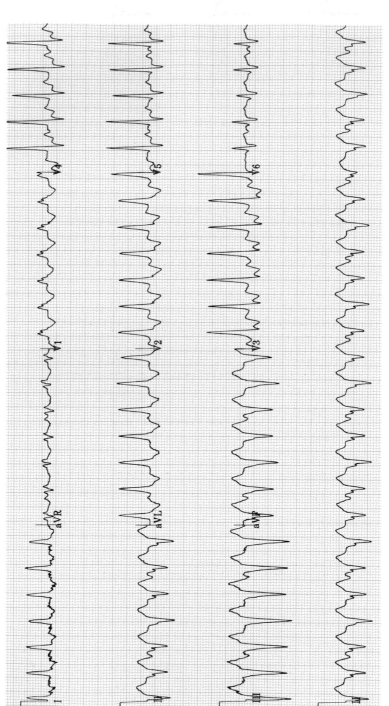

Figure 27.92

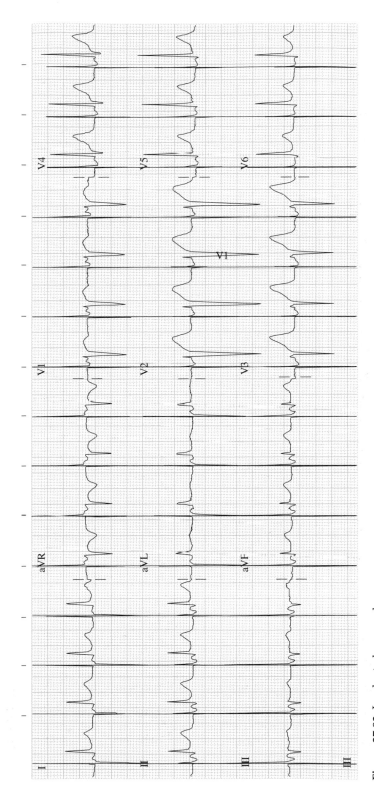

Figure 27.93 Implanted pacemaker.

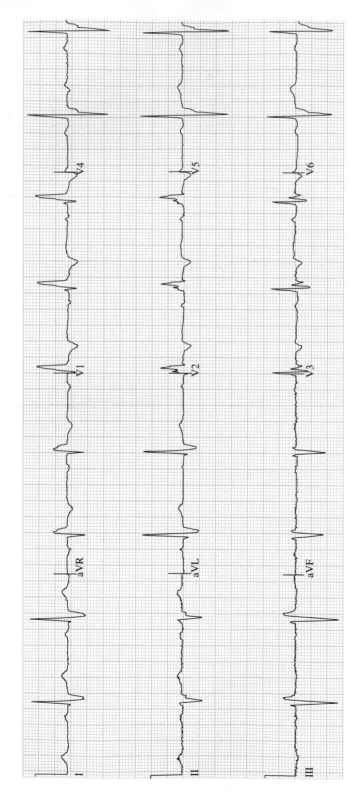

Figure 27.94

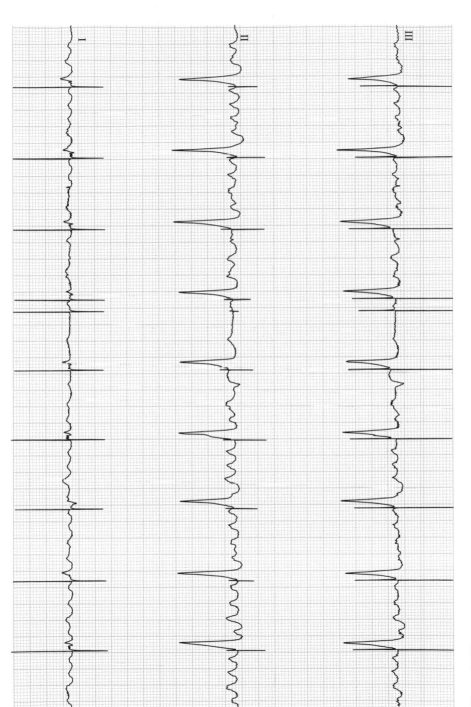

Figure 27.95

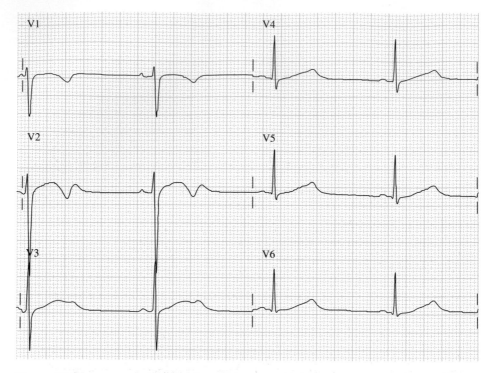

Figure 27.96

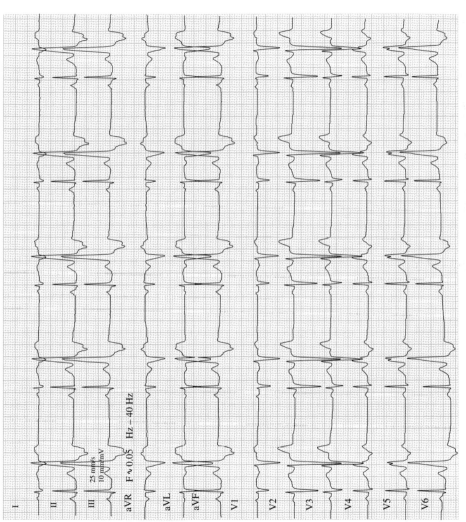

Figure 27.97

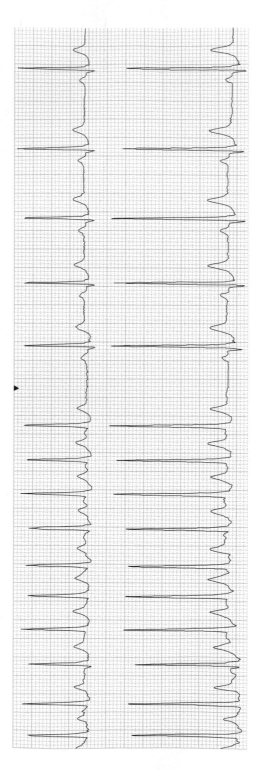

Figure 27.98 Ambulatory electro cardiography.

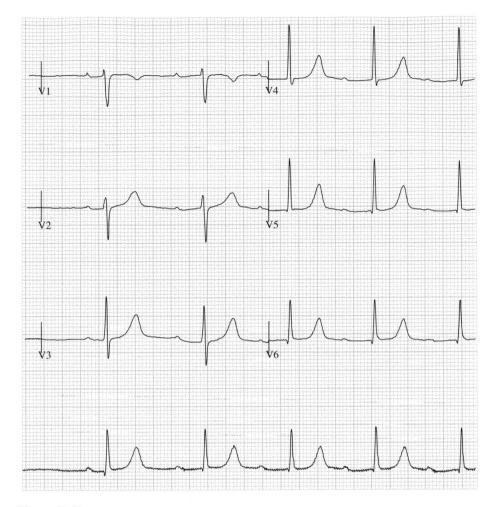

Figure 27.99

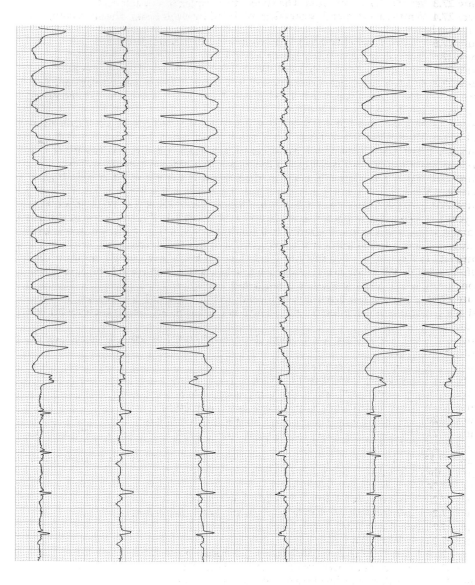

Figure 27.100

INTERPRETATIONS

Figure 27.1 Typical atrial flutter.

Figure 27.2 Sinus rhythm with ventricular trigeminy.

Figure 27.3 Ventricular tachycardia. The sixteenth complex is a fusion beat.

Figure 27.4 Ventricular demand pacemaker inhibited by sinus beats. The sixth complex is a fusion beat.

Figure 27.5 2:1 atrioventricular block with ventricular ectopic beats.

Figure 27.6 Monomorphic ventricular tachycardia.

Figure 27.7 Complete atrioventricular block with narrow ventricular complexes.

Figure 27.8 Atrial ectopic beat superimposed on T wave of fourth ventricular complex. There is a further atrial ectopic beat superimposed on the T wave of the fifth complex which is not conducted to the ventricles.

Figure 27.9 Non-sustained monomorphic ventricular tachycardia (with ventriculoatrial conduction) after single normal beat.

Figure 27.10 Atrial fibrillation with rapid ventricular response. The f waves are of low amplitude but the diagnosis is clear from the totally irregular ventricular rhythm.

Figure 27.11 After two normally conducted sinus beats there is right bundle branch block (lead V1).

Figure 27.12 (a) Normal sinus rhythm. (b) Typical atrioventricular nodal re-entrant tachycardia: there is an apparent secondary r wave in V1 which is not present during normal rhythm. It is due to retrograde atrial conduction. The very short ventriculoatrial conduction time indicates atrioventricular nodal re-entrant tachycardia.

Figure 27.13 The first, penultimate and last beats show sinus rhythm and Wolff–Parkinson–White syndrome. After the first beat there is an episode of atrial fibrillation during which all complexes are pre-excited.

Figure 27.14 Atrial ectopic beats superimposed on third and fifth ventricular T waves. First ectopic beat is not conducted; the second is conducted to the ventricles with left bundle branch block.

Figure 27.15 Sinus bradycardia with long QT interval and short episode of torsade de pointes tachycardia.

Figure 27.16 Mobitz II atrioventricular block.

Figure 27.17 Complete atrioventricular block.

Figure 27.18 Atrial synchronized ventricular pacing (VAT).

Figure 27.19 Atrioventricular junctional re-entrant tachycardia.

Figure 27.20 Ventricular bigeminy: inferior myocardial infarction.

Figure 27.21 The fourth ventricular complex is an interpolated ventricular ectopic beat.

Figure 27.22 Atrial demand pacing.

Figure 27.23 Twelve-lead ECG showing right ventricular outflow tract tachycardia. Sinus rhythm has returned at time of recording rhythm strip (II).

Figure 27.24 Termination of atrial fibrillation.

Figure 27.25 Atrial flutter. 2:1 atrioventricular conduction.

Figure 27.26 Atrial fibrillation with long pause in ventricular activity.

Figure 27.27 Atrial tachycardia with atrioventricular block.

Figure 27.28 Atrial fibrillation.

Figure 27.29 Ventricular tachycardia initiated by third ventricular ectopic beat.

Figure 27.30 Normal sinus rhythm: Left bundle branch block.

Figure 27.31 First-degree atrioventricular block. PR interval = 0.46 s.

Figure 27.32 Ventricular demand pacing at 40 beats/min. Ventricular ectopic after first paced beat. Last complex is a fusion beat.

Figure 27.33 Atrial flutter with complete atrioventricular block.

Figure 27.34 Junctional rhythm.

Figure 27.35 Atrial pacing. There are two ventricular ectopic beats which are of course not sensed by pacemaker.

Figure 27.36 Ventricular asystole after four sinus beats conducted with right bundle branch block.

Figure 27.37 Markedly prolonged QT interval caused by clarithromycin.

Figure 27.38 Junctional rhythm.

Figure 27.39 2:1 atrioventricular block. Single ventricular ectopic beat after third ventricular complex leading to subsequent PR prolongation due to concealed atrioventricular conduction.

Figure 27.40 Two paced ventricular beats preceded and succeeded by ventricular tachycardia.

Figure 27.41 Atrial flutter with high degree atrioventricular block.

Figure 27.42 Ventricular tachycardia with retrograde atrial activation. Sinus rhythm returns at end of ECG.

Figure 27.43 Two episodes of second-degree sinoatrial block.

Figure 27.44 Atrial fibrillation with rapid ventricular response.

Figure 27.45 Atrioventricular sequential pacing.

Figure 27.46 Left posterior fascicular ventricular tachycardia with independent atrial activity.

Figure 27.47 Single ventricular ectopic beat. First-degree atrioventricular block.

Figure 27.48 Junctional rhythm followed by sinus arrest and then sinus bradycardia.

Figure 27.49 Atrial fibrillation and complete atrioventricular block.

Figure 27.50 Ventricular trigeminy.

Figure 27.51 Termination of atrioventricular junctional re-entrant tachycardia.

Figure 27.52 Ventricular pacing with intermittent failure to capture.

Figure 27.53 Second-degree atrioventricular block with narrow ventricular complexes.

Figure 27.54 Sinus arrest followed by junctional escape beat.

Figure 27.55 Long RP short PR tachycardia which terminates just before end of trace. During tachycardia an inverted P wave precedes each QRS complex.

Figure 27.56 Atrial synchronized and then atrioventricular sequential pacing, i.e. DDD pacemaker.

Figure 27.57 P wave synchronized (VAT) pacing. The narrow QRS complexes is consistent with biventricular pacing.

Figure 27.58 Type A Wolff–Parkinson–White syndrome.

Figure 27.59 Ventricular tachycardia with fusion beats.

Figure 27.60 2:1 atrioventricular block deteriorating to third-degree atrioventricular block.

Figure 27.61 Atrial flutter; ventricular pacing.

Figure 27.62 Incomplete right bundle branch block. The third complex is an atrial ectopic beat, conducted with complete right bundle branch block.

Figure 27.63 Mobitz II atrioventricular block: there is 3:1 atrioventricular conduction.

Figure 27.64 Complete atrioventricular block, best seen in V1, and marked QT prolongation. (Patient presented with torsade de pointes tachycardia.)

Figure 27.65 Normal sinus rhythm. Apparent atrial fibrillation in some of limb leads due to patient tremor.

Figure 27.66 Fusion and capture beats indicate ventricular tachycardia: the ninth complex is a fusion beat and the thirteenth and seventeenth complexes are capture beats. Relatively narrow QRS complexes together with right bundle branch block and left axis deviation indicate left posterior fascicular origin.

Figure 27.67 Frequent unifocal ventricular ectopic beats.

Figure 27.68 Bifascicular block due to anterior myocardial infarction.

Figure 27.69 Onset of atrial fibrillation.

Figure 27.70 Complete atrioventricular block; narrow QRS complexes. QT prolongation = 0.6 s.

Figure 27.71 Sinus rhythm, marked QRS prolongation and ventricular bigeminy.

Figure 27.72 Multifocal ventricular ectopic beats: the third, fifth and eighth complexes. The first is an end-diastolic ectopic beat, the third initiates monomorphic ventricular tachycardia.

Figure 27.73 Atrial fibrillation with very long pause.

Figure 27.74 Right ventricular outflow tract bigeminy, then a salvo of right ventricular outflow tract ectopics initiates atrioventricular re-entrant supraventricular tachycardia.

Figure 27.75 Onset of atrial fibrillation after four sinus beats.

Figure 27.76 Type B Wolff–Parkinson–White syndrome (due to postero-septal accessory pathway).

Figure 27.77 Monomorphic ventricular tachycardia.

Figure 27.78 Brugada syndrome.

Figure 27.79 Ventricular pacing; atrial fibrillation. After the eighth paced ventricular complex there are two, not one, pacing stimuli preceding the next complex. This indicates the patient has a dual chamber mode switching pacemaker and for one cycle the pacemaker has failed to detect atrial fibrillation and therefore delivered an atrial stimulus.

Figure 27.80 Upper trace – atrioventricular sequential pacing. Lower trace – failure of ventricular capture.

Figure 27.81 First-degree atrioventricular block.

Figure 27.82 Atrial flutter and complete atrioventricular block.

Figure 27.83 Complete atrioventricular block.

Figure 27.84 Dextrocardia. The inverted but normally timed P wave in lead I indicates either arm lead reversal or dextrocardia: the latter is confirmed by the reversal of the normal chest lead sequence.

Figure 27.85 Atrial fibrillation; some broad QRS complexes due to aberrant conduction.

Figure 27.86 Lead aVF. Complete atrioventricular block due to acute inferior infarction.

Figure 27.87 Atrial fibrillation. QRS complex appearance strongly suggests Wolff–Parkinson–White syndrome.

Figure 27.88 Right bundle branch block.

Figure 27.89 Left anterior fascicular block and atrial fibrillation.

Figure 27.90 Sinus arrest after three normal beats. Ventricular ectopic beat after fourth ventricular complex.

Figure 27.91 Normal!

Figure 27.92 Ventricular tachycardia with direct evidence of independent atrial activity.

Figure 27.93 Atrial pacing. The inverted P waves in the inferior leads are due to a pacing site low in the right atrium.

Figure 27.94 Left anterior fascicular and right bundle branch block.

Figure 27.95 Mode switching pacemaker. During atrial fibrillation there is ventricular demand pacing. There is termination of atrial fibrillation after fifth ventricular complex which is followed by atrioventricular sequential pacing for one beat before atrial fibrillation returns and leads again to mode switching.

Figure 27.96 Marked QT prolongation. QT interval = 0.64 s. Notched T wave typical of LQ2 hereditary long QT syndrome.

Figure 27.97 Right ventricular outflow tract ectopia.

Figure 27.98 Paroxysmal atrial fibrillation.

Figure 27.99 Atrioventricular Wenckebach block.

Figure 27.100 Monomorphic ventricular tachycardia preceded by sinus rhythm. Close inspection reveals independent atrial activity.